CASE MANAGEMENT & SOCIAL WORK PRACTICE

Stephen M. Rose

State University of New York at Stony Brook

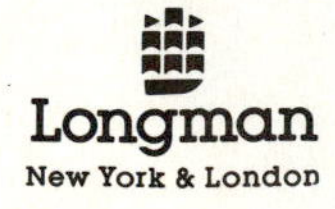

Case Management and Social Work Practice

Longman, 95 Church Street, White Plains, N.Y. 10601

Associated companies:
Longman Group Ltd., London
Longman Cheshire Pty., Melbourne
Longman Paul Pty., Auckland
Copp Clark Pitman, Toronto

Senior editor: David Estrin
Production editor: Till & Till, Inc.
Cover design: Renee Kilbride Edelman
Text art: Burman
Production supervisor: Anne Armeny

Library of Congress Cataloging-in-Publication Data

Case management and social work practice / [edited by] Stephen M.
Rose.—1st ed.

p. cm.

Includes bibliographical references (p.) and index.

ISBN 0-8013-0332-X

1. Medical social work. 2. Social case work. 3. Hospitals—Case management services. 4. Medical social work—United States.
I. Rose, Stephen M.
HV687.C37 1992
361.3′2—dc20 90-19563
CIP

1 2 3 4 5 6 7 8 9 10-MA-9594939291

Contents

Introduction: Case Management and Social Work Practice: History and Context

Social work and case management share two essential features. Both occur historically when the social structure of society creates "surplus" populations that cannot be integrated within existing resources and patterns of resource allocation (Gough, 1979; Ehrenreich, 1985). And *each has a dual practice responsibility—to individual clients or families,* on the one hand, and *for social reform,* for producing more supportive environments, on the other. Often, particularly in health and mental health settings, restrictive funding guidelines (see Azzarto, 1986, in Part IV) or conventional agency practice models limit or restrain these responsibilities (Rose & Black, 1985). Both case management and social work are confronted with problems of direction and assertiveness, with conflict over funding and legitimation in relation to advocacy and system change.

Establishing the mutuality of social work and case management through their dual practice commitments confronts the problems faced by each. Where is the primary obligation? Does it belong with vulnerable, devalued people, impoverished, sick, underserved or unserved by provider systems, without political assets and often isolated in their suffering? Or does it belong with the funding/provider system with its dual resources of money and legitimation? Can ways be developed to integrate the two interests, to serve the people without losing either the funding or legitimation that come with professional status? What role does professional status play in enhancing or obstructing the dual practice commitment of case management? The values and principles of the profession come very close to the espoused values of the client-driven advocacy/empowerment model of case management that will be discussed later on in this book. But, when it comes to implementation, can the same be said?

These questions and others related to them form the focus of this book. We do not intend to foreclose the questioning process, but to support it. The reason is clear: case management does belong in the realm or domain of social work, but not because we simply declare this to be self-evidently true [see the National Association of Social Workers' (NASW) Policy Statement, 1987, in Part I]. Social work *potentially* can best construct and implement a client-driven, systems-impact paradigm for case management practice (see Kisthardt and Rapp article in Part II and Part VI—"An Advocacy/Empowerment Model of Case Management for Social Work"). The stated values of human dignity and social justice, along with expressed commitments to clients' self-determination and to a dual focus on individuals or families and on social contexts, grant social work the right to leadership in case management policy and practice. Yet, paradigms integrating these values with a problem-defining theory and derived interventions are not universally acknowledged by the profession.

Potential exists in the legacy and values of social work which mandate an authentic psychosocial conceptual framework for practice. The authenticity, when implemented, demands that we design and construct professional relationships with clients which emphatically honor human dignity through commitment to active client involvement in producing individual and agency goals and directions. Clients, in this value-based perspective, have validity and potential for growth: "The question is not what kind of a life one has had, but what kind of a life one wants, and then bringing to bear all the personal and social resources available to accomplish this goal" (Weick et al., 1989, p. 353).

The pivotal point for success exists in building authentic relationships between case managers and clients, not in the efficiency of referrals to service providers. Intagliata grasps this point in stating the following,

> *Perhaps the most influential aspect of the case management process is the quality of the personal commitment that case managers develop toward their clients.* The case manager is the human link between the client and the system, and the only service provider concerned with and responsible for the whole client. (Intagliata, 1982, p. 660—italics in original; see Intagliata article in Part I)

The related mandate in professional social work, its commitment to transforming negative environments, challenging inequity in resource allocation, and opposing social injustice through both case and issue advocacy, elevates its potential for asserting leadership in defining case management functions. Thus, we see in the espoused values and commitments of the profession the interactive paradigm, advocacy and empowerment, each seen as a necessary dimension to a complete conceptualization of a practice model. Translating the stated conceptual framework into practice, as always, is a far more difficult and complex matter. Difficulties increase where social work education bifurcates methods training, separating clinical models from other interventions or from fields of practice. This emulates service providers' concepts of appropriate domain boundaries or practice models and can restrict advocacy activities or empowerment processes.

There are major problems in the profession that have to be confronted before social work can claim legitimate leadership in case management development and operations. Most models of case management agree that the role of case manager is diversified, tasks are multiple, and responsibilities range from the personally uninvolved "broker" of services (more typical of health care settings and the very recent growth of private practice case management, where the workers are employed by insurers) through advocate to primary therapist (Lamb, 1980; Harris & Bergman, 1987, in Part II).

Within the diversity of case management roles, five typical case management functions regularly appear: needs assessment; service or treatment planning; linking or referring; monitoring; and advocacy. Few constructions of case management leave out any of these five task areas, although the advocacy function rarely receives the same amount of time and attention as the other four when compared in most models. In fact, advocacy frequently evaporates when it comes to operationalizing its meaning and relating it to the other four functions. In some models, additional tasks are added including therapeutic interactions, case identification and outreach, or evaluation and documentation. The problems that arise, however, are not related to disputes about the functions or tasks of case management so much as they are rooted in the practice paradigms or conceptual frameworks that determine the way tasks are defined or operationalized, implemented, and prioritized.

The growing influence of clinical social work in mental health settings serves as an example. Johnson and Rubin's research on the views of clinical social workers found that "the level of importance assigned to monitoring, linkage and advocacy . . . was inversely related to the level of importance assigned to a psychodynamic orientation and to amount of experience in practicing psychotherapy. Moreover, social workers placed slightly more emphasis on psychodynamics than did nonsocial workers" (Johnson & Rubin, 1983, p. 52). Social workers' preferences directly related to the reason why social work is not clearly dominant in holding case management within its domain: "A large number of social workers in settings in which case management is appropriate appear to be indifferent to such work" (1983, p. 52).

Clinical models used increasingly in recent years by many social workers loom as obstacles to claiming or to preserving case management as a social work function. As Johnson and Rubin note, "social work clinicians seem to pay scant attention to interventions into social systems. Thus, workers seem to have abdicated the distinctive dual focus of social work, which could lead to a strong claim to leadership in case management . . ." (1983, p. 53).

Case management will be an expanding form of practice over the next decade and more. Mandated by such federal legislation as Public Law 99-660, case management has become inseparable from the funding and delivery of public services. Growing numbers of people are being brought into and sent forth from institutional care in hospitals, nursing homes, prisons, mental hospitals, and other tertiary care institutions. Institutional settings share in common two unpleasant facts: they are costly, and, for the most part, they are unable to produce a useful practice paradigm. Such a paradigm would provide for the supports and resources necessary to produce continuity of care; comprehensive, integrated care cutting across service domains of different sectors; and stable, supportive environments in community settings allowing clients to remain out of institutions.

Continued fragmentation within large provider systems and across different service delivery systems characterize the setting for case management practice. In service area after area, the demand for coordination, rationalization, and accountability promotes case management activity. In mental health, for example, all state mental health departments must develop a comprehensive mental health plan premised on the principles of community support systems (Stroul, 1989; Parrish, 1989). Case managers are the pivotal function in the entire design and are central to a statewide case management system to serve all people receiving substantial amounts of mental health services reimbursed by federal funding. Whatever its guiding model, the practice is seen as a focal point for assigning responsibility for individual clients, following them, and attempting to replace their use of the most costly forms of institutional care with coordinated, community-based care in more supportive environments.

The need for case management constitutes an indictment of existing organizational and interorganizational patterns of service design and delivery. Put somewhat differently, case management would not exist if there were integrated systems of care; comprehensive, integrated coverage across diverse organization sectors as income, housing, health/mental health/psychosocial rehabilitation/employment; or client-centered providers supporting people to identify their own needs and goals and negotiating systems to acquire or produce the resources required to live stable, positive lives in communities.

As a consequence of the absence of these social prerequisites, case management must become a system reform strategy with responsibility for direct practice with individuals and/or families.

Denial of either aspect of case management's dual focus on clients and on system reorganization inadvertently becomes a form of betrayal to the clients. The most common form of betrayal, failure to advocate for needed system interventions, obstructs the possibilities for clients' social development or capacity to gain independence from the service providing system. The economic and social context that forms the basis for most case management clients' lives demands advocacy either to arrange resources that clients need in a more responsive, coordinated manner or to produce vitally needed resources, such as safe, affordable housing, when none exist. These are the very areas where clinical social work has resisted intervening despite the fact that concrete needs structure and organize everyday life. While the psychodynamic paradigm (in any of its variations—e.g., "life cycle" theory) and its primary practice of psychotherapy are often perceived as the basis of status and legitimation within the profession, its overt manifestation frequently comes in the form of invalidating procurement of concrete resources as a desired professional task. Another common expression is assigning such tasks to nonprofessionals to preserve the professional aura of psychotherapy and desk-bound practice.

Social work has developed a number of case management models. Five of them are presented in this book, including four in Part II and the advocacy/empowerment model in Part VI. Each model must confront the dual responsibilities of providing direct services to clients and system intervention. The primary task facing the reader will be to evaluate how the different models stand in relation to the dual responsibilities. Further enriching the evaluative process will be the necessity to examine the models in the context of several formidable value differences. Among the most significant are the principles of self-determination or empowerment and the belief that all people can learn, grow, and develop. The self-determination or empowerment principle gets transformed into practice via the quality of involvement and participation clients have in setting their own goals, constructing their own needs assessment, and prioritizing those needs for action independent of the array of existing services offered by providers. The principle is articulated by Cnaan et al. as follows: "Individuals have the right and the ability to participate in making decisions regarding their lives and to do so on a regular basis. . . . The key issue is not to do things in the best interest of the client . . ." (1988, p. 65). Supporting clients to focus on their own strengths (see Kisthardt and Rapp in Part II), to feel validity in articulating their own desired directions and in setting forth their own direction plans or implementation varies considerably from assisting them in complying passively or adaptively to treatment or service plans defined by professionals for the client.

Central to the self-determination principle is a related one—that people can never be limited to what diagnostic categories project for them. Involvement in goal formulation, needs assessment, or decision-making necessitates seeing the client as a whole human being, not a patient or a disease category. It involves identifying and supporting strengths rather than imposing limitations (see Kisthardt and Rapp later). It requires promoting and supporting autonomy rather than acting for clients out of benevolent professionalism or simple expediency (see Collopy, 1988, in Part I).

Implementing empowerment as presented here changes the nature of the worker–client relationship. Workers are expected to relate to the client as a person participating in a voluntary partnership, not as a service consumer or manageable object whose relationship to the worker is shaped by providers' services or funding-stream limitations. Considerable problems can exist as a consequence, an observation made by Ozarin some years ago:

> It is almost impossible to achieve effective case management under most of the circumstances in the human services field where each agency views the client as a total case, although it is able to carry out only certain of the needed functions. Fundamental changes are needed, and this is difficult to achieve because present prerogatives and turfs of providers would have to be disturbed. (1978, p. 166)

Carol Austin's analysis of case management in long-term care indicates that providers often successfully thwart attempts to intervene in their domains. After systematic review of many projects, she concluded:

> Perhaps case management has enjoyed wide-spread acceptance because it has not been viewed as a systemic reform but as a function that can be incorporated into ongoing service delivery systems without changing structural relationships among providers. (1983, p. 17; see Part IV)

Accommodation to preexisting structural arrangements among providers brings with it a more subtle and previously documented dimension as well—at the level of shared paradigms or problem definitions and intervention methods (Rose, 1972; Warren et al., 1974; Rose & Black, 1985). Lourie captures this very point:

> The concept of case management has its central value in what is best for the client. The reason we haven't been able to make it work more effectively and more rationally is that its most effective realization runs counter to the baronial characteristics of service arrangements that professionals, guilds and interests create . . . it is clear that the arrangements are often more comfortable for the professionals and service interests than effective for clients. (Lourie, 1978, p. 163)

If we relate this notion to our discussion about clinical social work, we can see such professionalized conveniences in the consciousness and attitudes of the workers reluctant to validate clients through empowerment-based practice or to collaborate with them in advocacy activities designed to reform dysfunctional systems.

The interface between providers, especially within similar systems (e.g., mental health), allows for the common form of case management which we refer to as provider-driven. In this typical pattern of case management services, professional staff design treatment plans based more on the service providers' existing array of services and reimbursement formulas than on clients' active input. Case managers most often are assigned very large caseloads (40 to 60+) and are designated as the staff responsible for meeting clients' concrete needs through fulfilling the terms of the treatment plan. Concrete, material needs for such necessities as safe, affordable housing, income, or transportation commonly get devalued in these models, as do the case managers who work to fulfill them.

The predetermined package of services in most provider-driven models contains a common problem defining framework that is ideologically compatible among referring agencies. Frequently, providers have divided up the community turf and allocated different functional areas to particular agencies who legitimate one another's existence through referral patterns and their shared practice paradigm. The consistency of these interorganizational patterns was so prevalent in a multiagency, multicity study that Warren and his associates called it a "domain consensus pattern." They referred to the cohesiveness of problem defining practice paradigms among the providers as an "institutionalized thought structure" (Warren et al., 1974). The interaction of the domain consensus pattern and the institutionalized thought structure produces provider-driven models of case management which threaten neither.

Tacit agreement on individual defect models, implicitly neglecting the social context factors affecting clients' lives, and on therapeutic intervention modalities which devalue advocacy and systems intervention were central to the consensus. Provider-based models of case management devalue the tasks of linking, monitoring, and advocating around client-determined needs and securing necessary concrete resources. No one assumes overall responsibility for continuity of care or for clients' needs that fall beyond the paid services of providers and their mutually agreed on domains. Typically, these models foreclose all systems or issue advocacy, implying that there is no need for system reform or reorganization and certainly none for examination of prevailing practice models. As Lourie noted, it is a closed circle. To the extent that empowerment or self-determination are discussed, they represent provider-driven definitions of services or options, with clients being "empowered" to choose from among provider-defined menus.

Social work has participated in both client-driven and provider-driven paradigms. It has varied in its focus on the dual practice commitments described earlier. But social work still has the opportunity to seize leadership in case management development and infuse its leadership into the multiple service arenas where case management is present and expanding. However, internal obstacles and external barriers exist which require exploration. As already presented, the primary internal deterrent is the emphasis on individual defect explanatory paradigms and psychotherapeutic intervention coupled with the trend toward private practice. At the external level is the ongoing fiscal crisis and its impact on policies of the welfare state (Gough, 1979). These problems interact to produce a scenario that emphasizes cost containment through the reduced use of institutional settings in all service fields, the absolute need for alternative community-based support systems, and the urgent need for advocacy in both direct practice and policy, planning and program evaluation, all shaped by psychosocial conceptual frameworks.

Case management can become a service strategy to achieve the goals contoured by cost containment mandates while providing a data base for system impact. Where social work can grasp these political and economic priorities and their interaction, it will enhance its leadership potential. Where it does not grasp these priorities and continues to devalue public sector work and the clients who require it, there is good reason to believe that at least workers with a master's of social work (MSW) [and possibly those with a bachelor's degree in social work (BSW)] will be replaced by nurses or staff with less education and training. Finding adequate roles and functions within the psychosocial framework for all levels of social work personnel will be a major opportunity and challenge in coming years, provided appropriate conceptual frameworks are developed.

This book examines a number of the issues discussed in this chapter. Some of the articles cited here appear in the first section—"Creating a Critical Focus". Different case management models developed by social workers are presented in the next section along with two other articles designed to raise questions and discuss functional aspects of case management practice in mental health. Two other sections, on health care and long term care, address case management issues specific to those areas as well as the more general issues raised earlier. A section on research/program evaluation is included to develop a focus on system-impact and client-outcome variables. Finally, the volume concludes with an advocacy/empowerment model of case management practice to be used as a baseline for reflecting on values, goals, implementation processes, and outcomes of case management. It is hoped that this book will revitalize social work commitment to public sector practice, system reorganization, and leadership.

PART I

Creating a Critical Focus: Issues for Reflection

The first section of this book designates a number of themes to follow throughout the remainder of the volume. The four articles discuss case management functions, organizational and professional turf or domain issues, values and principles, and social work professional interests.

As the reader, your primary task in this section, reflecting on prevailing issues, anticipates an integration of these areas of importance. For example, all case management models delineate or specify tasks, roles, or functions. Rubin does an excellent job describing the case management skill areas and reviewing the literature that discusses and evaluates their overall effectiveness. The National Association of Social Workers (NASW) position statement mentions the tasks, articulates a number of issues, and establishes professional policy. But, as indicated in the introduction, the debate about case management's validity and legitimation rarely occurs in relation to its component tasks. Rather, the underlying values defining and shaping case management practice form the contentious material.

Intagliata develops a fine overview of case management practice. Although written about mental health care, his ideas can be generalized to other practice arenas. Note the attention paid by Intagliata to the concrete, material needs of the case management client and the necessity for advocacy. Intagliata identifies the basis for advocacy and the requisite administrative supports for its development. Use these concepts to assess the extent to which other case management models acknowledge and develop this area of activity.

Intagliata also describes the relationship between the case manager and the client as the central factor in producing positive client outcomes. The three objectives he specifies for case management all emphasize the systems focus for case management practice: producing continuity of care, enhancing accessibility and accountability of service systems, and improving service system efficiency. Aware of the dual focus of case management, he highlights three basic case management functions: remaining aware of the comprehensive needs of clients, linking clients to resources appropriate to their needs, and monitoring services to assure that they are effective. Advocacy at the client and systems or issue levels is discussed together with the necessity for supervisory and organizational backup.

Intagliata does not enter into a major controversy within mental health program development—the issue of client- versus provider-driven case management. His argument strongly implies a client-driven case management model as indicated by the references to services being appropriate to clients' goals and needs; to the tasks of monitoring and assessing provider performance; and to the inevitability of advocacy activities. But there is also the importance of linking and referring clients to services. How do criteria get established for deciding which providers' services are relevant and appropriate to a given client's needs? Who makes that decision? What supports exist for challenging providers on the appropriateness of their practice patterns or paradigms?

The mediating quality of Intagliata's work is found in his focus on the case manager–client relationship and its supports as the central concern. How well do the other authors maintain this focus? Where does primacy rest: with the relationship between worker and client or, more subtly, between the worker and his or her colleagues among the providers?

None of the value-based issues can be more significant than the commitment to clients' self-determination, autonomy, or empowerment. As the chapter by Collopy suggests, these values are complex and each case manager, like each social worker, has a moral responsibility to examine how to operationalize this professional principle in daily practice. Rhetoric, whether professional or organizational, is insufficient. How do different case management models view the client? Where does human dignity come into practice? Can diagnostic classification schemes and funding mechanisms that require their use permit workers to see clients as capable of participating in defining their own directions or needs? How are the commitments to clients as whole human beings actually reflected in what case managers do? What role is established, if any, for clients' active input into service plans? How are clients' family members to be involved, and what role do they play in relation to clients' autonomy? Can family members be included in positive roles while maintaining commitments to the clients' self-determination?

The dignity of the human being and the case management program's capacity to operationalize its definition of autonomy or empowerment interact. Empowerment has become a frequently used concept lately, but ambiguity about its meaning prevails. Collopy's work is practice-based, directed toward clarifying the meaning of autonomy as a living principle and commitment. How do the case management models presented in the later sections define their principles? What have they to say about the dignity of clients? What position do they take on the empowerment concept?

Can case managers automatically assume that clients will be validated as whole human beings because they are being offered services by a legitimated provider agency? To reply affirmatively suggests that clients derive validity and dignity through the providers. This issue requires careful reflection. Can the social development of clients or clients' growth and movement as people arise as the result of improving their service consuming abilities? How do we know whether available services are appropriate to the clients' goals? Or do automatic treatment or service planning mechanisms prescribe available services and assume their validity without regard to the individual client's goals?

How do clients' needs and agency services interface? If you are working or placed in a mental health or health agency, what do these places do about such issues as the need for safe, affordable housing? Are clients viewed differently in terms of their human value when they are assigned different diagnostic classifications? Is there any relationship between how your agency is funded and what boundaries it applies to its work with clients, to its approach to case management, or to its definition of advocacy?

Examining the value-based issues, the turf-based issues, and the paradigm-based influences in shaping case management practice purports to increase the conscious, active decision-making aspect of each case manager's work. It is assumed that reflection on these issues will produce a more active, more informed case manager. Quite obviously, the client-driven or the advocacy/empowerment approach is endorsed, but many other models have been included. What makes one model appear more or less effective? How can the criteria for making decisions such as this become more conscious and actively selected? How do the different models perceive the responsibility of the worker? All of these questions are part of the process of developing focus.

CHAPTER 1

Case Management

Allan Rubin

Case management is an approach to service delivery that attempts to ensure that clients with complex, multiple problems and disabilities receive all the services they need in a timely and appropriate fashion. It is a boundary-spanning approach in that, instead of providing a specific direct service, it utilizes case managers who link the client to the maze of direct service providers. These case managers are expected to assume ulitmate responsibility for seeing that the service delivery system is responsive to all the needs of each client. Case management has been used in various fields of practice, especially in mental health with the chronically mentally disabled, in the care of the aging and of those with physical or developmental disabilities, and in child welfare (Bedford & Hybertson, 1975; Fitz, 1978; Beatrice, 1979; Caragonne, 1980, 1981; Steinberg & Carter, 1983).

Although the emphasis in case management is on linkage, case managers in theory do whatever it takes—whether brokerage, advocacy, or resource development—to ensure that all client needs are met; they may even provide a missing service themselves. Holding one worker responsible for the overall fate of the client and for the responsivity of the entire service delivery system is a strategy for overcoming the neglect and fragmentation that are thought to typify the way in which myriad service providers have historically dealt with multiproblem or profoundly impaired clients. In other words, designating one person as the case manager is an attempt to ensure that there is somebody who is accountable and who is helping the client hold the service delivery system accountable, someone who cannot "pass the buck" to another agency or individual when and if services are not delivered quickly and appropriately (Miller, 1983).

GROWTH AND AIMS

Little was known about case management before the mid-1970s (Platman et al., 1982). Its emergence as a distinct concept was linked to the growth of human service programs during the 1960s. Public funding for those service programs was provided largely through categorical channels, resulting in a network of services deemed "highly complex, fragmented, duplicative and uncoordinated" (Intagliata, 1982, p. 655). As different programs emerged to offer specialized services or to serve narrowly defined target groups, the perception developed that persons with multiple problems and needs were not being served adequately by disconnected programs dealing with narrow aspects of their problems. For example, an elderly client might need cash supports from one source, housing from another, nutritional services from a third, care for physical or mental impairments from a fourth or fifth, social interaction and support from a sixth, and so on.

During the early 1970s, the Department of Health, Education and Welfare funded a series of demonstration projects to test various approaches to improving the coordination of federal service programs at the state and local levels (Mittenthal, 1976; Morrill, 1976). These "service integration" projects featured such techniques as "client-tracking systems, information and referral mechanisms, one-stop service centers, specialized management information systems, interagency planning and service delivery agreements, computerized resource inventories, and management reorganization projects" (Intagliata, 1982, p. 656). Most projects also featured case managers, called "system agents," who were expected to coordinate resources for clients and be accountable for their appropriate passage through the service system.

Another force giving rise to the growth of case management was the deinstitutionalization movement, particularly in the fields of mental health and developmental disabilities. After the discovery of psychotropic drugs in the mid-1950s mental health systems began moving people from institutional to community settings in the belief that, with the ability of these drugs to inhibit their symptomatology, these clients would benefit from being in the community, which was thought to be less restrictive and more humane than institutions. The expansion of community-based human service programs during this period fostered this belief. However, during the 1970s evidence accumulated indicating that previously institutionalized individuals with profound, multiple needs did not always fare well in the community. They often lived in squalor and were rejected and perhaps victimized by their neighbors. Although aftercare was comprehensive in some localities, in most it was not. In many places human service agencies, even community mental health centers that were established to offset institutionalization, responded inadequately to the plight of the formerly institutionalized (Arnhof, 1975; Kirk & Therrien, 1975; General Accounting Office, 1977; Lamb, 1979a; Mechanic, 1980).

As the literature began to expose these problems, the field began to learn that the mere presence in the community of expanded categorical services did not mean that those services would be utilized. It also learned that community settings would not necessarily be less restrictive or more humane than the protected institutional environment (Bachrach, 1980, 1981), particularly for individuals whose profound impairments and unresponsiveness to conventional treatment approaches favored by professionals but geared to less impaired clientele made them unattractive to some community-based agencies and practitioners (Hogarty, 1971; Lamb, 1976; Rubin & Johnson, 1982). These clients often are unable or unmotivated to negotiate an unresponsive service delivery system themselves (Test, 1979). Research has shown that many of them, even with adequate community-based care, will be in and out of institutions throughout their lives (Talbott, 1978).

Consequently, a service component termed case management was recommended in an effort to accomplish the following objectives: (1) ensure continuity in care across services at any given point or over time (for example, as the individual moves between the institution and community through cycles of relapse and recovery); (2) ensure that services will be responsive to the full range of the person's needs as these needs change over time, perhaps throughout the person's life if necessary; (3) help these individuals gain access to needed services, overcoming obstacles to accessibility associated with eligibility criteria, regulations, policies, and procedures; and (4) ensure that the services that are provided match the client's needs, are provided in a proper and timely fashion, and are not inappropriately duplicative (Intagliata, 1982).

During the late 1970s, the National Institute of Mental Health funded demonstration projects in 19 states to implement and test its services integration concept, which was termed the community support system (CSS) (Turner, 1977; Turner & TenHoor, 1978; Turner & Shiffren, 1979). The CSS concept included the allocation of special coordinating power and authority to a specified agency at the local level. This "core CSS agency" would assess the needs of the chronically mentally ill in its area, negotiate interagency linkages and agreements for providing all needed support services, and develop new service components to connect existing gaps in the service network. A keystone of the CSS approach was the case manager, whose coordination efforts were empowered by the formal set of contracts that were negotiated by the core agency and that bound providers to deliver the specified services to the case manager's clients. During the same period, Congress (P.L. 94–103 and P.L. 95–602) mandated that service integration mechanisms featuring case managers be provided to deinstitutionalized developmentally disabled persons, and the Joint Commission on Accreditation of Hospitals (1979) established the requirement that community mental health services provide case management. By 1984, Johnson (1984) reported that 36 states required case management in their mental health services and that an additional 12 states recommended it.

CORE FUNCTIONS

Although the term "case management" grew in response to recent forces, it is not a new concept. It has antecedents in the knowledge bases of vocational rehabilitation, public health nursing, and social work (Platman et al., 1982; Miller, 1983). In social work the parallels are strongest in theories of generalist social work practice, which emphasize boundary spanning by developing resource systems, linking people to resource systems and making those systems more accessible and responsive to people's needs, and enhancing the coordination of resource systems (Minahan, 1976). Some authors from other disciplines consider case management "a well-established social work technique" (Schwartz, Goldman, & Churgin, 1982, p. 1006). Miller (1983) considers case management "part of the history of the profession of social work" (p. 6).

The range of case management functions varies depending on such contextual factors as the characteristics of the target population, environmental constraints, the type of agency employing the case manager, caseload size, and the nature of the service delivery system (Intagliata, 1982; Intagliata & Baker, 1983). For example, the extent to which case managers become engaged in linking clients to existing services as opposed to creating the needed services may depend on the range of services already available. This variation notwithstanding, four basic functions—assessment, planning, linking, and monitoring—appear in almost every description of case management and are deemed essential regardless of context.

Assessment

Case managers are expected to remain aware of their clients' comprehensive needs as well as their current and potential strengths and weaknesses. They are expected to be familiar with, although not necessarily directly involved in, the initial intake and assessment. They are expected to stay in close regular contact with direct service staff to ensure that their information is comprehensive and up to date. They are also expected to remain in regular contact with their clients so as to observe changes in client capabilities and needs. This includes a recurring evaluation of the amount of support currently and potentially available to the client, such as through natural helping networks and informal support systems. The case manager has been called "the only provider in the system whose responsibility is being aware of the 'whole' client" (Intagliata, 1982, p. 660).

Planning

Case managers may be expected to develop an overall case plan for each client. It should include provision for services the client might need day or night. It should focus on the progression of services to be provided over time and on the linkages among them and between them and the informal support system. In case management, planning is done early. In deinstitutionalization, for example, the case manager does not wait until the client has left the institution and entered the community-based agency to begin assessment and planning. Instead, an awareness of the community resources for a given client is part of the discharge planning process, and the case manager is the one practitioner who assumes responsibility for ensuring that the plan is implemented in a timely fashion and as intended. The assumption of this responsibility has been deemed the core, overarching principle of case management (Intagliata, 1982; Miller, 1983). To enhance their contribution to case planning, case managers maintain a complete roster of service agencies and organizations in the community, know what services each provides and its policies and procedures, supply information to case planners on available resources, and interpret the purpose and function of the case plan to service providers (Gerhard & Dorgan, 1983).

Linking

Case managers are expected to link clients to the services and entitlements that are available to meet their needs. This includes referring or transferring clients to all required services and informal support networks. It also includes helping clients overcome barriers to utilizing the required services or receiving entitlements. Such barriers may include eligibility requirements or restrictive regulations and policies. Some generic agencies, for example, may be reluctant to serve clients with particular disabilities, such as the mentally ill or developmentally disabled. More subtle barriers might include practitioners who informally resist serving the chronically and profoundly disabled, perhaps by delays in follow-through or by a lack of enthusiasm or persistence in working with these less articulate clients who do not respond well to conventional therapies. To overcome these barriers, case managers sometimes have to function as case advocates for their clients, particularly those clients whose profound impairments make them unable to speak for themselves. (Advocacy is often listed as an additional, separate function of case management.)

Case managers therefore establish and maintain contact with service providers and maintain formal and informal relationships with administrative personnel who can facilitate referrals (Gerhard & Dorgan, 1983). However, this does not mean that the case manager always must bear the brunt of advocating directly with external agencies. In more difficult situations (for example, those not responsive to informal interpersonal negotiation), case managers might enlist the support of supervisors or administrators in their own agency or seek the help of legal aid services or of agencies set up to provide advocacy services for specified target populations, such as the National Association for Retarded Citizens. Although the type of advocacy most often undertaken is case advocacy—interceding on behalf of an individual client—this function can also lead to class advocacy in response to documented service deficiencies detected through the accumulation of case advocacy efforts involving numerous clients.

Not all barriers to linkage come from service providers. Sometimes clients resist being served or drop out of service. Some are unable to utilize services unless appropriate supports are provided (Test, 1979). For example, some profoundly impaired clients recently discharged from the institutions may need transportation assistance to keep appointments or may forget to take their prescribed medications. To be effective, linkers need to remain aware of these contingencies and ensure that the appropriate emotional or tangible supports are provided to help clients do their part toward implementing the case plan. Nevertheless, the case manager respects a client's right to refuse treatment.

Monitoring

Case managers are expected to monitor continuously the services provided to their clients. This requires ongoing contact with clients and service providers to ensure that appointments are kept and that appropriate and effective services are provided with minimum delay. This contact is often face to face and includes visits with the client while the service is being provided. Firsthand contact is thought to enhance the quality of the feedback and to improve the case manager's relationship with service providers and clients and therefore his or her ability to influence them. Implicit in the monitoring function is an evaluation function in which the case manager systematically rates and records progress toward attaining the objectives each component of the service plan is designed to attain. Information gained from monitoring can lead to reassessment and the development of new plans or linkages.

Other Common Functions

As the link between the client and the service system—the persons ultimately responsible for seeing that the client's needs are met—case managers are often not able to pass the buck. They often function as trouble-shooters and are expected to be ready to perform whatever role it takes to ensure that their clients receive appropriate, coordinated, and continuous care despite the inadequacies of the service system (Miller, 1983). As noted earlier, case managers at times deliver a service, secure advocacy services, or become directly involved in creating needed services. This might involve developing natural support systems.

Outreach is another common role. Case managers are often expected to identify eligible clients, and they may have to invest time in finding clients and encouraging them to utilize services. Such outreach often must be persistent and aggressive and include home visits. Case managers cannot remain office-bound or deem their clients "unmotivated" and therefore neglect them when they fail to keep appointments or are hard to locate. This relates to a most critical and controversial issue—the degree to which case managers themselves provide direct services to clients.

To some extent, the direct service function of case management may be inescapable. For example, the case manager may provide the one stable relationship the client can rely on—a relationship that endures and provides continuity as the client moves back and forth across institutional, community, and agency boundaries. This relationship can be rewarding and reassuring to individuals devalued by society, and perhaps by other human service practitioners. It also can give them a sense of stability and hope and enhance the case manager's capacity to motivate clients to utilize services or comply with case plans, for example, by taking their medications.

When other direct service staff are unavailable, the case manager may be responsible for performing some of their functions. This might include training clients in basic living skills, such as those required for personal hygiene, using public transportation, or household management. For example, the case manager might also help clients shop for groceries or might transport them to a needed service if no other arrangements can be made. Case managers may have to provide crisis intervention when unexpected changes in the environment overwhelm clients, particularly those, such as formerly institutionalized psychiatric patients, whose ability to cope is impaired and whose social adjustment is tenuous. Case managers are not necessarily expected to function as therapists or to aid clients directly in resolving crises, but they do need to provide personal support and be on hand to refer and perhaps accompany the client to a crisis intervention service provider. In this connection, case management services are expected to be available around the clock; in some sites case managers are on call 24 hours a day (Intagliata & Baker, 1983, p. 83).

ROLE ISSUES AND AUTHORITY

Case management was conceived as a boundary-spanning function. It was intended primarily to coordinate and monitor the efforts of multiple service providers, not to create another group of specialized direct care staff. Yet case managers are expected to be prepared to depart from their boundary-spanning role to fulfill their ultimate responsibility for ensuring that clients' needs are met in the face of incomplete service delivery systems.

Some find it difficult to envision how case managers can properly and effectively implement their assessment, planning, and linking functions without performing direct care tasks and utilizing specialized direct service knowledge and skills (Lourie, 1978; Lamb, 1980; Intagliata, 1982; Miller, 1983). For example, case managers working with the chronically mentally disabled may need to recognize early signs of decompensation or unmanageable stress and to understand the likely psychological effects of various environmental circumstances. They may have to use their relationship with the client to motivate and secure client compliance with the discharge plan. In view of this, Lamb (1980) argues that it is difficult for the case manager to possess the requisite psychological knowledge of the client outside the context of the therapeutic relationship. Lamb therefore believes that the clients' therapists should be their case managers, although he adds the qualification that the type of therapy he envisions is supportive and ecologically oriented, not in-depth psychotherapy.

In view of the breadth of the case management role, Lamb further argues that good case management and good direct service provision are inseparable. If case management functions are part of the normal duties of a conscientious caseworker and if extensive direct service skills and involvement are necessary for a case manager to assess needs adequately and ensure that they are met, then why add another layer (the case manager) to the already complex system of services and communication? Instead, why not simply deal directly with direct service providers who fail to perform case management functions?

Others point out that the foregoing conceptions overlook the authority of case management. The case manager has the ultimate authority for the case. In theory, this authority separates real case management from the referral, linkage, and coordination functions of direct service providers who are part of a professional treatment team. In this view case managers are distinguished by their *empowerment* to negotiate on behalf of consumers (R. E. Dorgan, personal communication, April 19, 1983).

However, the degree of empowerment of case managers has not always been as much as was envisioned in the original community services system concept. The authority case managers have varies widely in different localities and service delivery systems. Ross (1980) and Caragonne (1981) have identified different models of case management, ranging from situations in which case managers or their agencies have minimal authority over provider programs to those in which the authority is more comprehensive.

Some believe that the extent of the case manager's authority is the most critical factor influencing the effectiveness of case management. Various ways have been proposed to enhance the case manager's authority with service providers (Schwartz, Goldman, & Churgin, 1982). One way is to increase the formality and clarity of policies, procedures, and agreements that provide case management authority in and between agencies. Another is through fiscal control, by giving case managers discretion over the funds needed to purchase specific services for individual clients. A third way recognizes the importance of informal authority and informal working relationships and focuses on the case manager's credibility with administrators and clinical service providers. Will they accept the case manager as a peer and perhaps as an ally?

Or will they reject the case manager as an intruder, perhaps one who is clinically unsophisticated or otherwise not qualified? One suggestion for enhancing the informal clout of case managers has been to provide them with adequate agency resources, such as office space and secretarial support, so as to signify the importance the agency attaches to their work. Another suggestion calls for locating case managers in clinical service units. Most attention concerning the informal authority of case managers, however, has been focused on their professional status.

STATUS AND TRAINING

Just as programs vary in the scope they assign to the case management role and the amount of autonomy and authority they give case managers, there is variation in the level of education reported for case managers. It ranges from a high school diploma to a doctoral degree and may depend on what a given program expects the case manager to do (Intagliata, 1982). Prior experience may influence education requirements. One system, for example, employs as case managers for the chronically mentally ill either individuals with bachelor's degrees plus extensive experience in working with psychiatric patients in state institutions, or individuals with master's degrees in social work or counseling but without prior contact with these clients (Baker, Jodrey, & Morrell, 1979).

Most programs require case managers to have a bachelor's degree (Intagliata, 1982). However, concern has been expressed as to whether that is sufficient in view of the range of activities case managers may need to perform without supervision and the difficulties they may have in establishing credibility with administrators and other professionals, who may denigrate them as "paraprofessionals" (Schwartz, Goldman, & Churgin, 1982; Intagliata, 1982; Johnson & Rubin, 1983; Bagarozzi & Kurtz, 1983). At the same time, doubt exists about the willingness and enthusiasm of more highly educated professionals, MSWs included, when faced with the less prestigious functions case managers frequently perform, such as transporting clients to an appointment or accompanying them on a shopping trip (Schwartz, Goldman, & Churgin, 1982; Intagliata, 1982; Johnson & Rubin, 1983). There is also concern that highly qualified case managers may be prone to burnout more quickly than case managers without advanced degrees, who may not be as likely to perceive the less prestigious duties as beneath them (Intagliata, 1982).

Doubt has been expressed as to whether any level of formal education can adequately prepare a person to perform competently the full range of case management roles. Some wonder whether it is realistic to expect any worker, regardless of prior education and training, to be able and willing to blend diagnostic and therapeutic understanding and skills, political savvy in overcoming bureaucratic rigidity, the ability to develop formal resource systems and informal helping networks, rehabilitation skills, and patience in helping clients achieve minute and simple changes in their basic living skills (Johnson & Rubin, 1983).

In view of the scope of the case management role and the potential for role ambiguity and conflict, orientation and in-service training are deemed essential for case managers, regardless of their professional level (Intagliata, 1982; Bagarozzi & Kurtz, 1983). Orientation sessions could focus on the full range of functions and responsibilities the case management role entails, the rationale for the role, and the values that guide it. Case managers would be helped to understand that their clients often have disabilities that severely limit their ability to progress and that the goal of case management for these clients is to improve the quality of care they receive and enhance the quality of their lives, not to attain any dramatic improvement in their level of functioning. Lamb (1979b) has warned that without a realistic conception of what they can accomplish with their clients, case managers will experience frustration and burnout as a result of their overreaching expectations.

The components of in-service training vary, depending on prior education and experience. They might include information on assessing and understanding client disabilities, common psychotropic medications and their side effects, the range of local services and client entitlements available, legal rights of clients, and record keeping. They might also include skill development in relating to clients, goal setting, problem solving, crisis intervention, and advocacy.

Attention has been given not just to the level of education and training recommended for case managers, but also to the preferred academic disciplines. Conclusive empirical data are lacking as to which disciplines offer the best preparation for case management. Most case managers have been educated in a human services discipline, but there is no clear consensus that any one human services discipline offers the best preparation. The fields most commonly cited as likely to offer good preparation are social work, public health nursing, vocational rehabilitation, and human services generalist practice. Which, if any, level or type of preparation best prepares individuals to perform case management roles skillfully, enthusiastically, and effectively remains a key question for future research. Conceivably, such research might find that the answer varies, depending on the range of functions, expectations, level of autonomy, and organizational supports the case manager has in a given setting.

CASELOAD AND SUPERVISION

The literature identifies a number of additional factors that may influence how case management services are delivered. One factor is caseload size. Research reviewed by Intagliata (1982) found that a large increase in caseload size may impair the quality and effectiveness of case management services by reducing the case managers' contact with clients and predisposing them to respond to crises rather than anticipate problems and help clients plan ahead. It also might predispose them to do things for clients instead of helping clients become more independent.

Likewise, heavy caseloads often diminish the opportunity to build close relationships with clients and increase the propensity to wait for clients to take the initiative to make contact instead of reaching out to them. Estimates of the ideal caseload size vary, depending on client attributes, their geographic proximity to one another, and the case manager's competencies. Suggested estimates for an individual case manager working with chronic psychiatric clients have ranged from a low of 15 to a high of 30. The typical caseload size for these clients appears to range from 25 to 35 (Intagliata & Baker, 1983).

Some have recommended that comprehensive case management responsibilities might be better assigned to a case management team instead of individual case managers (Kirk & Therien, 1975; Test, 1979; Turner & TenHoor, 1978; Intagliata, 1982). The members of the team may all be case managers, or the team might comprise a single case manager along with other professionals, such as a psychiatrist, nurse, psychologist, or social worker. It is argued that a team would increase staff availability to provide continuous coverage, add viewpoints for managing difficult problems, and avoid the isolation that can lead to burnout of the individual case manager.

Another factor affecting case management services is how case managers are supervised. Concern about supervision stems in part from the potential for role ambiguity and role conflict and the consequent need to monitor the activities of case managers, which might depart from what is expected of them. Caragonne (1981), for example, found that many supervisors were not aware that the pattern of activities of the case managers they supervised differed markedly from their prescribed roles. Supervision is also cited as an important source of recognition and support, encouraging case managers to experience a sense of value in their work. Such a sense of value is often difficult for case managers to derive given the limited potential for improvement in the social functioning of many of their clients and the relatively low value that others sometimes attach to the case manager's work. In view of this, adequate supervisory support is deemed essential in sustaining the motivation of case managers and preventing burnout (Caragonne, 1981; Intagliata, 1982; Intagliata & Baker, 1983).

RESEARCH AND CRITICAL ANALYSES

Evidence is accumulating on the potential efficacy of case management programs. In a rigorous and often cited experiment, Stein and Test (1980) evaluated a community-based service program that incorporated case management principles as part of a comprehensive approach to respond to the needs of the chronically mentally disabled. The program effectively maintained clients in the community without worse consequences than occur in institutionalization; the consequences measured were client symptomatology, self-esteem, social functioning, quality of life and life satisfaction, burden to family or community, and program cost. King, Muraco, and Wells (1984) reported a quasi-experimental study that also had results favoring the effectiveness of case management services. In addition, three experimental evaluations found case management effective in reducing the cost of caring for those who are aged, physically ill, or disabled (Boone, Coulton, & Keller, 1981; Akabas, Fine, & Yasser, 1982; Davies, Ferlie, & Challis, 1984). Not every study of the impact of case management has had positive results, however. Coulton and Frost (1982), for example, found that the receipt of case management services had no effect on the extent to which the elderly utilized mental health services. Ozarin (1978) and Miller (1983) reviewed the evaluative research on the effectiveness of case management programs.

Caution must be exercised in interpreting the meaning of evaluations of case management programs and generalizing from them. Case management program evaluated experimentally are often implemented under ideal conditions, perhaps as part of a much broader system of service provision geared exclusively to the unique needs of disabled clients and not compromised by such factors as insufficient support, insufficient empowerment of case managers, or critical gaps in service availability. A stiffer test of the case management concept is not how well it works when accompanied by a comprehensive package of direct service provisions targeted to the needs of the disabled, but how well it works when it stands alone as a boundary-spanning strategy for dealing with an inadequate service delivery system that contains programs unresponsive to the needs of the target population. Given the limitations in the public funding of social welfare programs, a critical issue is whether the impact of case management on a weak service delivery system is sufficient to justify redirecting scarce funds to it from existing direct care provisions (Morris & Lescohier, 1978). In other words, is there a net improvement in client care by transferring resources from other services into a boundary-spanning function?

In this connection, it is important to realize that not everyone who is called a case manager performs most of the core case management functions. Conversely, not everyone who performs some case management functions is called a case manager. Some programs hire "case managers" merely to assist the primary clinician with routinized, mundane activities or to provide concrete services or linkage without any authority (Intagliata & Baker, 1983). Other programs assume that each client's primary clinician also serves as case manager and therefore call every clinician a case manager and assume that every client has a case manager (Kurtz, Bagarozzi, & Pollane, 1984).

This confusion has prompted some to liken the term "case management" to a Rorschach test on which is projected any image one wishes (Schwartz, Goldman, & Churgin, 1982), or to "question whether case management is simply a new term for social work" (Bagarozzi & Kurtz, 1983, p. 13). Lourie (1978) argues that all human service agencies dealing with individual or family social, physical, or mental disability subscribe to and claim to practice case management. Lamb (1980) claims that good therapy must include case management. In theory at least, generalist social work practitioners, no matter whether they are called case managers or something else, are supposed to be prepared to perform assessment, planning, linkage, brokerage, and advocacy functions in a boundary-spanning context. Bachrach (1983) argues that merely designating staff members as case managers is no guarantee that case management aims will be achieved:

> If a system of care is turly responsive to the needs of chronic mental patients, it is prima facie evidence that de facto case management exists, whether or not there are people called case managers. (p. 100)

That serious deficiencies in society's care of its profoundly disabled and unwanted citizens can be overcome through service integration strategies, without a much greater expenditure of public resources, can be a seductive notion to those who resist such expenditures or feel that they will not be forthcoming. It dates back over a hundred years to an era when the Charity Organization Society was viewed as a remedy for deficiencies in the voluntary welfare system. Morris and Lescohier (1978) equate the current popularity of case management with this notion. They cite fiscal incentives as more powerful than the efforts of case managers in motivating agencies to modify their services. They note that greater agency responsivity to the clients of case managers requires taking resources away from other demands on these agencies that they may feel better equipped to meet. Rather than use scarce funds to add case managers to the service delivery system, they argue, would not a greater impact be achieved by reserving these funds as incentives to modify agency practices or to create new services?

Process research on case management programs has shown that "case managers' actual activities are shaped ultimately by the constraints of the environments within which they work, not by their formal job descriptions" (Intagliata, 1982, p. 670). This research has also found that even when case managers strive to implement their role as intended, they may lack the authority needed to accomplish their objectives. Based on his review of this research, Intagliata (1982) recommended more research to evaluate and improve the implementation of case management programs. Additional experimental studies also are needed on the outcomes of alternative case management models in different kinds of service delivery systems. The results of such research may help determine whether case management remains a viable strategy or succumbs to the criticisms that it cannot be implemented properly and that its costs might be better spent in directly filling gaps in existing services rather than through a boundary-spanning mechanism.

REFERENCES

Akabas, S. H., Fine, M., & Yasser, R. 1982. Putting secondary prevention to the test: A study of an early intervention strategy with disabled workers. *Journal of Primary Prevention*. 2(2):165–187.

Arnhof, F. M. 1975. Social consequences of policy towards mental illness. *Science*. 188(6):1277–1281.

Bachrach, L. L. 1980. Is the least restrictive environment always the best? Sociological and semantic implications. *Hospital and Community Psychiatry*. 31(2):97–103.

Bachrach, L. L. 1981. Continuity of care for chronic mental patients: A conceptual analysis. *American Journal of Psychiatry*. 138(11):1449–1456.

Bachrach, L. L. 1983. New directions in deinstitutionalization planning. In L. L. Bachrach (Ed.), *New Directions in Mental Health Services: Deinstitutionalization*. San Francisco: Jossey-Bass, pp. 93–106.

Bagarozzi, D. A., & Kurtz, L. F. 1983. Administrators' perspectives on case management. *Aretê*. 8(1):13–21.

Baker, F., Jodrey, D., & Morell, M. 1979. *Evaluation of Case Management Training Program: Final Report*. New York: New York School of Psychiatry.

Beatrice, D. F. 1979. *Case Management: A Policy Option for Long-Term Care*. Washington, DC: Health Care Financing Administration, Department of Health, Education & Welfare.

Bedford, L., & Hybertson, L. D. 1975. Emotionally disturbed children: A program of alternatives to residential treatment. *Child Welfare*. 54(2):109–115.

Boone, C. R., Coulton, C. J., & Keller, S. M. 1981. The impact of early and comprehensive social work services on length of stay. *Social Work in Health Care*. 7(3): 65–73.

Caragonne, P. 1980. *An Analysis of the Function of the Case Manager in Four Mental Health Social Services Settings*. Austin: University of Texas School of Social Work.

Caragonne, P. 1981. *A Comparative Analysis of Twenty-Two Settings Using Case Management Components*. Austin: University of Texas School of Social Work.

Coulton, C., & Frost, A. K. 1982. Use of social and health services by the elderly. *Journal of Health and Social Behavior*. 23(12):330–339.

Davies, B. P., Ferlie, E., & Challis, D. 1984. *A Guide to Efficiency—Improving Innovations in the Social Care of the Frail Elderly*. Canterbury, England: Personal Social Services Research Unit, University of Kent.

Fitz, J. 1978. *Case Management for the Developmentally Disabled: A Feasibility Study Report*. Raleigh: North Carolina University Center for Urban Affairs and Community Services.

General Accounting Office. 1977. *Returning the Mentally Disabled to the Community: Government Needs to Do More* (HRD-76-152). Washington, DC: Author.

Gerhard, R. J., & Dorgan, R. E. 1983. The case manager: A vehicle for consumer continuity. Unpublished manuscript.

Hogarty, G. 1971. The plight of schizophrenics in modern treatment programs. *Hospital and Community Psychiatry*. 22(7):197–203.

Intagliata, J. 1982. Improving the quality of community care for the chronically mentally disabled: The role of the case management. *Schizophrenia Bulletin*. 8(4):655–674.

Intagliata, J., & Baker, F. 1983. Factors affecting case management services for the chronically mentally ill. *Administration in Mental Health*. 11(2):75–91.

Johnson, P. J. 1984. A survey of state-level emphasis on case management. Manuscript under review for publication, University of North Carolina School of Social Work, Chapel Hill.

Johnson, P. J., & Rubin, A. 1983. Case management in mental health: A social work domain? *Social Work.* 28(1):49–55.

Joint Commission on Accreditation of Hospitals. 1979. *Principles for Accreditation of Community Mental Health Service Programs.* Chicago: Author.

King, J. A., Muraco, W. A., & Wells, J. P. 1984. *Case Management: A Study of Patient Outcomes.* Columbus: Ohio Department of Mental Health, Office of Program Evaluation and Research.

Kirk, S. A., & Therrien, M. E. 1975. Community mental health myths and the fate of former hospitalized patients. *Psychiatry.* 38(3):209–217.

Kurtz, L. F., Bagarozzi, D. A., & Pollane, L. P. 1984. Case management in mental health. *Health & Social Work.* 9(3):201–211.

Lamb, H. R. 1976. Guiding principles for community survival. In H. R. Lamb (Ed.), *Community Survival for Long-Term Patients.* San Francisco: Jossey-Bass, pp. 1–13.

Lamb, H. R. 1979a. The new asylums in the community. *Archives of General Psychiatry.* 36(2):129–134.

Lamb, H. R. 1979b. Staff burnout in work with long-term patients. *Hospital and Community Psychiatry.* 30(6):396–398.

Lamb, H. R. 1980. Therapist-case managers: More than brokers of services. *Hospital and Community Psychiatry.* 31(11):762–764.

Lourie, N. V. 1978. Case management. In J. A. Talbott (Ed.), *The Chronic Mental Patient.* Washington, DC: American Psychiatric Association, pp. 159–164.

Mechanic, D. 1980. *Mental Health and Social Policy.* Englewood Cliffs, N.J.: Prentice-Hall.

Miller, G. 1983. Case management: The essential services. In C. J. Sanborn (Ed.), *Case Management in Mental Health Service.* New York: Haworth Press, pp. 3–16.

Minahan, A. 1976. Generalists and specialists in social work—implications for education and practice. *Aretê.* 4(2):62.

Mittenthal, S. 1976. Evaluation overview: A system approach to services integration. *Evaluation.* 3(1,2):142–148.

Morrill, W. 1976. Services integration and the Department of Health, Education and Welfare. *Evaluation.* 3(1,2):52–55.

Morris, R., & Lescohier, I. H. 1978. Service integration: Real versus illusory solutions to welfare dilemmas. In R. C. Farri & Y. Hasenfeld (Eds.), *The Management of Human Services.* New York: Columbia University Press, pp. 21–50.

Ozarin, L. 1978. The pros and cons of case management. In J. A. Talbott (Ed.), *The Chronic Mental Patient.* Washington, D.C.: American Psychiatric Association, pp. 165–170.

Platman, S. R., et al. 1982. Case management of the mentally disabled. *Journal of Public Health Policy.* 3(3):302–314.

Ross, H. 1980. *Proceedings of the Conference on the Evaluation of Case Management Programs, March 5–6, 1979.* Los Angeles: Volunteers for Services to Older Persons.

Rubin, A., & Johnson, P. J. 1982. Practitioner orientations toward serving the chronically disabled: Prospects for policy implementation. *Administration in Mental Health.* 10(3):2–12.

Schwartz, S. R., Goldman, H. H., & Churgin, S. 1982. Case management for the chronic mentally ill: Models and dimensions. *Hospital and Community Psychiatry.* 33(12):1006–1009.

Stein, L. I., & Test, M. A. 1980. Alternative to mental hospital treatment. *Archives of General Psychiatry.* 37(4):392–397.

Steinberg, R. M., & Carter, G. W. 1983. *Case Management and the Elderly.* Lexington, MA: Lexington Books.

Talbott, J. A. (Ed.). 1978. *The Chronic Mental Patient.* Washington, DC: American Psychiatric Association.

Test, M. 1979. Continuity of care in community treatment. In L. Stein (Ed.), *Community Support Systems for the Long-Term Patient.* San Francisco: Jossey-Bass, pp. 15–23.

Turner, J. C. 1977. Comprehensive community support systems for severely disabled adults. *Psychosocial Rehabilitation Journal.* 1(1):39–47.

Turner, J., & Shiffren, I. 1979. Community support system: How comprehensive? In L. Stein (Ed.), *Community Support Systems for the Long-Term Patient.* San Francisco: Jossey-Bass, pp. 1–13.

Turner, J. C., & TenHoor, W. J. 1978. The NIMH Community Support Program: Pilot approach to a needed social reform. *Schizophrenia Bulletin.* 4(3):319–349.

CHAPTER 2

Case Management in Health, Education, and Human Service Settings

National Association of Social Workers

BACKGROUND

Case management has been uniquely a social work role for more than 100 years. Social work is the only profession in which education and training maintains a dual focus on the client and the environment, enabling the client to utilize agency services and linking and coordinating agency services to meet client need. Within the past 10 years, policymakers have appropriated case management tasks and assigned them to nonprofessionals in the interest of cost containment. It is our obligation to our clients to arrest a movement that deprives clients of professional psychosocial assessment, skilled counseling, mediating interventions with service providers at each stage of the process, and advocacy efforts that will increase client options.

Case management is an approach to service delivery whereby clients with complex, multiple problems and disabilities efficiently receive all necessary services. Case management is a facilitative process within the framework of assessment, planning, linking, monitoring, and advocacy. Components of case management have been a traditional part of social work practice since the days of Mary Richmond, who stressed the importance of case coordination. Since the mid-1970s, case management has increased in popularity in the delivery of social services to clients with complex situations that place them at risk of diminished capacity. Case management services have been used in many practice fields, including chronic mental disability, aging, physical and developmental disabilities, and child welfare.

Case management is the link between the client and the service delivery system. It is a process based on several tenets and functions, which include but are not limited to:

Functions of assessment, planning, linking, and monitoring services

Recognition that a trusting and enabling relationship is needed to expedite the utilization of services along a continuum of care and to promote, restore, or maintain the independent functioning of clients.

Advocacy on behalf of clients to ensure that clients receive appropriate and continuous care despite inadequacies of the service system

Assurance that clients of health and human service systems receive the prescribed services, treatment, and care

At the center of service delivery systems is the case manager. The case manager's activities are aimed primarily at enhancing the quality of life of the client in the community, serving as a client representative, keeping individuals from being overlooked, making the system work consistently and coherently for the client, and, from a clinical perspective, reducing the client hospitalization rate and length of stay, should hospitalization become necessary.

Social work concepts, especially in the generalist social work theoretical practice model, emphasize four processes:

1. Enhancing the developmental, problem-solving, and coping capacities of people
2. Promoting the effective and humane operation of systems that provide resources and services to people
3. Linking people with systems that provide them with resources, services, and opportunities
4. Contributing to the development and improvement of social policies

Accordingly, the social worker as a case manager will establish a helping relationship, assess client needs and available resources, select problem-solving interventions, and help clients to function. Professional values regarding the recognition of the inherent worth and capacity of the individual, the individual's right to self-determination, and the right to confidentiality along with the National Association of Social Workers (NASW) *Code of Ethics* interact with the tenets of case management.

With the underlying interaction of the person and the environment in case management and social work, it is appropriate that the profession of social work take an active role and leadership position in advancing case management.

STATEMENT OF ISSUES

Social workers are the primary providers of case management services to many health education and human service systems. The case management model evolved and developed from the concepts and practices of promoting the social welfare of individuals, groups, and populations. Inherent in social work practice is the organization of resources to resolve immediate problems of society, community, family, and the individual as the practitioner (or case manager) seeks solutions and strategies to reduce the risk of further harm.

The generic model for case management service delivery grew from the experience and expertise of professional social workers involved in all aspects of health education and human services programs—that is, service delivery, planning, evaluation, research, and policy development. Recently, we have witnessed an emergence of case management models in a variety of human and health service settings—including those for the chronically mentally ill, substance abusers, and, most recently, people with acquired immune deficiency syndrome. With this, we see a movement toward the use of persons other than social work professionals in the design, development, implementation, and administration of case management services. Other professionals are cognizant of the concepts of case management, its cost-effectiveness (as demonstrated through evaluation research), and its potential efficacy in organizing resources for delivery of human services.

Only the professional social worker receives the rigorous education and training required to provide and administer case management services. Furthermore, professional licensing and certification demands that the professional social worker demonstrate a thorough knowledge of concepts and practices required by case management model applications. The demonstration of this knowledge involves not only the successful completion of cognition tests but a demonstrated ability to apply this knowledge in actual practice. Social workers, therefore, represent the primary source of experience and expertise in case management; a profession with a tradition of promoting minorities, women, the disabled, and the recovered into its ranks of management, research, and direct service; and the only professional occupation that requires all practitioners to obtain professional education and training in the concepts of case management and to demonstrate an ability to apply these concepts successfully before recognition as social work professionals.

We believe the quality of case management services is highly dependent upon the professionals responsible for applying the model, organizing the resources for clients services, and evaluating the outcome. We also believe there is sufficient supply of experienced social work professionals to plan, manage, and evaluate case management service models and applications. The demand for experienced professionals depends in part upon how well their peers advocate representation of the social work profession in all aspects of case management service administration and delivery.

POLICY STATEMENT

NASW strongly urges the use of professional social workers in all aspects of case management service delivery. NASW views the use of qualified social work professionals in case management as the primary means of assuring the quality and comprehensiveness of client services. The use of social work professionals also assures that approaches to case management are applied effectively and appropriately.

The emergence of case management applications in health education and human services management requires that NASW support the use of professional social workers in the delivery, planning, and evaluation of services. In settings where case management models are used, NASW recommends that organizations and institutions employ professional social workers as service managers and providers.

NASW strongly urges organizations to recruit, select, and retain professional social workers to assume responsibility for case management services. In less populous geographic regions and rural areas and in cases where an organization is unable to hire and retain adequate numbers of professional social workers and social work managers, NASW recommends that organizations use qualified and experienced social work professionals to act as consultants until such time that others can be recruited to serve as principals in case management service delivery.

NASW strongly urges schools of social work at the baccalaureate and graduate level to include in their curriculum the specific knowledge, methods, and techniques of the case management model.

NASW encourages adequate compensation of case managers in order to attract the best qualified and trained professional social workers in case management.

NASW Standards and Guidelines for Social Work Case Management for the Functionally Impaired should be recognized as the standard for professional case management practice.

CHAPTER 3

Improving the Quality of Community Care for the Chronically Mentally Disabled: *The Role of Case Management*

James Intagliata

Although case management is not a new idea, it has gained increased popularity in the human services field in recent years, particularly as a mechanism for improving services delivery to chronically mentally disabled persons.[1] To appreciate the case management concept, it is useful to begin by examining some of the factors underlying its current popularity.

The pressing need for case management has emerged in response to two major forces that have radically changed the human services environment over the last two decades. The first of these is the rapid expansion of human service programs that took place throughout the 1960s and continued into the 1970s. As a result of this expansion, the overall availability of services increased significantly. Because public funding for these programs was provided primarily through narrow categorical channels, however, the network of services that has resulted is highly complex, fragmented, duplicative, and uncoordinated. Countless individual programs have been developed to provide extremely specialized services or to serve narrowly defined target groups. While these factors interfere with service accessibility for all potential users, the barriers are particularly burdensome for those persons whose complex problems require them to engage in multiple, disconnected programs in order to get the assistance they need.

[1] The term "mentally disabled" is used here to refer to both the chronically mentally ill and the mentally retarded.

This situation was recognized by many professionals, even during the early 1960s. For example, the President's Panel on Mental Retardation (1962) expressed concern about the ease with which consumers could secure needed services. According to this panel, the concept of a "continuum of care" was a critical consideration for service system planners and involved:

> The selection, blending and use in proper sequence and relationship, the medical, educational and social services required by a retarded person to minimize his disability at every point in his life span. . . . A continuum of care permits fluidity of movement of the individual from one type of service to another while maintaining a sharp focus on his unique requirements. The ongoing process of assuring that an individual receives the services he needs when he needs them and in the amount and variety he requires is the essence of planning and coordination.

Unfortunately, the networks of services in most areas have not developed with the planning or coordination necessary to ensure quality care for consumers. For example, Test (1979) notes that most professionals' familiarity with continuity of care consists of a variety of cliches that describe its absence. It has, in fact, become commonplace to use such terms as "the fragmented system," or to refer to the patients who "fall through the cracks" or "become lost in the system."

In response to these problems increasing attention has been given to the concept of services integration, especially by federal, state and local levels of government. In the early 1970s, the Department of Health, Education and Welfare recognized the need for improved coordination of its own programs at state and local levels, and proposed a legislative initiative, the Allied Services Act, to facilitate integration of services. The Department also began a series of demonstration projects—the Services Integration Targets of Opportunity (SITO) grants—to test various services integration techniques at the state and local levels.

Under the SITO grants numerous service integration techniques were developed and demonstrated, including client-tracking systems, information and referral mechanisms, one-stop service centers, specialized management information systems, interagency planning and service delivery agreements, computerized resource inventories, and management reorganization projects (Mittenthal, 1976; Morrill, 1976). The one additional feature that was common to most of the SITO projects was creation of the role of "systems agent," operationally a case manager, who was expected to coordinate system resources for individual clients and to be accountable for successful client transit of the system. Thus, the widespread use of case managers as part of SITO efforts directed increased attention to the case management concept.

A second force that has radically changed the human services system, and that has also contributed to the current popularity of case management is deinstitutionalization. Before the movement toward deinstitutionalization, many thousands of mentally disabled persons were served in large public institutions. Though the institutions themselves were frequently characterized by overcrowding and dehumanizing conditions, the institutional model nevertheless offered the potential to meet all resident needs "under one roof" and thus provide reasonable continuity of and clear accountability for care (Kirk & Therrien, 1975).

When mentally disabled persons were released from institutions, however, responsibility for their care and support generally became diffused among several agencies and levels of government. The roles and responsibilities of these agencies and specific actions that needed to be taken to meet the special needs of deinstitutionalized persons were not clearly defined, understood, or accepted (General Accounting Office, 1976, p. 24). As a result, deinstitutionalized persons were forced to depend for their support on a complex, uncoordinated network of community service agencies.

Although many people could manage such a situation reasonably successfully given sufficient persistence and patience, the mentally disabled, whose own abilities to cope are significantly impaired, were generally incapacitated by it. Thus, most did not receive the services they needed, either because the services did not exist or because they were unable to obtain them on their own (Test, 1979). The negative consequences of failing to provide adequate and appropriate community care to deinstitutionalized persons have received widespread attention in recent years (Lamb & Goertzel, 1977; General Accounting Office, 1976; Bassuk & Gerson, 1978; Segal & Aviram, 1978; Willer, Scheerenberger, & Intagliata, 1978). In response, a number of important initiatives have been developed to address the special needs of this population.

To meet the needs of the chronically mentally ill living in the community, the National Institute of Mental Health (NIMH) has developed the conceptual framework for a comprehensive network of required services—the "community support system" (CSS)—and has provided funds to operationalize this concept through demonstration projects in 19 states and the District of Columbia (Turner, 1977; Turner & TenHoor, 1978; Turner & Shiffren, 1979). The positive aspects of this comprehensive support approach for dealing with schizophrenic populations have been highlighted by Mosher and Keith (1980) in their review of psychosocial treatment strategies. At least 10 different potential elements of community support programs have been identified as part of the CSS concept. However, case management is considered to be the key element since it provides the mechanism for coordinating all system efforts.

There has also been considerable attention given to the need for better integration of the services provided to deinstitutionalized mentally retarded persons. In recognition of the need for better coordination of the community-based care of this population, specific services integration mechanisms were mandated by Congress in the Developmentally Disabled Assistance and Bill of Rights Acts of 1975 (D.D. Act, P.L. 94–103) and 1978 (D.D. Act, P.L. 95–

602). In the 1975 version, there is a requirement that each client be assigned a "program coordinator" responsible for implementing the person's individual habilitation plan and attending to the "total spectrum of the person's needs." The 1978 version specifically mandates that coordination be achieved by the delivery of "case management services" to all eligible persons. These services are to involve an ongoing relationship between the clients and an agency or provider to ensure access to and coordination of all social, medical, educational, and other needed services.

In summary, the rapid expansion of human service programs created a sprawling, fragmented network of services. The subsequent attention given to the difficulties experienced by consumers in general, and the deinstitutionalized mentally disabled in particular, has led to the current widespread interest in services integration techniques, especially case management.

THE CONCEPT OF CASE MANAGEMENT SERVICES

Numerous definitions of case management have appeared in the human services literature in recent years. Though they vary somewhat, their common theme suggests that case management is a process or method for ensuring that consumers are provided with whatever services they need in a coordinated, effective, and efficient manner. The specific meaning of case management, however, depends upon the system that is developed to provide it. In turn, the particular characteristics of the system are shaped by the context in which it is expected to operate. The characteristics that more fully define case management systems include objectives, ideology, functions, and structural elements.

Objectives

A variety of objectives have been associated with case management efforts. Perhaps the most fundamental of these is to enhance the *continuity of care* provided to clients. Test (1979) suggests that continuity of care in fact, has two dimensions. The first is cross-sectional such that, at any given time, the services provided to an individual are comprehensive and coordinated. The second dimension is longitudinal, and necessitates that the system continue to provide comprehensive, integrated services over time, as well as be responsive to ongoing changes in the person's needs. This longitudinal dimension is particularly critical when case management systems are intended to serve populations whose disabilities are not only significant but also lifelong. Thus, to ensure continuity of care, case management efforts must take both of these dimensions into account.

Other objectives frequently associated with case management are the enhancement of *accessibility* and *accountability* within the service system. As mentioned previously, the current human services system comprises multiple categorical programs, each with its own eligibility criteria, regulations, policies, and procedures. As a result, clients are likely to experience significant difficulties in gaining access to many of the services they need. Case management with its provision of a designated agency or service provider to assist clients in negotiating the system is thus intended to make services more accessible. Another consequence of the fragmented character of the service system is that it becomes exceedingly difficult to assure accountability when multiple agencies are involved in meeting a client's needs. Case management is intended to enhance accountability by designating a single person or agency as responsible for the overall effect of the system (Baker & Northman, 1981).

One final objective of case management is to enhance the *efficiency* of service delivery within the system. In the absence of case management it is frequently reported that clients either fail to receive the services that match their needs or, if they receive services, they are provided in an improper sequence or untimely fashion. Thus, the potential positive effects of available services are greatly diminished. By fixing responsibility for developing and implementing a coordinated service plan on a single person or agency, however, case management is intended to improve the efficiency of the service system.

This objective of enhanced efficiency is sometimes equated with that of reducing costs for service delivery. While, in theory, case management might reduce costs within the system, in practice, case management often results in the identification of more client needs and the delivery of more services (Mittenthal, 1976; Morrill, 1976). Thus, while the specific services delivered to clients may be more cost-effective, it does not necessarily follow that total service costs per client will be reduced by case management.

Ideology

To understand the case management concept, it is also important to be aware of the ideology or belief system that accompanies it. The following components typically characterize this ideology:

The planning and implementation of service plans must be responsive to the fact that individual clients are unique, each with their own set of strengths and needs.

The services and supports provided to clients must vary over time in their type and intensity if they are to continue to fit the changing configuration of each client's strengths and needs.

The level of support provided to clients should match the degree of their individual deficit. Clients should be encouraged to function as independently as they can.

> The commitment of case management services to clients must be open-ended. It is a support that must be made available around-the-clock and throughout the lifespan according to clients' needs.

If those designing a case management system wish it to operate according to these principles, care must be taken to design and scrutinize all aspects of the system so that they are taken into account (Jessing & Dean, 1976). The subsequent discussion of the functions and structures of case management systems will illustrate how these aspects of case management ideology are, in fact, operationalized.

Functions

Case management is frequently presented as a process comprised of multiple functions without specifying the persons or structures responsible for carrying them out. According to Agranoff (1977), the five basic functions of a case management system include:

Assessment of client need
Development of comprehensive service plan
Arranging for services to be delivered
Monitoring and assessing the services delivered
Evaluation and follow-up

These five functions—assessment, planning, linking, monitoring, and evaluation—in fact appear in almost every description of a case management system, regardless of its context.

There are additional functions, however, that are considered to be important components of some case management systems. While some of these functions might be subsumed under Agranoff's five basic functions, a number of them clearly expand the role to be played by a case management system. The additional functions that appear most frequently in case management systems are outreach, direct service provision, and advocacy.

The appropriate range of functions for a case management system varies with the context. Acknowledging this, Ross (1980) offers three different models for case management programs designed to serve elderly persons in need. Table 3-1 presents the set of functional components associated with each of the three models. According to the author, the major difference among them is the increasing amount of control over provider agencies that is exercised in the coordination model and the comprehensive model. This multimodel conceptualization is offered not to suggest that the more comprehensive models are necessarily more effective, but rather to illustrate that there is a range of options to consider when designing or implementing a case management system.

TABLE 3-1. THREE MODELS FOR CASE MANAGEMENT PROGRAMS

Minimal Model	Coordination Model	Comprehensive Model
Outreach	Outreach	Outreach
Client assessment	Client assessment	Client assessment
Case planning	Case planning	Case planning
Referral to service providers	Referral to service providers	Referral to service providers
	Advocacy for client	Advocacy for client
	Direct casework	Direct casework
	Developing natural support systems	Developing natural support systems
	Reassessment	Reassessment
		Advocacy for resource development
		Monitoring quality
		Public education
		Crisis intervention

Source: Ross (1980).

Structural Elements

While it is useful to describe case management systems in terms of goals and functions, one must ultimately discuss the specific structural characteristics that are required to enable such systems to function effectively. Though the functions that define case management do not necessarily require that one create a role for a person termed "case manager," this is by far the most common structural characteristic of case management systems.

Case manager. The need for a human services generalist worker whose function is to coordinate services for the individual client has been recognized since the early 1960s (Intagliata, 1978). The concept of an expeditor (case manager) was adapted by Reiff and Reissman (1965). Since that time, various labels have been used for this role including: case manager (the term to be used here), integrator, expeditor, broker, ombudsman, advocate, primary therapist, patient representative, personal program coordinator, systems agent, and continuity agent, to name but a few.

Case managers are the most critical components in the case management system. They serve as the human link between the client and the system. In collaboration with other providers case managers ensure continuity of care to clients by ultimately determining the services, environments, providers, and duration of service that will be of greatest advantage to the consumer. In addition, the case manager has the responsibility for ensuring the achievement of the highest possible level of social, economic, and physical integration of consumers.

Specifying the particular functions performed by case managers is not a simple task. Although great care is often taken to define the scope of activities that case managers engage in, the reality is that substantial differences typically exist between officially mandated patterns of case manager activity and actual patterns of service (Caragonne, 1979). The reason for this is that someone thrust into the case manager role must function essentially as a troubleshooter, confronting and resolving a wide range of problems, many of which are unpredictable. More specifically, case managers have the unenviable task of assuring that clients receive appropriate, coordinated, and continuous care from service systems whose design provides for none of these features. As a result, persons acting as case managers must be ready to play whatever role the situation may require—outreach worker, broker, advocate, counselor, teacher, community organizer, planner, or administrator (McPheeters, 1974; Turner & Shiffren, 1979).

Undoubtedly, the comprehensiveness and intensity of the role that case managers assume should be tailored to fit the particular needs of the client populations being served. The case manager functions that are judged to be essential when serving one type of client may be elective or even inappropriate for another. However, three functions must be viewed as essential for case managers regardless of their clientele.

The first and perhaps most basic role that must be played by case managers in any system is *to remain aware of the comprehensive needs of their clients.* This means that case managers must be aware of, though not necessarily directly involved in, the initial intake and assessment of their clients. If these functions are assigned to other workers in the system, it is important that case managers be in close contact with them so that there is no slippage in the communication of crucial information. The assessment of client needs must be an ongoing process that does not stop after initial formal intake sessions. Thus, regardless of the role that case managers play during intake, they must stay in regular contact with their clients, remaining sensitive to and observant of changes in their clients' needs. This activity is crucial because the case manager is the only provider in the system whose responsibility is being aware of the "whole" client.

A second basic function is *to link clients to services* that will meet their needs. To do this case managers must be aware of the resources that are available to their clients. These resources include both services and entitlements (e.g., food stamps, Medicaid). To be effective linkers, it is also important that case managers function as advocates for their clients. Though individual service plans may call for referral of clients to certain services, there may be barriers that inhibit clients from actually receiving them. Potential barriers include service agencies' restrictive regulations and policies or the reluctance of many generic providers to serve clients with particular disabilities (e.g., mental illness, mental retardation). In addition, it should be noted that it is sometimes the clients themselves who resist being served or "drop out" of service. While respecting clients' individual rights to refuse treatment, case managers should actively encourage clients to help maintain their motivation for treatment. This is especially true for adults with severe and chronic mental or emotional disorders (Turner & Shiffren, 1979).

The responsibility to link clients to services does not require that case managers also be responsible for making the professional clinical decisions about which services are appropriate to meet their clients' needs. If, however, the development of an individual service plan is conducted by another professional or team of professionals, it is crucial that the case manager, as well as the client, be actively involved in the process. Involvement of the case manager has several important benefits: (1) it acquaints the case manager with the rationale and expectations for the treatment prescribed, (2) it allows the case manager an opportunity to inform clinical treatment staff about the local availability and adequacy of the services being considered, and (3) it provides the case manager with an opportunity to serve as the client's advocate, raising questions about specific decisions or making alternative suggestions.

The third essential function of case managers is *to monitor the services being provided to clients.* The most basic aspect of the monitoring process is to ensure that the agreed upon services are being received. This means that case managers must have ongoing contact with both clients and their service providers to ensure that appointments are being kept. In addition, the case manager must be responsible for assessing the appropriateness and effectiveness of the services provided. To do so, the case manager must not only keep in contact with the client and service provider but, if feasible, also visit with the client while the service or program is actually being provided. This kind of firsthand contact often provides valuable feedback otherwise missed. If case managers are not given the authority to change clients' treatment plans, then there must be effective mechanisms enabling them to communicate their observations to those persons who do make these decisions.

While the three activities of assessing, linking, and monitoring are the essential elements of the case manager's role, the "process" of carrying out these activities also requires consideration. *Perhaps the most influential aspect of the case management process is the quality of the personal commitment that case managers develop toward their clients.* The case manager is the human link between the client and the system, and the only service provider concerned with and responsible for the whole client. Individual case managers thus provide a mechanism for personalizing the service delivery system. The human relationships that develop between case managers and clients should be considered a fundamental strength of the case management model, and case management programs should be structured to facilitate and capitalize on this process.

While the essential aspects of the generic case manager role have been described, case managers who are expected to meet the needs of special populations, such as the mentally disabled, must assume more intensive and comprehensive client responsibilities. The special needs of mentally disabled persons necessitate that effective case management systems provide clients with such additional supportive services as:

Assistance with managing problems of daily living
Crisis intervention
Individual level advocacy
Systems level advocacy

However, while case managers ought to have some role in providing these types of special support, the extensiveness of each of these additional case-management functions necessitates that certain aspects be delegated to other direct care staff, supervisory or administrative level staff of the agency providing case management, other specialized service agencies, and even consumer groups. A brief discussion of each of the additional supportive services will illustrate the considerations involved.

Case managers for the chronically mentally ill are commonly expected *to assist their clients with the management of simple life activities and practical daily problems.* In New York State, for example, case managers of CSS clients often provide their clients with the assistance or encouragement they need for the proper maintenance of their personal hygiene or individual households. Other supporting activities might include helping clients prepare a grocery list, accompanying them on a shopping trip, or transporting clients to a needed service if no other arrangements can be made.

Although case managers can be expected to provide some of the support that clients may need in managing daily activities, they clearly cannot meet all of their clients' direct service needs in this area. If system developers are not sensitive to this issue, there is the risk that case managers who are hired for the purpose of coordinating and monitoring the efforts of multiple direct service providers will themselves become another group of specialized direct care staff. Thus, systems planners might assign the responsibility of teaching clients community living skills to direct care staff who have special expertise in doing so. For clients who need continuous and intensive support in negotiating the community, other types of special service providers can be used.

Weinman and Kleiner (1978), for example, employed lay persons to act as enablers for chronic mental patients living in the community. These persons spent several hours each day with their individual clients teaching them basic community living skills, escorting and introducing them to services and resources in the community, and acting as a liaison to gain the understanding and support of neighbors and local merchants for their clients. This program was highly successful in facilitating clients' adjustment to the community and is an example of the way that case manager functions can be extended and provided more intensely through the use of specialized ancillary staff.

Another important case management function is *crisis intervention*. The need for this type of support is particularly critical for those clients whose abilities to cope with living stresses are impaired or deficient. For example, the adjustment to community living made by many formerly institutionalized psychiatric patients is quite tenuous. Significant crises may be precipitated by unexpected changes in the environment, even events that seem trivial to persons with a "normal" level of coping ability. If such crises are not managed in a timely fashion, they can easily lead to significant deterioration in clients' levels of functioning and perhaps to their rehospitalization.

Because of their frequent ongoing contact with clients, case managers are likely to encounter such crisis situations. At the minimum, they must be prepared to provide clients with personal support. However, case managers need not be expected to function as therapists or to assist their clients directly in resolving the crisis. Instead, it may be more appropriate for them to refer or accompany the client to a crisis intervention team or agency.

Individual client advocacy is yet another important case management function, since some agencies may be resistant to providing entitlements or services to chronically disabled persons. In many situations such barriers can be overcome by the case manager through informal interpersonal negotiation (Riffer & Freedman, 1980). However, in more difficult cases it may be necessary for case managers to enlist the support of supervisory or administrative level staff within their own agency or even to make use of more formal channels to advocate for clients. This may involve seeking the assistance of legal aid services or of agencies that traditionally provide advocacy services for clients in need (e.g., Mental Health Associations, Associations for Retarded Citizens). In fact, because of administrative barriers and conflicts of interest, citizen groups and legal advocates rather than formal service providers are often in the best position to provide certain types of advocacy (Governor's Interagency Task Force, 1979).

Thus, while individual client advocacy is an important case management function, it cannot be delegated solely to case managers. As with other functions, there may be a need to involve other levels of agency personnel or specialized providers of services in order to provide clients with the degree of support required.

A final case management function to be considered here is *systems level advocacy*. In the course of trying to assure that clients receive continuity of care, it is inevitable that case managers will identify gaps in the service system. In other words, the system to which they are attempting to link their clients is likely to be incomplete. Needed services will simply not be available. The role of case managers in such a situation is, at a minimum, to document the gap and make their supervisors aware of the situation. However, there is a need for more direct action if the situation is to be alleviated. This is another example of a case management function that must involve key actors in addition to case managers. The intervention that is required to develop new service resources must take place on a system level.

In order to facilitate systems level change it may be appropriate for case managers to begin by banding together not only to document the unmet need as a group but to act as a catalyst stimulating others to act (Horejsi, 1978). These others may be the group of clients who have a similar unmet need or the agencies that may be responsible for planning, funding, and implementing the needed services within the locale. If continuity of care is to be provided to clients, case management activities must take place at many levels within the system.

Thus far, this discussion of structures needed to provide effective case management has focused primarily on just one element, the case manager. The individaul in this role has the responsibility for the coordination of services at the individual client level. While this level of coordination is essential, the effectiveness of the case manager's efforts is constrained by the degree of support provided for case management at higher levels within the system. Thus, in order for a case management system to operate effectively there must be other formal structures for assuring coordination and linkage of services on a systems level.

Core agencies. Although there are many possible approaches for assuring the systemic integration of services for given target populations, almost all of these involve the allocation of special coordinating power and authority to a specified agency at the local level. The President's Commission on Mental Health (1978, p. 65), for example, recommended that "state mental health authorities, in consultation with local authorities, designate an agency in each geographic area to assume responsibility for assisting the chronically mentally ill from that area." Consistent with this suggestion, NIMH, in its contracting for the development of community support systems, expects state mental health agencies to specify a "core CSS agency" in each planning area to act as a convenor and catalyst in assuring that the comprehensive needs of the CSS population are met. More specifically, this core agency is responsible for the assessment of the needs of the CSS population, the negotiation of the interagency linkages and agreements necessary to provide all needed support services including case management, and the development of new service components to remedy any gaps in the existing service network (Turner & Shiffren, 1979).

The importance of establishing this type of structure as part of an effective case management system cannot be overemphasized. One of the major lessons learned from services integration efforts thus far has been that compliance with the coordination efforts of case managers depends on a formal set of contracts that bind providers to deliver specified services to case-managed clients (Mittenthal, 1976; Ross, 1980). The core agency for a given locale is the most appropriate negotiator of such contracts. However, it can negotiate and implement such agreements effectively only if it has real enforcement power. Such power can result from the control of funds to purchase services from other providers, legislation or guidelines that require providers to respond to case manager requests, or the core agency being designated to serve as the single entry point into the entire local provider system.

Another important role that can be played by a core agency is to take responsibility for the development of new service components. While a major function of case managers is to link clients to services, they cannot perform it effectively if needed services do not exist. Thus, one of the very real constraints that case managers face is the adequacy of the service system in which they operate. If the system needs to be moved, a core agency is likely to be a far more effective change-agent than is the case manager. Nevertheless, even a core agency is unlikely to function effectively in this role unless it is explicitly empowered with the authority or responsibility for local system development.

Summary. Case management is a complex function. If effective continuity of care is to be provided for clients, coordination must take place at many levels within the system. Among the many possible structural elements that could be developed to implement case management, two have been specified as essential. The first is the case manager who provides coordination and integration of services at the client level. The second is the core agency which is responsible for coordination and linkage of programs at the local systems level. The specific details that must be considered when implementing the overall case management system are considered below.

CASE MANAGEMENT IMPLEMENTATION

Systems Level Issues

Federal. In order for case management systems to function effectively, they need to be supported at all levels of governance within the service system. The federal level has already expressed clear support for the development of coordinated case management services for mentally disabled individuals. For the chronically mentally ill, federal support for the case management concept has taken the form of financial support of NIMH Community Support Program demonstration efforts, all of which have case management as a key service component. Further, as already discussed, federal support for the provision of case management services to the developmentally disabled has actually taken the form of a legislative mandate (P.L. 95–602). Ultimately, however, it is up to the states to respond by designing and actually operationalizing case management systems.

State. At the state level, the first step that needs to be taken in building a case management system is to fix responsibility for the program in a single agency of state government. Organizational structures for case management systems must be statewide in order to ensure uniformity and equity in the services delivered to those in need (Lippman, 1976). However, the decision of which agency should assume responsibility and authority for providing case management services to the mentally disabled will vary from state to state.

In states that have separate departments to serve particular subgroups of mentally disabled persons, it is generally preferable for case management to be provided by the department most familiar with the given target population. However, since effective case management systems inevitably require the cooperation of all providers of human services, such a lead agency must coordinate its efforts with the activities of other specialized departments within state government. In New York State, for example, the Office of Mental Health has played the lead role in developing and managing the CSS services that are being provided to chronic psychiatric patients living in the community. However, the Governor's Interagency Task Force has been formed to bring together the various human service departments that relate to CSS clients in order to enable them to serve these clients better.

One subcommittee of this task force deals specifically with case management services since they are such an essential component of the overall system. This subcommittee comprises representatives from the Office of Mental Health, Department of Social Services, Office of Vocational Rehabilitation, Office for Aging, and Office of Mental Retardation/Developmental Disabilities.

> Its purpose is to improve the practice of case management functions, finding out which agencies are currently fulfilling those functions and making recommendations which will reduce duplication and enhance efficient and effective delivery of case management services to CSS clients. (Governor's Interagency Task Force, 1979, p. 1)

Such an interagency coordinating body is essential when case management services are delegated to an agency that serves just a particular population or provides only specific service functions. However, the need for such a mechanism may be somewhat less in those states in which the total responsibility for providing human services is assigned to a single, generic agency. Clearly, the nature of the existing human services organizational structure at the state level will be the primary determinant of how case management efforts are organized and administered. Nevertheless, it is also possible to alter organizational structures for case management purposes.

One example of such an alteration would be to create a totally new generic state level agency whose sole responsibility is the case management of human services clients. This model offers the advantage of avoiding a potential conflict of interest by separating case management from the provision of services. However, it may result in a style of case management that is not as individualized to clients as that which could be provided by agencies intimately familiar with the specific needs of their specialized target groups. In addition, the fiscal expenditures required for the creation of an entirely new department are likely to be substantial. Given the current climate in which resources for human services are shrinking, it is thus probably more realistic to build case management systems into the structures that presently exist.

Local. Regardless of the option that is chosen, once a state level agency has assumed responsibility for case management of a particular client population (e.g., mentally ill, developmentally disabled), this agency must then develop a plan for fixing the responsibility of case management in selected agencies at the local level. The primary consideration in selecting these agencies is that there be a single agency defined as responsible for each geographic subarea of the state. Further, since these "core agencies" provide the primary responsible mechanism for service integration within their regions, they must be chosen on the basis of their demonstrated leadership capacity.

Most case management programs have encouraged flexibility in determining the types of agencies that should assume the leadership role at the local level. The core service agencies designated for the NIMH Community Support Program developed for the chronically mentally ill vary from public hospitals to community mental health centers, to county social service agencies (Turner & Shiffren, 1979). Core service agencies designated to serve this same population in New York State include county departments of mental health, general county hospitals, family services agencies, and even state psychiatric centers. The regional centers that provide case management services to mentally retarded persons in California include existing service or advocacy organizations, hospitals, and some nonprofit corporations developed specifically to assume the coordination role played by a regional center (Lippman, 1976). The use of different models for the core agency is an important feature of case management systems since the factors that contribute to an agency's effectiveness in the leadership role vary greatly from one locale to another.

While the agencies assigned the core agency role may have no problems in exercising leadership, it is a good idea to provide formal mechanisms to facilitate their coordinating efforts. The most essential of these is to provide them with "purchase of service" power so that they can more easily gain the cooperation of a variety of the local human service agencies in providing services to clients served by the case management system (Washington, Karmen, & Friedlob, 1974; Ross, 1980).

In addition, the use of a local level counterpart to the state level interagency task force described above might be considered. More specifically, local interagency cooperation could be facilitated if the core agencies were to form interagency committees composed of those agencies within their area whose services would be required in order to meet the comprehensive needs of clients (New York State Office of Mental Health, 1978). Such a local interagency committee could be a useful forum for negotiating which roles would be performed by whom and for identifying gaps in the services available to the target population of interest. Thus, the core agency can use this committee to strengthen its capacity for carrying out its charge to provide comprehensive coordinated services to clients and to ensure that the entire range of services needed by clients is available.

Another method for strengthening the capacity of local core service agencies to coordinate care for clients is to designate these agencies as the single entry point into the service system in their geographic areas. This, in fact, is a model that has been used for serving the mentally retarded in California (i.e., Regional Centers) and that was recommended for use in serving the developmentally disabled in New Jersey (Lippman, 1976). The model has distinct advantages over that of a core agency which must rely on multiple outside agencies to refer the clients who are eligible for or in need of case management.

One final consideration is crucial in the development of a statewide case management system and requires coordination between planners at the state and local levels. This consideration regards the completeness of the various local service systems within which case managers must work. Since case management is primarily a service linking and coordination function, its impact ultimately depends on the availability of the needed services. If some clients need to live in a supervised residence in order to adjust successfully to the community, and no such residences are available, providing them a case manager will not solve their problem. Although case management can assist clients in getting the maximum continuity of care available from a given service system, case management cannot be expected to be a sufficient intervention in a system which is missing fundamental direct service components. Thus, the development of needed services must, in some cases, precede or at least be contemporaneous with the development of a case management system if it is to operate as intended.

Client Level Issues

Just as core agencies are responsible for sevice coordination at the system level, case managers are responsible for integration at the client level. In most cases, it is probably a good strategy for case managers to be a part of the core agency. Provided that the core agency has been given adequate authority and power, this close relationship enhances the ability of case managers to gain the cooperation of other service providers within the area. However, for a variety of reasons, some core agencies may choose to contract with another local service agency to provide case manager services. For example, this might be a good strategy for avoiding a potential conflict of interest when the core agency itself is a major provider of direct services to clients.

Regardless of where case managers are located, they are the key to the quality and the effectiveness of any case management system. While core agencies may provide the support and authority to facilitate interagency coordination, it is the individual case managers who must interact with a wide range of individual service providers in order to make the coordination actually take place for individual clients. Given the centrality of the role of the case manager in case management systems, it is important to consider how various aspects of the job design and context affect case manager effectiveness.

Case Manager Status

Perhaps the most essential aspect of the job design of the case manager role is the status that the case manager is given. One question frequently raised in this regard is whether the case manager should be a professional or a paraprofessional level worker. Since the demarcation between these two categories may vary from one human services discipline to another, however, it is probably more useful to discuss specific aspects of individuals' preparation for the role, including their educational background and previous job experience.

The important aspects of educational background are the type and level of academic degree obtained. In general, case managers have typically been individuals with education in a human services field. Some persons would suggest, however, that training in some human service disciplines may be more relevant to the case manager role than that of others. For example, individuals who have been trained to be aware of how to use various providers of human services in order to meet clients' needs (e.g., social workers, human service generalist workers) are likely to be better prepared to act as case managers than persons whose training has been focused primarily in a given discipline (e.g., psychology).

In addition to type of education, however, there is also the factor of level of education. The educational level reported for case managers in various programs described in the human services literature ranges from high school diploma (McPheeters, 1974) to doctoral degree (Altshuler & Forward, 1978). Depending on what is expected of the case manager, individuals anywhere within this range can function effectively.

The impact of level of education on job functioning will also interact to a great degree with the specific job experiences of the individuals involved. For example, case managers for chronic psychiatric patients in New York State include both persons who do not have college degrees but who have had extensive experience in working with these patients in state psychiatric facilities and persons who have masters level degrees in social work or counseling but who have had no prior contact with chronic psychiatric clients (Baker, Jodrey, & Morell, 1979). Clearly, each type of worker brings different strengths to the case manager's role. Which strength is more important is not clear, since there is empirical evidence that level of education and number of years' experience in the specific problem field both seem to strengthen case manager effectiveness (Berkeley Planning Associates, 1977).

In most systems, case managers are required to have no more than a B.A. level degree, which affords them a paraprofessional status. This fact has a number of consequences. First, it limits the range of activities that case managers can perform without supervision. In addition, due to their paraprofessional status case managers may have difficulty in establishing credibility with the professionals to whom they must relate in coordinating client care. While there is some evidence to suggest that the case managers can effectively resolve this problem over time (Baker, Intagliata, & Kirshstein, 1980), they may occasionally require additional backing and support from their core agency.

Because of these problems, some program administrators might feel that it would be better to use professionals for the case manager role. However, while professionals may be capable of functioning more independently as case managers, they are likely to be unwilling to devote time to many of the important but "less professional" services which paraprofessional case managers frequently provide to clients (e.g., transportation to an appointment, assistance in filling out forms to secure entitlements, visiting a day program to observe client activity). For example, Caragonne (1981) found that many case managers in mental health settings spent extensive amounts of time providing direct services to clients (e.g., counseling, assessment) and neglected such key case management functions as linking, referral, follow-up, and evaluation. Further, since professionals are overqualified for many important case manager duties, they may "burn out" more quickly than paraprofessionals (Dormady, 1980). Finally, an important economic consideration is that the use of professional level case managers would greatly increase the costs of any sizable case management effort.

These various considerations would suggest that the most cost-effective alternative may be to hire paraprofessionals to perform the essential case manager functions of linking and monitoring. The other important case management functions of assessing and planning could be performed by these individuals to the extent to which they are capable but should ultimately be the responsibility of professional level clinician supervisors. Before making any final decisions regarding the degree of discretion and authority that paraprofessional case managers should be given in their activities, however, it should be noted that case managers attach great importance to autonomy in their jobs (Caragonne, 1980). Further, their job satisfaction reportedly increases as they are given greater freedom and discretion in carrying out their role responsibilities (Graham, 1980). There is no evidence that one particular level of autonomy is ideal, but it is advised that the degree of autonomy given to case managers must be matched to the expectations that were established when they were recruited for the role and that it be adjusted over time to reflect their increasing competence.

Training/Preparation. The development and implementation of a case manager training program should be viewed as an essential component in the building of any effective case management system. Regardless of the professional level of the individuals being hired as case managers, it is important that they approach their role with a clear understanding of their functions and responsibilities. Further, in order to provide a consistent and equitable statewide case management program, it is important that all case managers be given similar orientation and preparation for the job.

In considering the development of a statewide training package for case managers, it is essential to build in a great deal of flexibility in its implementation. The people who will be assuming the case manager positions will undoubtedly vary widely in the knowledge, skills, and competencies that they bring to their job. A useful strategy is to design a training program as a series of self-contained learning modules (Baker, Jodrey, & Morell, 1979). In this way, those trainees who can demonstrate their preparation in a given area need not complete that specific module.

The statewide training package should focus on the basic aspects of the case manager role. It should include modules that present the rationale for the case management process and make explicit the values that are intended to guide the activities of case managers. These are modules that should be required for all trainees regardless of their prior job experience. Additional modules should provide basic information in such key content areas as the nature of mental illness or mental retardation (e.g., causes, definitions, associated consequences, limitations), common medications and their side effects, the local availability of specific services and the entire range of available client entitlements (e.g., SSI, food stamps), clients' legal rights, and the record-keeping responsibilities of case managers. Training should also include modules that deal with the process of case management. These should focus on teaching case managers skills for relating to clients, setting goals, solving practical problems, knowing how and when to intervene in crisis situations, and advocating effectively for clients.

In training case managers for working with chronically mentally disabled clients, it is also important to help trainees appreciate that the nature of the disabilities of many of their clients will severely limit their ability to progress behaviorally. Lamb (1979) has noted that unless staff who work with this client population have a realistic conception of what they can expect to accomplish, staff frustration and burnout are inevitable. Case managers must accept that enhancing the quality of clients' lives rather than increasing their level of independent functioning is a reasonable and appropriate treatment goal for this population.

In addition to considering the training content, it is also important to consider how the training can be implemented most effectively. One suggestion made by several authors who have evaluated case manager training programs is that care should be taken to avoid assigning complete caseloads to case managers until they have completed their training (Amadio, 1976; Baker, Jodrey, & Morell, 1979). While it is useful to have some actual client responsibilities during training so that trainees can apply what they are learning, there are indications that too much client responsibility interferes with learning. To avoid this problem, it may be desirable to conduct training intensively over a short period rather than to extend it in small segments over a longer period.

A final consideration is that while a basic statewide training program should be developed to prepare case managers for their role, plans should also be made to provide continuing education to case managers. An initial time-limited, intensive training program simply cannot be expected to meet all case managers' training needs. As with most positions, case managers will not really know what they need to know until they have been on the job for a while. Thus, either at the state or local level, continuing education sessions should be planned. Further, case managers themselves should be assessed periodically in order to determine the most important areas of training need so that continuing education sessions remain relevant and useful.

Supervision. The type and extent of supervision that is appropriate for case managers depends upon the range of functions that they are assigned and on the level of individual selected for the role. If experienced professional level case managers are hired, they certainly will not require the extent of supervision appropriate for a paraprofessional or less experienced individual in the same role. However, since most programs are likely to use paraprofessional level persons to fill this challenging role, it is extremely important to plan to provide them with adequate support and supervision.

Those assigned as case manager supervisors should perform several important functions. First, they must monitor the performance of case managers in a thorough, ongoing fashion. In addition to meeting regularly with individual case managers to discuss their caseload activities, it may be useful for supervisors to observe or even assist their case managers in working with certain clients. While one might assume that case management supervisors in all settings would routinely conduct such activities, the findings of Caragonne (1981) suggest otherwise. Specifically, she reported that many of the supervisors and program administrators at the 22 case management sites studied did not have accurate perceptions of the scope, extent, and pattern of their own case managers' activities. Further, it was exactly in those sites where supervisors were most out of touch with their case managers' activities that the case managers departed most drastically from their defined roles.

A second important aspect of the supervisory role is the staff development function. Supervision should include an ongoing commitment to the continuing education of case managers. Part of this education might be informal and consist of something as simple as encouraging case managers to develop a habit of generating multiple alternative strategies for dealing with clients' problems before taking action. However, it is also appropriate for supervisors to consider providing some more formal continuing education sessions to case managers. These sessions can be designed to be either didactic or experiential and should focus on specific content areas in which the case managers themselves feel a need for more background.

A third, and perhaps the most important, function of the supervisory role is to provide case managers with needed individual support. Graham (1980) found that the provision of consistent supervisory feedback and support to case managers of chronic psychiatric patients was associated with greater case manager work motivation. Apparently, case managers need such support in order to maintain an ongoing sense of the value of their work and the extent to which it is appreciated. Further evidence of the importance of providing supportive supervision to case managers has been provided elsewhere. Specifically, Baker, Intagliata, and Kirshstein (1980) reported that case managers identified regular supervision as an essential activity for preventing "burnout." They described good supervision as providing them with an opportunity to "vent their frustrations with their clients and the system" and to receive support for their efforts. Further, Caragonne (1979) found that case management sites where supervision consisted more of supportive, enabling activities rather than of monitoring and control were also the sites where case managers exhibited less antagonism toward management, lower levels of absenteeism and stereotyping of clients, and, in general, fewer overall symptoms associated with case manager burnout.

Clearly, the role of the case manager supervisor is a very significant one. Establishing such an upper level case management related position not only provides case managers with an opportunity to receive needed support and back-up, but also offers case managers the possibility of upward job mobility. While such a position would provide just part of a case management career ladder, any efforts along these lines enhance the likelihood of case managers remaining with the system after they have significantly increased their expertise.

Individual versus Team Case Management

Those implementing the case manager concept for chronic psychiatric patients living in the community have indicated that comprehensive responsibility for clients might be more appropriately assigned to a case management team than to individual case managers (Gittelman, 1974; Kirk & Therrien, 1975; May, 1975; Altshuler & Forward, 1978; Turner & TenHoor, 1978; Test, 1979). This team comprises a group of individuals who, together, are responsible for the case management functions of assessing, linking, and monitoring to assure continuity of appropriate care to clients. The individuals on this team may all be case managers or might include a case manager along with a variety of professionals from different disciplines (e.g., psychiatrist, nurse, psychologist, social worker).

According to Test (1979), the advantages of a team structure are that it provides (1) more continuous coverage and coordination since the unavailability of a single case manager does not incapacitate the client; (2) better planning based on the availability of more points of view for managing difficult problems, a factor especially important for maintaining energy and creativity in working with chronic clients; and (3) a way to avoid the isolation that may lead to burnout of the individual case manager who must face tedious, seemingly endless, and emotionally draining problems alone.

A recent report on the case management efforts at one of the NIMH Community Support System demonstration sites in New York State provides some support for Test's (1979) position. Specifically, Reagles and Sheets (1979) reported that after a year of using the individual case management model to serve caseloads of chronic psychiatric patients, two significant problems had surfaced. These were the overwhelming burden of responsibility leading to staff burnout and the dysfunctional phenomenon of clients becoming overly dependent on case managers. In response to these problems the program has switched to a group case management model in which the ultimate responsibility for individual clients' care rests with an interdisciplinary team rather than one case manager.

While the team model of case management may not be appropriate or feasible in all programs, those using an individual case manager model must pay serious attention to the need to provide case managers with adequate support. If case managers are not included as part of an interdisciplinary treatment team, then it is essential that the case managers themselves be organized either formally or informally for the purpose of mutual support. One possibility is to designate them as a distinct formal organizational entity, the "case management unit." Whether or not such a unit is formed, there is a need to provide mechanisms that facilitate the regular interaction of case managers as a group. Examples would include daily morning meetings, weekly supervision sessions and periodic training sessions.

Caseload Characteristics

A major factor influencing the style and effectiveness of services offered by case managers is the number of clients for whom they are responsible. It is a simple fact that as the number of clients assigned to a given case manager increases, the amount of time the case manager can potentially devote to each individual client decreases. Graham (1980) confirmed this relationship in his study of case managers who were serving varying sized caseloads of chronic psychiatric patients in New York State. He reported that as caseload size increased, case managers *did not* increase the number of clients seen each week. Thus, the frequency with which individual clients were seen by case managers decreased with increasing caseload size. This relationship is extremely important to consider because there is evidence that the quality of case management services is strongly related to the intensity of contact between client and case manager (Berkeley Planning Associates, 1977).

Increasing caseload size can affect not only the amount or frequency of case managers' contact with clients but also the nature and quality of client contact. In a study of case management being provided to chronic psychiatric patients, also in New York State, Baker, Intagliata, and Kirshstein (1980) indicated that the increase from caseload sizes of approximately 15 clients to as many as 30–50 clients had a significant impact on case managers' working styles. In addition to the inevitable consequence of having less time for each client, case managers reported that:

> Their efforts with clients had become primarily reactive rather than proactive such that the majority of their time was consumed responding to crises rather than anticipating problems and helping clients to plan ahead for them
>
> They were always "on the run" and no longer had the chance really to get to know their clients and their needs
>
> In order to save time, they had begun increasingly to do things for clients instead of helping clients become more independent
>
> Their frequency of contact with clients was increasingly being determined by clients taking the initiative to contact them rather than vice versa (i.e., "the squeaky wheel gets the oil")
>
> The amount of time they were required to spend simply documenting their efforts with clients was consuming an increasingly alarming portion of their time that otherwise might be spent with clients

Clearly, these are troublesome developments that potentially, if not immediately, threaten the quality and effectiveness of their case managers' efforts.

Undoubtedly, caseload size is an extremely important factor shaping case management. However, determining ideal caseload size is a difficult task. The number of clients that a case manager can serve effectively will vary depending on the mix of clients' levels of functioning (acute/chronic needs), the degree to which clients live close together or in scattered locations, and the competencies of individual case managers. Lannon (1979) reported that case managers serving chronic psychiatric patients tended to give more attention and service to those individuals who had poor community living skills or who exhibited behavior management problems. Graham (1980) indicated that case managers who serve specialized groups of clients tend to have different work patterns than those serving mixed caseloads. Specifically, he reported that case managers serving only psychiatric clients living in family (foster) care homes spent significantly less time in direct client contact than did case managers assigned a mix of clients living in varied community residential settings.

Clearly, a variety of client characteristics affect case management activities, independent of caseload size. However, it is useful to discuss at least estimates of reasonable caseload levels based on actual program experience. For chronic psychiatric patients being served in community support system programs in New York State, suggested estimates for an individual case manager's load have ranged from a low of 15 clients (Reagles & Sheets, 1979) to a high of 30 (Baker, Intagliata, & Kirshstein 1980). On the other hand, those reporting the use of the case management team model for a similar client population describe team member/client ratios ranging from 1/4 (Test, 1979) to 1/10 (Reagles & Sheets, 1979).

Regardless of the client population being served, determining ideal caseload size ultimately depends on the type of case management that program planners intend to offer. If, for example, case managers are expected to provide clients with support only when they are in crisis, they may be able to handle caseloads of 40–50 clients. However, if case managers are expected to assess clients' needs, develop treatment plans, link clients to services, monitor clients' progress, attend to needs of clients' families, and update treatment plans in an ongoing fashion, caseloads of 20–30 clients are likely to be more appropriate.

The actual caseload size that is ideal for serving any client group should be determined on a program by program basis. Thus, as part of the planning for developing a case management program, it may be wise to set caseload sizes conservatively low at first and then, if all goes well, gradually increase them while monitoring the consequences. In this fashion, the decision to set fixed caseload sizes can be made more empirically and rationally.

Other Contextual Factors

There are two additional contextual factors that can have a significant impact on how case managers perform their functions. The first of these is the degree to which the existing range of services available to clients meet their comprehensive needs. A number of studies of case managers' activities (Caragonne, 1979; Baker, Intagliata, & Kirshstein, 1980; Graham, 1980) have indicated that case managers' activities are significantly shaped by the service system in which they operate. If, for example, there are relatively few services available, case managers spend relatively little time linking clients to services. Further, when certain important support services are unavailable, case managers are likely to devote their own time either to providing or creating the needed services. These results are important for program planners to consider. They indicate that case managers' actual activities are shaped ultimately by the constraints of the environments within which they work, not by their formal job descriptions.

The other contextual factor that deserves consideration is that the local agencies that assume responsibility for providing case management in their respective regions are each likely to develop somewhat unique case management programs. Though efforts may be made at a state level to give programs essential structural and ideological uniformity, the implementation of these guidelines at the local level is ultimately shaped by the unique local contexts.

Factors that result in interprogram variation include the differences between regions in population make-up, geography, availability of support services, history of interagency cooperation and competition, and case management ideologies of the individual core agencies. Thus, a statewide case management effort typically comprises the activities of a variety of somewhat unique case management programs. While monitoring mechanisms to ensure a certain amount of program uniformity and equitable quality care for clients are desirable, local flexibility in program implementation should be not only tolerated but encouraged. This flexibility enables programs to be tailored to meet both local and individual needs.

SUMMARY AND RECOMMENDATIONS

The design, development, and implementation of a statewide case management program for the chronically mentally disabled is a complex task that requires the coordinated efforts of human services providers at all levels of the system. Consequently, the level of difficulty facing those charged with this task depends upon the degree to which the structures and actors within the system facilitate cooperation and collaboration. However, since the need for case management has resulted, at least in part, from the lack of coordination and cooperation within the system, the development of case management services will inevitably be hindered by significant barriers.

Perhaps the easiest solution would be to start over by designing, building, and installing a completely new human services system into which case management services could be neatly incorporated from the very beginning. Unfortunately, this is not a realistic option. Instead, planners must develop case management programs that can be "fit into" existing service systems. They must build upon the system components that provide potential for enhancing service coordination and continuity while working around those elements that create service fragmentation. In addition, some new mechanisms and structures for ensuring coordinated continuous care will need to be designed and implemented. In each case, the end result must be a case management program that reflects the unique strengths and needs of the system of which it is a part.

A number of suggestions and recommendations for the effective implementation of case management systems have been discussed here. The major considerations can be summarized as follows:

The development of a case management system should begin with a thorough assessment of client needs and the service resources that currently exist to meet them. Plans must be made to begin to fill identified service gaps. Case management alone cannot be expected to solve the problems created by incomplete, inadequate service systems.

The responsibility for providing case management services to a given population of mentally disabled persons should be delegated to a single agency at the state level. If this agency specializes in serving this particular client group, steps must be taken to involve representatives from all other relevant human service agencies at the state level in the process of planning and implementing case management services.

The agency responsible for case management services at the state level must delegate case management authority and responsibility to "core agencies" at the local level. These core agencies must be responsible for establishing interagency cooperation in their locales and for providing case management services. To create reliable human services networks in their regions, core agencies must be supported with formal mechanisms for enhancing cooperation (e.g., purchase of service authority, legislation).

Case managers are the most important service providers in a case management system. While they do not perform all case management functions, they are the human link between the client and the system. They assure that clients are receiving all the services they need, in the amount and at the time they are needed. To function effectively, case managers must be provided with adequate training, supervision, and ongoing support.

Evaluation and Research Needed

To enhance the quality of case management services, there is also a clear need to give far greater attention to conducting systematic ongoing evaluation of and research on case management systems. Two types of evaluation efforts should be considered. In the early phases of program development, it is important that evaluation be conducted and focus on measuring program implementation. Information that is produced from this phase of evaluation can provide system planners with formative feedback that can be used to keep program development "on track" or to modify or reshape program design if deemed necessary. These process evaluation efforts should help to pinpoint how case management services are provided and the factors that seem to affect their delivery. This information is important if administrators or providers are to understand or replicate the results of any case management program.

Once case management programs are functioning as intended, it is appropriate for evaluators and researchers to shift their focus to measuring program outcomes or benefits. Examples of outcomes that should be studied include the extent to which the various objectives of case management services, described earlier in this article, have actually been met. These include enhancing the continuity and comprehensiveness of care, improving the accessibility of services to clients, and increasing the efficiency (i.e., cost effectiveness) with which needed services are provided.

In addition to assessing the extent to which case management enhances the effective functioning of an extant service system, it would also be useful to evaluate the impact of those direct services which case managers provide to their own clients, often as a means of filling in gaps in the service system. Further, since as described previously, the case manager is the important *human* connection between the client and the system, it would be useful to assess how having such a personal advocate affects clients' feelings about themselves and their responsiveness to the services to which their case managers link them.

In addition to evaluating a number of aspects of the process and outcome of case management, there is also a need for research to determine how a large number of important contextual variables exert their influence on both case management processes and outcomes. In general, these factors can be grouped into four major categories. The first category includes the individual characteristics that case managers bring with them to their jobs. These characteristics include age, level of education, relevant work experience, and their expectations about the job. A particular research question that should be addressed regards the relative influence of case managers' education, experience, and personal qualities on their work activity patterns and overall effectiveness.

The second category of variables includes the characteristics of the clients who are served. These characteristics include age, functional skill level, level of maladaptive behavior, institutionalization history (degree of chronicity), and current diagnosis and symptomatology. Important research questions in this category relate to how client characteristics affect the frequency of case manager contact, the total amount of case managers' time expended, and the specific nature of the assistance which case managers provide to their clients.

A third category of variables comprises the characteristics of the case managers' job design and work environment. These characteristics include the breadth of role responsibilities, degree of job autonomy, size of client caseload, the individual vs. team model of case management, and the type and quality of supervision provided. One important researchable issue in this area is the optimum number and types of disabled persons in a caseload. Other important research questions relate to identifying the factors that enhance work motivation, reduce burnout, and increase overall job tenure and effectiveness among case managers.

A fourth and final category comprises characteristics of the broader services network within which case managers must function. These characteristics include the degree of service availability, the extent of interagency cooperation, and the type, if any, of core agency functioning within the locale. Important research questions in this area involve the assessment of how the extent of cooperation and connectedness between key agencies influences the case management process and what types of core-agency models work best to enhance case management effectiveness.

A number of exploratory studies (Lannon, 1979; Baker, Intagliata, & Kirshstein, 1980; Graham, 1980; Ross, 1980; Caragonne, 1981) of factors that affect case managers' activities and effectiveness have already been conducted, and their results have been discussed elsewhere in this article. However, much important research remains to be done. Each of the categories of variables described deserves more extensive attention and a variety of research methods can prove useful. These include case study approaches as well as experimental and quasi-experimental designs. Further, to gain a better overall sense of the relative importance of and interactions between the major categories of variables outlined, complex multivariate research designs will eventually be required. Nevertheless, ongoing work in this area is essential. Without solid empirical information on case management, program development can only continue to take place in a haphazard fashion.

The importance of research on case management should not be minimized. Given the present economic and political climate in which available funding for human services programs is shrinking significantly, case management programs will be particularly vulnerable since they provide indirect services to clients. If a choice has to be made between using funds for case managers or for work skills training programs for clients, it is likely that the more direct client services will be funded. Thus, if case management programs are to remain viable in the 1980s, it is crucial that program administrators have the information that is needed to demonstrate their value and effectiveness.

The development of case management systems is an ambitious undertaking. However, there is good reason to believe that the outcome will be worth the effort. Evaluations of service integration projects have reported that the use of case teams and case manager linkages leads to increases in the accessibility, comprehensiveness, and volume of services provided to clients (Baker & Northman, 1981). Caragonne (1979) came to similar conclusions and in addition, reported that the use of case managers led to more effective packaging of client service plans, documented gaps and duplications in service networks, and generally promoted organizational responsiveness to consumer needs. Although this evidence is encouraging, it is important to acknowledge that many questions about the most effective methods for providing case management services remain unanswered. At present, like many aspects of the human service field, case management is more art than science. Thus, as we proceed to implement case management systems for the chronically mentally disabled, we must remain open to learning and change.

REFERENCES

Agranoff, R. 1977. Services integration. In W. F. Anderson, B. F. Frieden, & M. J. Murphy, (Eds.), *Managing Human Services.* Washington, DC: International City Management Assoc.

Altshuler, S. C., & Forward, J. 1978. The inverted hierarchy: A case manager approach to mental health services. *Administration in Mental Health.* 6:57–58.

Amadio, J. B., (Ed.). 1976. *An Evaluation of the Jackson County Integrated Human Services Delivery Project.* Murphysboro, IL: Jackson County Health Department, 342-A North St., September.

Baker, F., Intagliata, J., & Kirshstein, R. 1980. *Case Management Evaluation: Second Interim Report.* Buffalo, NY: Tefco Services, Inc.

Baker, F., Jodrey, D., & Morell, M. 1979. *Evaluation of Case Management Training Program: Final Report.* New York: New York School of Psychiatry, September.

Baker, F., & Northman, J. E. 1981. *Helping: Human Services for the 80s.* St. Louis: The C. V. Mosby Company.

Bassuk, E. L., & Gerson, S. 1978. Deinstitutionalization and mental health services. *Scientific American.* 238:46–53.

Berkeley Planning Associates. 1977. The quality of case management process: Final report (Vol. III). In U.S. Department of Commerce, National Technical Information Service. *The Evaluation of Child Abuse and Neglect Projects 1974–1977.* Washington, DC: The Department of Commerce.

Caragonne, P. 1979. Implications of case management: A report on research. Presentation at the Case Management Conference, Buffalo, NY, April 6.

Caragonne, P. 1980. *An Analysis of the Function of the Case Manager in Four Mental Health Social Services Settings.* Report of the Case Management Research Project Austin, TX.

Caragonne, P. 1981. *A Comparative Analysis of Twenty-two Settings Using Case Management Components.* Report of the Case Management Research Project, Austin, TX.

Dormady, J. M. 1980. New York State Board of Social Welfare case management concept paper. (Draft) Albany, NY, April.

Gittelman, M. 1974. Coordinating mental health systems: A national and international perspective. *American Journal of Public Health.* 64:496–500.

General Accounting Office. 1976. *Returning the Mentally Disabled to the Community: Government Needs to Do More.* Comptroller General's Report to the Congress, Washington, DC.

Governor's Interagency Task Force on Mental Health Community Support Systems. 1979. *Subcommittee on Case Management: Final Report.* Albany, NY, December 1.

Graham, K. 1980. The work activities and work-related attitudes of case management personnel in New York State Office of Mental Health community support systems. Unpublished dissertation, Albany NY.

Horejsi, C. 1978. *What Is Case Management? Foster Family Care: A Handbook for Social Workers*. Missoula, MT: University of Montana.

Intagliata, J. 1978. The history and future of associate degree workers in the human services. In K. Nash, M. Lifton, & S. Smith, (Eds.), *The Paraprofessional: Selected Readings*. New Haven, CT: Center for Paraprofessional Evaluation and Continuing Education, pp. 206–215.

Jessing, B., & Dean, S. 1976. Case advocacy: Ideology and operation. In L. Baucom, & G. Bensberg, (Eds.), *Advocacy Systems for Persons With Developmental Disabilities*. Lubbock, TX: Research and Training Center for Mental Retardation.

Kirk, S. A., & Therrien, M. E. 1975. Community mental health myths and the fate of former hospitalized patients. *Psychiatry*. 38:209–217.

Lamb, H. R. 1979. Staff burnout in work with long-term patients. *Hospital and Community Psychiatry*. 30:396–398.

Lamb, H. R., & Goertzel, V. 1977. The long-term patient in the era of community treatment. *Archives of General Psychiatry*. 34:679–692.

Lannon, P. B. 1979. Functional assessments and service utilization patterns of clients within New York State community support systems. Presented at the Pennsylvania Evaluation Network Conference, Philadelphia, November.

Lippman, L. 1976. Three examples of case management advocacy. In L. Baucom, & G. Bensberg, (Eds.), *Advocacy Systems for Persons with Developmental Disabilities*. Lubbock, TX: Research and Training Center in Mental Retardation, pp. 167–176.

McPheeters, H. L. 1974. Theme III: Optimal continuity of care—Second faculty presentation. In *Creating the Community Alternative: Options and Innovations* (Proceedings of a conference). Philadelphia, PA: Horizon House Institute, March.

May, P. 1975. Adopting new models for continuity of care: What are the needs? *Hospital and Community Psychiatry*. 26:599–601.

Mittenthal, S. 1976. Evaluation overview: A system approach to services integration. *Evaluation*. 3:142–148.

Morrill, W. 1976. Services integration and the Department of Health, Education, and Welfare. *Evaluation*. 3:52–55.

Mosher, L. R., & Keith, S. J. 1980. Psychosocial treatment: Individual, group, family, and community support approaches. *Schizophrenia Bulletin*. 6:10–41.

New York State Office of Mental Health. 1978. *Request for Proposal: Community Support System Services*. Albany, NY.

President's Commission on Mental Health. 1978. *Report to the President From the President's Commission on Mental Health*. Vol. I. Washington, DC: Superintendent of Documents, U.S. Government Printing Office.

President's Panel on Mental Retardation. 1962. *A Proposed Program for National Action to Combat Mental Retardation*. Washington, DC: Superintendent of Documents, U.S. Government Printing Office.

Reagles, S., & Sheets, J. 1979. Hutchings Psychiatric Center second year CSP project report. In S. Steindorf, (Ed.), *Second Year Community Support Program Progress Report*. Albany, NY, October.

Reiff, R., & Reissman, F. 1965. The indigenous nonprofessional. *Community Mental Health Journal*. Monograph Suppl. No. 1.

Riffer, N., & Freedman, J. 1980. *Case Management in Community Based Services. A Training Manual*. Albany, NY: New York Office of Mental Health.

Ross, H. 1980. *Proceedings of the Conference on the Evaluation of Case Management Programs (March 5–6, 1979)*. Los Angeles: Volunteers for Services to Older Persons.

Segal, S. & Aviram, V. 1978. *The Mentally Ill in Community-Based Sheltered Care*. New York: John Wiley & Sons.

Test, M. 1979. Continuity of care in community treatment. In L. Stein, (Ed.), *Community Support Systems for the Long-Term Patient*. San Francisco, CA: Jossey-Bass. pp. 15–23.

Test, M. A., & Stein, L. I. 1977. Use of special living arrangements: A model for decision making. *Hospital and Community Psychiatry*. 28:608–610.

Turner, J. C. 1977. Comprehensive community support systems for severely disabled adults. *Psychosocial Rehabilitation Journal*. 1:39–47.

Turner, J., & Shiffren, I. 1979. Community support system: How comprehensive? In L. Stein, (Ed.), *Community Support Systems for the Long-Term Patient*. San Franciso, CA: Jossey-Bass. pp. 1–13.

Turner, J. C, & TenHoor, W. J. 1978. The NIMH community support program: Pilot approach to a needed social reform. *Schizophrenia Bulletin*. 4:319–349.

Washington, R. O., Karmen, M., & Friedlob, A. 1974. *Second Year Evalulation Report (SITO) of the East Cleveland Community Human Services Center*. Cleveland, Case Western Reserve University, February.

Weinman, B., & Kleiner, R. J. 1978. The impact of community living and community member intervention on the adjustment of the chronic psychiatric patient. In L. Stein, & M. A. Test, (Eds.), *Alternatives to Mental Hospital Treatment*. New York: Plenum Press, pp. 139–162.

Willer, B., Scheerenberger, R. C., & Intagliata, J. 1978. Deinstitutionalization and mentally retarded persons. *Community Mental Health Review*. 3:1–12.

CHAPTER 4

Autonomy in Long Term Care

Some Crucial Distinctions[1]

Bart J. Collopy

Within long term care, few ethical issues prove more problematic than those involving personal autonomy. When care impinges on the freedom and independence of the elderly, as it frequently does, a nettlesome question arises: Should the self-determination of the elderly or the decisions and standards of caregivers have priority? Beneath this question lurk primal philosophical and experiential tensions: between freedom and best interest, self-determination and dependence on others, individual choice and the pressures of collective care. When these tensions are resolved chiefly by caregivers and chiefly in favor of best interest, dependency, or collective concerns, the result can be ethically ironic. Care can slide toward control, not from malevolence but simply from the dynamic of powerful and resourceful professionals interacting with vulnerable and resource-weak clients.

Furthermore, precisely when care is beneficient, intrusions upon autonomy can go unchecked, unscrutinized, even unobserved behind the curtain of good intentions. Helping interventions are often judged by the motivations and goals of the helpers, not by the preferences and life projects of those helped (Buchanan, 1981; Gaylin et al., 1981; Veatch, 1981). In short, beneficient intentions can breed unchecked authority over those who are served or helped. To the extent, therefore, that it fails to pursue rigorous examination of autonomy issues, the long term care profession risks conceptual and philosophical naivete about its own ethical foundations.

[1] Research for this article was supported by a grant from The Retirement Research Foundation, Park Ridge, IL.

DEFINING AUTONOMY

Although the etymological roots of autonomy suggest the compact definition *self-rule* (autonomos), the conceptual contents of such a definition belie its neatness. As Beauchamp and Childress (1983) pointed out, autonomy is rich in paraphrase, loose in definition. It translates into a whole family of value-laden ideas: individual liberty, privacy, free choice, self-governance, self-regulation, moral independence. Focusing on just this latter paraphrase, Dworkin (1978) suggested seven different meanings for moral independence. In similar fashion, Thomasma (1984) suggested five different types of freedom which function within the ambit of autonomy.

With an eye to this conceptual plasticity, in the following discussion autonomy is defined as a notional field, a loose system of inter-orbiting concepts that trace out the varied paths of self-determination. Accordingly, autonomy is understood as a cluster of notions including self-determination, freedom, independence, liberty of choice and action. In its most general terms, autonomy signifies control of decision-making and other activity by the individual. It refers to human agency free of outside intervention and interference.

The scope of such agency is, of course, quite varied. It includes the freedom to shape long range goals and purposes, to determine life priorities and commitments, to control the content and direction of personal history. In more particular terms, it includes the freedom to manage the short range, ad hoc aspects of life, the mundane realities that measure self-determination on a day-to-day basis. It should be noted, too, that in this definition the autonomous person is not a lone, isolated, atomistic agent making decisions without ties to other people, social institutions, and traditions of thought and action (Callahan, 1984; Cohler, 1983; Dworkin, 1976, 1978; MacIntyre, 1981). Finally, autonomy does not require that an individual be master of all circumstances or be entirely untouched by outside influence and constraint. Even the autonomous person knows the bounds of time and space, history and biology, society and personality. Thus, truly autonomous decision-makers recognize and respond to external determinations, precisely by freely choosing and accepting them.

TENSIONS AND POLARITIES WITHIN AUTONOMY

A good deal of attention has been paid to paternalism as an external threat to autonomy (Childress, 1982b; Dworkin, 1972, 1983; Reamer, 1982, 1983; Van De Veer, 1986). But autonomy is an internally problematic concept, bristling with distinctions and polarities that can be ethically perplexing even in settings where professionals are committed to client self-determination. By way of preview, Table 4-1 indicates six such polarities, the ethical risks they create for client autonomy, and potential responses to these risks from caregivers.

As exploratory probes these polarities do not offer the only possible conceptual mapping of autonomy, nor do they reveal immediate solutions to the complex problems of autonomy in long term care. They can be used, however, to suggest directions for research, policy formulation, and canons of practice. Accordingly, the following explication and analysis of these polarities offer practical case illustrations, as well as focal questions about philosophy of practice and research agendas in long term care.

Decisional Autonomy and Autonomy of Execution

Decisional autonomy, as the name implies, consists in the ability and freedom to make decisions without external coercion or restraint. Autonomy of execution consists in the ability and freedom to act on this decisional autonomy, that is, to carry out and implement personal choices.

In full measure, autonomy should be decisional and executional. But it is not always so. Decisional autonomy can exist without the ability or freedom to execute decisions. Individuals can be intellectually and volitionally autonomous, and yet be incapacitated, constrained, or otherwise prevented from acting. For the elderly in long term care, this is, then, a pivotal distinction. With advancing frailty, autonomy of execution frequently shrinks or disappears completely. Consequently, if autonomy is defined principally in terms of execution, the frail elderly will be relegated to nonautonomous status. But autonomy is a broader concept and includes decisional modes which can remain quite intact, even when execution becomes limited or dependent on others.

The distinction between decisional autonomy and autonomy of execution is ethically critical, therefore, because it provides an incremental and conservationist mapping of self-determination. It challenges unitary, act-oriented, all-or-nothing notions of autonomy. It contends that loss of physical performance does not automatically signal or justify loss of decisional autonomy. In fact, as the outward reach of autonomy shrinks, its inner decisional core becomes a last and therefore most crucial preserve of self-determination. From an ethical perspective, then, loss of execution argues for greater protections for decisional autonomy, precisely because the physically dependent elderly are increasingly vulnerable to external coercion. The following case indicates how such coercion may develop.

Case 1. Mrs. A., 79 years old, shares a two family house with her married son and family. She is quite frail and needs assistance in a number of daily life activities and tasks instrumental to them. She cannot dress herself without assistance, cannot do her laundry, shopping, or most of her cooking. She has

TABLE 4-1. POLARITIES WITHIN AUTONOMY: RISK AND RESPONSE IN LONG TERM CARE

Polarity	Inherent Risks	Possible Correctives
Decisional vs. Executional: having preferences, making decisions vs. being able to implement them or carry them out	Decisional autonomy too easily abrogated whenever autonomy of execution is diminished or lost	Enabling the elderly to continue making decisions in activities (ADL, IADL) where they need assistance
Direct vs. Delegated: deciding or acting on one's own vs. giving authority to others to decide/act for one	Only direct autonomy fully recognized and respected; delegation effectively reduced to surrender or forfeiture of autonomy	Developing norms for delegation of decisions/activity to caregivers; developing explicit, mutually acceptable maps of what authority is retained by the elderly, what delegated to caregivers
Competent vs. Incapacitated: reasonably and judgmentally coherent choice/activity vs. that which exhibits rational defect or judgmental incoherence	Labeling of the elderly as incapacitated because of: (1) the sheer difficulty and complexity of competency assessments; (2) decisions made by the elderly which challenge institutional goals, professional expectations, societal norms	Avoiding global and perfunctory judgments of incompetency; recognizing the often partial, context-specific nature of competency; respecting elderly individuals own norms for what constitutes reasonable, logical, or coherent choice
Authentic vs. Inauthentic: choices/actions which are consonant with character vs. those which are seriously out of character	Defining autonomy solely in terms of rationality; ignoring or overriding the elderly individual's own personal values, moral career, goals, and motivations in favor of caregivers' value system	Developing an understanding of and protective response to the value histories of elderly clients; documenting a value inventory to aid caregivers in identifying authentic choices (particularly those which are highly idiosyncratic)
Immediate vs. Long Range: present of limited expressions of autonomy vs. future or wide-ranging expressions	Defining autonomy only in terms of a rigid rights perspective which unquestioningly allows immediate freedom to work against long-range autonomy; conversely, defining autonomy only in terms of long-range considerations, thereby giving wide latitude to paternalistic intervention and interference	Admitting the inherent tensions between immediate and long-range autonomy; recognizing that for the elderly long-range considerations may often be secondary to immediate ones; developing a calculus of care that counterbalances present/limited with future/global autonomy
Negative vs. Positive: choice/activity that claims a right only to noninterference vs. that which claims positive entitlement, support, capacitation	Defining autonomy only in terms of noninterference, thereby encouraging a laissez-faire response to harmful choice and behavior; defining autonomy in positive terms that do not recognize scarcity of resources; defining enhancement as a license for intervening in spheres where the elderly themselves want only a noninterfering commitment of their autonomy	Developing balanced interplay between positive and negative notions of autonomy; admitting and protecting the primacy of the negative definition (noninterference); moving beyond this minimum to explore caregiver obligations to enhance autonomous choice and activity among the elderly.

regular homemaker assistance, and her daughter-in-law gives her a good deal of daily help.

Even though she depends on this assistance, Mrs. A. has become increasingly frustrated and depressed by its effect on her independence. She feels that her daughter-in-law treats her like a child as she helps her dress and, automatically, chooses clothes for her every day. In addition, because Mrs. A. depends on others for shopping and meal preparation, she feels she has lost even more control over her daily life. She swings between arguing with her caregivers and depressively accepting their ministrations. In her view, care comes at a biting price. "My helpers have taken over," she says.

As suggested here, loss of autonomy can slide inexorably from execution to decision making. When frail elderly are no longer able to act independently in certain spheres, they can lose decisional control over those spheres. From an ethical vantage point, this suggests a number of questions for future research and conceptualizing, as well as for ethical guidelines and policy: Within the dynamics of care, is physical dependency interpreted as a sign of decisional dependency? Is loss of autonomy presumptively extended from levels of execution to levels of decision making? Are there specific zones of autonomy in which this is most likely to happen for the frail elderly (e.g., autonomy with regard to medication and medical treatment, autonomy in daily life style and schedule, autonomy with regard to finances, living arrangements, personal care)?

Direct and Delegated Autonomy

Direct autonomy is a matter of unmediated, hands-on agency. In such autonomy, long term care patients decide and act as individual, independent, self-sufficient agents with strong authorial control over their choices and actions. In delegated autonomy, on the other hand, individuals freely accept decisions and activities supplied for them by others. Here, care recipients authorize others to make decisions and carry out activities in their place. They no longer stand alone but instead depend on the agency of surrogates and sustainers.

If this distinction is not recognized, autonomy is liable to be understood in direct terms only. In such an understanding, delegation is seen as surrender or forfeiture of autonomy. All decision-making or activity given over to others therefore constitutes dependency, evidence of ineffectual or failed autonomy. Although such a definition would narrow the scope of autonomy in any setting, it is particularly straitening within long term care. It suggests that to remain autonomous the elderly must steadfastly resist any delegation of decisions or activity to others. In a world of direct autonomy only, the elderly are therefore left with a stark choice: loss of autonomy or lone and unsupported autonomy.

In contexts fixated on direct autonomy, the elderly must perform with high autonomy or else be relegated to the ranks of the nonautonomous. Such oversimplification can, however, be checked by notions of delegated autonomy. For the frail elderly, self-determination may be supported and survive longer when there are opportunities to delegate certain activity and decisions to others. When delegation is recognized as a valid form of autonomy, the elderly are clearly positioned as agents and active participants, indeed as authorizers of the circumstances and processes of care. Moreover, caregivers become not merely managers of care but true surrogates, supportive proxies, for their elderly clients. Thus, delegated autonomy directs attention to the inherently moral dimensions of long term care: its reciprocal nature, its response to vulnerability, its highly charged interplay between power and frailty, control and freedom (Childress, 1982a; May, 1975, 1982).

The notion of delegated autonomy does not, of course, solve the ethical problems of autonomy in long term care. Transference of agency to others is fraught with potential misunderstandings between the elderly and their caregivers. Indeed, delegation of autonomy can be injurious to personal freedom and independnece, not only within institutions (Bennett, 1963; Goffman, 1960), but within any setting where autonomy is pre-empted by those who provide care. Consider, for example, the following cases.

Case 2. Mr. B., a 72-year-old widower, has not fared well since his wife's death. He does not eat properly, misses doctors' appointments, and fails to take his blood-pressure medication regularly. He cares less and less about personal grooming and appearance. Troubled by this downhill course, his daughter finally prevails upon him to move in with her, her husband, and their two teenage sons.

Things do not go well, however. Mr. B. argues frequently with his two teenage grandsons, begins drinking heavily, is often withdrawn and reclusive. He regularly refuses to eat with the family, snacking instead on crackers and sardines in his room. His daughter claims that he is more trouble than her two teenage sons. "I feel he is deteriorating right before my eyes, and I can't get him to do anything about it." Finally, she confronts him with an accumulated list of grievances about his behavior. "This is my home, and I won't stand by and just let you fall apart," she tells him. "If I want to fall apart, I will. I'm not one of your children," he retorts.

Case 3. Mrs. C. and Mr. D., both of whom have lost their spouses, have been residents in the same nursing home for a number of years. Unable to manage independently outside the home, they are, nonetheless, mentally alert and emotionally robust. In the course of the last 2 years they have developed a close and intimate relationship, one that becomes highly problematic when a nurse's aide, coming unexpectedly into Mrs. C.'s room, finds them in bed together.

Word of the discovery spreads, and a senior staff member confronts the two, telling them that their behavior is inappropriate. Mr. D. keeps angry silence, refusing to discuss the matter at all. Mrs. C. tells the staff member that her relationship with Mr. D. is none of the staff's business, that their privacy should be respected. "The home is not in charge of our sexual relations," she says.

Mrs. C.'s son, who pays for part of his mother's care and visits her weekly, learns of the incident from a staff member. He reacts very negatively and goes to the home's administrator demanding that Mr. D. be "kept away" from his mother.

Both of these cases exhibit conflicts about the autonomy of the frail elderly and the authority of those who care for them. From the caregivers' vantage point, entry into a care setting can imply that the elderly have surrendered to others a determining role in certain areas of personal choice and behavior. The elderly, on their part, may feel that they retain direct control, that they have delegated very little of this autonomy to others. The resulting conflict suggests some leading questions for both theory and practice: Can long term care develop a well-defined, feasible principle of delegated autonomy? What ethical problems result when delegation of authority remains assumed, tacit, global, not negotiated mutually by the elderly and their caregivers? When should delegation of authority be mandated by the necessities of care and when should it be determined by the elderly themselves?

Competent and Incapacitated Autonomy

This is the most highly sanctioned and widely discussed distinction in the area of autonomy. Competent autonomy is choice or behavior that is informed, rationally defensible, and judgmentally effective in choosing appropriate means to desired ends. Incapacitated autonomy consists in choice or activity that is substantially uninformed, unreasonable, or judgmentally unsound. The distinction is crucial because incapacity, when it leads to harmful choice, provides defensible grounds for intervening in the choice and behavior of the elderly.

The interrelation of competency and autonomy is treated extensively in a separate section of this supplemental issue. Thus, it is sufficient, perhaps, to indicate that the principal ethical challenge involves determining when the exercise of autonomy is so incapacitated that others may justifiably intervene. For the elderly in long term care, this determination can be absolutely definitive for autonomy, as suggested by the following case.

Case 4. Mrs. E., 82 years old, has been a resident in a nursing home for 4 years. An alert, relatively vigorous and active woman, she has recently undergone surgery for the removal of a malignant ovarian tumor. Her surgery and post-surgical convalescence prove to be more protracted, painful, and emotionally draining than she had anticipated. After surgery she begins a chemotherapy regimen, but she experiences extreme nausea and weakness from the first treatment. She refuses to continue with chemotherapy, telling her son. "First, the awful surgery, and now this. I've never been so sick. I don't want any more chemo. If the cancer comes back, I'll deal with it."

Her physician and others try to convince her to continue with the treatment, but she remains adamant. "It makes sense for younger people, but not for me." Mrs. E's son is very troubled by this decision. He tells the physician that he thinks his mother's decision is tragically unreasonable. He urges that everything possible be done to change her mind and even asks whether there is some way they can "press" his mother into continuing with chemotherapy. In response, the physician arranges a psychiatric consult for Mrs. E.

As this case illustrates, refusal of care easily serves as the decisional gate for challenges to competency (Drane, 1985). But if the social, institutional, and professional canons which determine "indicated" care are not checked by the principle of self-determination, competency can come to mean little more than obedience to the value system of caregiving institutions and professions. In such a situation, the elderly run the risk of being judged decisionally incapacitated simply by being sharply and singularly individual, by being decisionally irregular. On the other hand, if idiosyncratic and harmful decisions are automatically honored under the rubric of autonomy, there is real danger that truly incapacitated choice and behavior will work grievous harm to the elderly.

Given the import of the competency versus incapacity distinction on the autonomy of the elderly, the long term care profession faces a number of pressing questions: Are the ethical problems connected with assessments of competency fully admitted and examined? Is there sufficient attention to the problems of borderline competency, intermittent and context-specific competency? In cases where refusal of care instigates doubts about competency, is reasonableness defined as a client-centered norm? In such cases, are professional, institutional, and other communal biases clearly held in check?

Authentic and Inauthentic Autonomy

Competency has long been the standard measure for determining when, on psychological, philosophical, and moral grounds, autonomy has a valid claim against intervention. But competency is not the only factor used to define and enforce this claim. Although autonomy obviously includes rationality and judgmental coherence, it goes far beyond this. In full measure, autonomy is the active expression of human identity, intention, and history. Thus, any thoroughgoing discussion must move beyond issues of rational competency to those which involve the wider repertoire of the self: individuality, character, personal integrity and coherence.

Authenticity moves beyond rational mechanisms to the characterological elements of autonomy: issues of life history, moral career, value priorities and dispositions, relational and ideological commitments, decision-making habits, precisely as all of these are rooted in personal identity, integrity, and responsibility (Dworkin, 1976). Authentic autonomy therefore consists in choices and behavior that are deeply in character, that flow from past moral career and ethical style, as well as from present values and immediate self-shaping. Inauthentic autonomy consists in choices and activities that are seriously out of character, discontinuous with personal history and present values, lacking self-possession and self-understanding.

Although authenticity widens the conceptual and empirical scope of autonomy, it does not make autonomy any more tractable from an ethical point of view. In long term care, for example, elderly individuals may express their deepest selves, act in utmost accord with their personal history and values, and yet make choices which caregivers find ambiguous, harmful, unacceptable and, therefore, dilemma-ridden. Conversely, the elderly may, under coercion, behave quite reasonably by common standards, and yet be acting in sharp discord with their authentic selves.

To make judgments about authenticity, then, caregivers must give careful attention to elderly individuals' moral careers, their past preferences, commitments, and value priorities, as well as their present motivations, options, and situations (Donchin, 1984; McCullough & Wear, 1985). Obviously, judgments about authenticity can probe autonomy on levels that are not as publicly available as those revealing competency (which explains, perhaps, why competency tends to be the primary norm in testing autonomy). Furthermore, the moral-psychological components of authenticity are mutable and historical. Authenticity can be built from a shifting history of decisions and choices, consents and refusals. It can involve alteration as well as constancy, wavering as well as decisiveness, tentative inchings and trials, and all manner of consonance between past and present (Cassell, 1978; Childress, 1982b).

Distinguishing between authentic and inauthentic autonomy can be, therefore, quite daunting. But the very recognition of this challenge is salutary. It prevents authenticity from being employed as a handy device either for quickly overriding idiosyncratic choices or underwriting harmful ones. Simply because authenticity is not readily available to scrutiny and easy assessment, it protects autonomy by building cautions around it. But those cautions can create ethical tension and perplexity, as is, perhaps, demonstrated in the following cases.

Case 5. Mr. F. is 72 years old and suffers from Parkinson's disease. He had always been a proud, highly independent, self-sustaining individual, but since the death of his wife 2 years ago, he has had to depend more and more on his two married daughters and their families for assistance and care. He has a close and warm relationship with all of them, and they very willingly respond to his needs, but he feels that he has become increasingly burdensome to them.

After much brooding about this, Mr. F. tells his oldest daughter that he has decided to sell his house and disperse all his capital to his grandchildren, keeping only enough to support himself in a small apartment until he can qualify for Medicaid. At that time he will apply for admission to a nursing home and so cease being a burden to his daughters and their families.

His daughter protests, but Mr. F. tells her that he has pondered all his options carefully. His plan is eminently reasonable and carefully calculated. That it is, she admits, but it is also very disturbing. To her mind, the plan represents a terrible surrender, a self-wounding, for this proud and independent man. She cannot imagine her father living in a small apartment, spending down into poverty, finally entering a nursing home bereft of resources. "It's just not him," she says to herself.

Case 6. Mrs. G., 83 years old, has been a resident at a nursing home since she suffered a serious stroke 6 years ago. Within the last year she has become increasingly frail and noncommunicative, and a bout with pneumonia, necessitating a 2-week hospital stay, leaves her only more frail.

Upon her return to the nursing home, the staff finds that Mrs. G. refuses all solid food. Sustained mainly by liquid nourishment which she intermittently takes, she continues to grow weaker. She becomes more quiet and withdrawn, almost never speaks, except to say "hello" or "thank you" to the staff who care for her. Mrs. G.'s daughter visits almost daily. Her mother smiles and greets her. She holds her daughter's hand, listens to her, but rarely says anything in reply. On one occasion when her daughter asks her why she doesn't talk, or eat, or respond more actively, Mrs. G. simply responds: "There's no need."

After some hard reflection, Mrs. G.'s daughter decides that her mother has chosen to accept death and struggle no longer to extend her life. The daughter speaks to a nurse who has cared for her mother for a number of years. "I think my mother has reached the point where she is waiting, willingly, for her death. If she continues to refuse food, I don't want her to be forced to eat or artificially fed." The nurse feels that Mrs. G.'s daughter has read the situation correctly. She also knows that, according to usual practice, the nursing home will very soon undertake intravenous feeding of Mrs. G. She sees potential conflict ahead, but for the time being she says nothing.

In both of these cases, the question of intervention hinges on notions of authenticity. For Mr. F.'s daughter, the possibility that her father's decision is deeply out of character could be grounds for intervening against the plan he has so single-mindedly and rationally proposed. In this case authenticity would pull against competency. The characterological oddness of Mr. F.'s plan, its failure to fit who he is and has been, would undercut its logic and rationality. But because authenticity and rationality do not mesh, any decision (to accept Mr. H.'s plan or to intervene against it) will face ethical risk and ambiguity. In case 6, Mrs. G.'s daughter faces the possibility that her mother's refusal to eat represents an authentic choice about the end of her life. If this is so, then the claims of her autonomy should not be summarily overridden. Those responsible for her care face probing questions and difficult weighing of options and responsibilities. If Mrs. G.'s refusal to eat is authentic, and if she is competent (her silence and withdrawal are not automatic denials of this), then her autonomy looms large as a value to be respected and protected.

In dealing with ethical dilemmas involving authenticity and inauthenticity, a number of focal questions might prove helpful: Are the controversial choices or troublesome behavior of the frail elderly scrutinized not only for reasonableness, but also for authenticity? Does authenticity protect choices that appear unreasonable but are idiosyncratically personal? Conversely, do signs of inauthenticity warn that individuals may be under coercion because they are acting against their own personal history and values? How thorough are attempts to understand the value history, personal goals, life plan, and present motivations of the elderly whose autonomy is at stake? Is authenticity recognized as an added empowerment to competency, so that interventions against competent and authentic decisions are faced with exceedingly grave burdens of justification?

Immediate and Long Range Autonomy

The ethics of long term care is frequently complicated by conflict between immediate and long range autonomy. Immediate autonomy refers to present freedom or freedom in a specific, limited sphere of choice and behavior. Long range autonomy is a matter of future freedom or wide-ranging, global areas of decision-making and action.

It is the very nature of autonomy that individuals are able, ironically, to choose against themselves. Present choice can delimit or thwart future choice; autonomous action in one area of life can foreclose on such action in another area. This opposition is, of course, a chief incentive to paternalistic intervention. To the extent that long term care professionals are primarily committed to long range autonomy for the elderly, immediate choice or behavior which threatens this autonomy will seem ripe for well-intentioned intervention (Weiss, 1985).

Furthermore, those who define long range autonomy (in many cases, not the elderly but their caregivers) will, in the very act of definition, determine the grounds for intervening in immediate choice. For example, if the ultimate goal of medical treatment is long range autonomy (Komrad, 1983), then patient resistance or noncompliance can be viewed as merely an immediate and short range expression of autonomy. The future and more comprehensive goals or care can easily override such specific and narrow expressions of autonomy.

On the other hand, if the moral force or autonomy is primarily housed in its immediate forms, that is, in present choice, then every autonomous choice and act creates moral constraints against intervention (Nozick, 1974). The major weakness of this position is that it can nullify social responsibility for destructive choices and acts. It does this precisely by its act-centered framework, its atomistic definition of autonomy. In such a definition, the contradictions and harm of autonomous choice are simply the risks of private responsibility. Thus, if this definition protects autonomy, it also isolates it, creating very short moral linkage between caregivers and their clients. For long term care practitioners, this presents particular problems, because it can create a kind of laissez-faire attitude, a passive, uninvolved model of moral agency for caregiving.

The tension between immediate and long range autonomy derives, in large measure, from competing conceptualizations. Long range autonomy envisages self-determination as a final, ultimate good. In immediate autonomy, on the other hand, self-determination is perceived as an instrumental, immediate right (Nozick, 1974). Thus, the opposition between the two is formal and structural. Given the elemental nature of this opposition, it is important to sustain the tension between immediate and long range autonomy, rather than release it by giving priority to one over the other. A case example illustrates the problem.

Case 7. Mr. H., 83 years old, is in a nursing home where he is recuperating from a hip fracture. He receives physical therapy but is making very slow progress in his ability to walk. One evening, trying to maneuver the few steps from the wheelchair to his bed, he falls. He is not hurt, but the next day he gets up from his wheelchair and falls again. Told not to leave his wheelchair without assistance, he persists in his short journeys. After a third fall in which he suffers a cut on his head, the decision is made to restrain him in the wheelchair. Mr. H. reacts vigorously against this, constantly pulling at the restraint and pleading with staff, even with visitors, to untie him.

Mr. H.'s son initially accepts the protective rationale offered for the restraint, but when his father continues to be agitated by the restraint he finally goes to the charge nurse and asks that the restraint be removed for the sake of his father's freedom. The nurse tells him that this would be a mistake. "If he falls again and really hurts himself, what freedom will he have? You should consider his long term status. He might be restrained now, but it's only for the sake of his future mobility."

In this case, caregivers intervene against present autonomy in the name of future or long range autonomy. Yet neither the priority nor the substance of long range autonomy is defined by the elderly client. Mr. H. seems to prefer risk-laden independence now rather than more secure independence later. His caregivers, following their own value systems, define independence in terms of future, fuller, and fall-free mobility. But although their view, that long range autonomy trumps immediate autonomy, creates ethical conflict, the reverse prioritization is by no means free of ethical problems. If immediate autonomy is granted strict priority over long range autonomy, then caregivers can remain unconcerned about choices that work against long range autonomy. Mr. H. can simply take his own chances at walking and falling.

Rather than opt, programmatically, for either immediate or long range autonomy, the surer ethical course might be for caregivers to admit dilemma and ethical bind, to struggle with the moral equivalent of Mr. H.'s physical restraint. Again, some exploratory questions might indicate the nature of this restraint and the ethical deliberations it would provoke. Within the dynamics of care is the immediate freedom of the elderly protected against absorption into long range autonomy (especially as defined and imposed by caregivers)? Conversely, are the elderly protected from isolation and unconcern when they choose immediate paths that diminish future autonomy? Do conflicts between immediate and long range autonomy provide an opportunity for everyone involved (the elderly, their families, and their caregivers) to realize how they are all entangled in the coils of mutual responsibility and freedom, of shared conflicts and crossed intentions?

Negative and Positive Autonomy

This last binary description of autonomy is developed from the philosophical discussion of rights and liberty. Such discussion commonly distinguishes between negative claims to noninterference and positive claims to entitlement (Beauchamp & Childress, 1983; Fried, 1978; Young, 1986). Accordingly, a negative liberty or right is a claim against invasion and interference. It prevents restraint, forbids coercion and control, and builds barriers around spheres of agency. Bluntly put, it announces that an individual agent should be left alone.

A notion of negative autonomy, developed along similar lines, would forbid interference or intervention in an individual's self-determination. It would oblige others to stand back, not to overrule, block, or even meddle in the free choice and action of an individual. In effect, negative autonomy would set off human agency as something posted against trespass, even beneficient and well-intentioned trespass.

On the other hand, with positive liberties and rights, claims are levied for empowerment, for support and enhancement beyond the negative minimum of noninterference. A positive right proclaims entitlement, obliges others not simply to stand back and refrain from interference, but to step forward and provide resources, to offer instrumental means. Consequently, positive autonomy could be used to assert a claim to opportunity, to assistance and resources that would operationalize choice and enable it to reach at least some minimal potential. Given a positive definition, response to autonomy becomes a matter of advocacy, of mounting barricades to press freedom forward, not merely building barricades to protect its present forms.

Within the long term care system, positive notions of autonomy involve a much more comprehensive, interactive, and time-consuming process than do negative notions (Gadow, 1979, 1980). In contrast to the dictum-like guideline of negative autonomy ("do not interfere"), positive definitions of autonomy raise a wide-ranging series of questions about how elderly individuals ought to be supported and strengthened in their autonomous choices and actions. The tensions between these quite different notions of autonomy can be exemplified by a case example.

Case 8. Mr. J., in his late seventies, has been in a nursing home for 2 years. Three months ago, weakened from a bout with pneumonia, he was given a wheelchair as a temporary means of mobility. As matters turned out, he adapted very well to the wheelchair, finding that it meant certain prerogatives and special attention from staff. In fact, he so valued these "rewards" that he showed little inclination to walk on his own, as his recuperation progressed.

At present, Mr. J. routinely refuses to go to physical therapy sessions, and most staff members have begun to treat him as wheelchair-bound. In fact, moving him about by wheelchair is in many ways less troublesome than trying to get him to walk even a few steps. Mr. J.'s wife, who visits him daily, presses the staff to get him back on his feet. She is very distressed that more isn't being done to make him ambulatory. The staff explains that her husband cannot be physically coerced or intimidated into walking. Moreover, they do not see his wheelchair status as a serious problem.

In this case Mr. J.'s caregivers contend that he should be left alone. His wife, on the other hand, holds a strongly positive view of autonomy, one that requires staff members to draw out and enlarge her husband's dormant mobility. In this latter view, respecting autonomy goes beyond mere nonintervention to active involvement and encouragement. Caregivers ought to call autonomy forward, ought to prompt and capacitate self-dependence, particularly when an individual is passive and unduly dependent on others. Thus, in the case of Mr. J., caregivers are especially obligated to encourage independence because the reward system of the institution may have induced and encouraged his nonmobility. (Those who advance positive notions of autonomy would be very sensitive to instances of iatrogenic dependency, to learned helplessness that might go unchallenged by those applying only negative definitions of autonomy.)

But if negative notions of autonomy can be used to justify care that is noninvolved, nonresponsive, and minimally custodial, positive notions of autonomy are also ethically problematic. Are there, for example, any limits to entitlement? To what lengths must staff go in efforts to rehabilitate an uncooperative Mr. J.? Given scarce resources and multiple, competing claims on them, caregivers cannot face absolutely open-ended obligations. Autonomy might be an ever-expanding possibility in the life of an individual, but it cannot be used to levy limitless obligations on others. An additional problem with positive autonomy is that it can encourage interference with the choice and behavior of the elderly in the name of enhancing autonomy. Thus, in the name of expanding autonomy, caregivers might be prompted to intervene quite freely in client choices which they consider too narrow and limiting.

The two extremes which threaten autonomy (non-interference that constitutes neglect and care that constitutes control) can be checked by cautionary questions: Are the risks of negative autonomy fully recognized (i.e., isolation and separation of the elderly; noninvolvement on the part of caregivers)? At the same time, are positive definitions of autonomy scrutinized for unrealistic, promissory notions of entitlement, for the risk that caregivers might too readily intervene in the name of enhancing client autonomy?

CONCLUSION

Autonomy can be a source of persistent and serious ethical conflict between the frail elderly and those institutions, agencies, and individuals who provide care to them. To the extent that care subordinates or suppresses autonomy, its benefits come at dubiously high cost of human individuality and freedom. To the extent that individuality and freedom run counter to the dictates of care, autonomy can seem an ambiguous benefit.

Steering a course through this underlying dilemma is more than a matter of good will. Autonomy is a philosophically complex and ethically problematic value, thick with distinctions, polarities, and interpretive variation. Kept in full view, this multiplicity of elements reveals the range and fertile dynamics of self-determination. Fixation on a particular aspect or interpretation of autonomy can lead, however, to a narrow constraining or tyrannical enlargement of this value. To avoid both extremes, long term care theory, research, and practice must develop the fullest possible account of autonomy, its conceptual and empirical complexity, its relative priority as a value, its conflictual potency and pervasiveness.

REFERENCES

Beauchamp, T., & Childress, J. 1983. *Principles of Biomedical Ethics.* New York: Oxford University Press.

Bennett, R. 1963. The meaning of institutional life. *The Gerontologist.* 3:117–125.

Buchanan, A. E. 1981. Medical paternalism. In M. Cohen, T. Nagel, & T. Scanlon (Eds.), *Medicine and Moral Philosophy.* Princeton, NJ: Princeton University Press.

Callahan, D. 1984. Autonomy: A moral good, not a moral obsession. *Hastings Center Report.* 14:40–42.

Cassell, E. 1978. Self-conflict in ethical decisions. In H. T. Engelhardt, Jr. & D. Callahan (Eds.), *Morals, Science and Sociality.* Hastings, NY: Hastings Center.

Childress, J. 1982a. Metaphors and models of medical relationships. *Social Responsibility: Journalism, Law, Medicine.* 8:47–70.

Childress, J. 1982b. *Who Should Decide: Paternalism in Health Care*. New York: Oxford University Press.

Cohler, B. J. 1983. Autonomy and interdependence in the family of adulthood: A psychological perspective. *The Gerontologist*. 23:33–39.

Donchin, A. 1984. Personal autonomy, life plans, and chronic illness. In D. H. Smith (Ed.), *Respect and Care in Medical Ethics*. Lanham, MD: University Press of America.

Drane, J. F. 1985. The many faces of competency. *Hastings Center Report*. 15:17–21.

Dworkin, G. 1972. Paternalism. *The Monist*. 56:64–84.

Dworkin, G. 1976. Autonomy and behavior control. *Hastings Center Report*. 6:23–28.

Dworkin, G. 1978. Moral autonomy. In H. T. Engelhardt & D. Callahan (Eds.), *Morals, Science and Socialty*. Hastings, NY: Hastings Center.

Dworkin, G. 1983. Paternalism: Some second thoughts. In R. Sartorius (Ed.), *Paternalism*. Minneapolis, MN: University of Minnesota Press.

Fried, C. 1978. *Right and Wrong*. Cambridge: Harvard University Press.

Gadow, S. 1979. Advocacy nursing and new meanings of aging. *Nursing Clinics of North America*. 14:81–91.

Gadow, S. 1980. Medicine, ethics, and the elderly. *The Gerontologist*. 20:680–685.

Gaylin, W., Glasser, I., Marcus, S., & Rothman, D. J. 1981. *Doing Good: The Limits of Benevolence*. New York: Pantheon.

Goffman, E. 1960. Characteristics of total institutions. In M. R. Stein, A. J. Vidich, & D. M. White (Eds.), *Identity and Anxiety: Survival of the Person in Mass Society*. Glencoe, IL: Free Press.

Komrad, M. S. 1983. A defense of medical paternalism: Maximizing patient autonomy. *Journal of Medical Ethics*. 9:38–44.

McCullough, L., & Wear, S. 1985. Respect for autonomy and medical paternalism reconsidered. *Theoretical Medicine*. 6:295–308.

MacIntyre, A. 1981. *After Virtue*. Notre Dame, IN: University of Notre Dame Press.

May, W. F. 1975. Code, covenant, contract, or philanthropy? *Hastings Center Report*. 5:29–38.

May, W. F. 1982. Who cares for the elderly? *Hastings Center Report*. 12:31–37.

Nozick, R. 1974. *Anarchy, State, and Utopia*. New York: Basic Books.

Reamer, F. 1982. *Ethical Dilemmas in Social Service*. New York: Columbia University Press.

Reamer, F. 1983. The concept of paternalism in social work. *Social Service Review*. 57:254–271.

Thomasma, D. C. 1984. Freedom, dependency, and the care of the very old. *Journal of the American Geriatrics Society*. 32:906–914.

Van De Veer, D. 1986. *Paternalistic Intervention: The Moral Bounds of Benevolence*. Princeton, NJ: Princeton University Press.

Veatch, R. 1981. *A Theory of Medical Ethics*. New York: Basic Books.

Weiss, G. 1985. Paternalism modernized. *Journal of Medical Ethics*. 11:184–187.

Young, R. 1986. *Personal Autonomy: Beyond Negative and Positive Liberty*. New York: St. Martin's Press.

PART II

Case Management in Mental Health

Social Work Contributions, Concepts, and Questions

Case management in mental health catapulted into prominence in 1978 with the development of the Community Support Program (CSP) within the National Institute of Mental Health (NIMH). Arguing that traditional and contemporary providers had abandoned responsibility for the thousands of institutionalized people being discharged from state hospitals, Judy Turner and Bill TenHoor of NIMH designed a comprehensive CSP. The role of case manager in the new policy initiative was prominent: Case managers coordinated the rest of the component parts and attempted to make them responsive to clients' needs (Turner & TenHoor, 1978).

Implicit in the construction of CSP was an indictment of the provider system: Prevailing practice paradigms and system boundaries were honored at the expense of a very vulnerable client group. The CSP, like case management in general, can be seen from both a provider-driven and a client-driven perspective. The provider-driven view presumes that the primary role of case manager derives from the treatment or service plans prepared by professional staff: responsibilities include providing linkage to the existing service delivery agencies; monitoring to assure patients' medication compliance and attendance at the activities specified by the provider's treatment plan; and providing transportation to assure concrete needs get attended. Advocacy applies only to case-by-case issues, restricted to such activities as assuring Medicaid eligibility.

In the very common provider-driven framework for mental health case management, the *appropriateness of services to clients' goals and needs is equated with the availability* of services offered; assessing the *effectiveness of services is reduced to measuring the efficiency* of service delivery; the quality or *outcome of services in clients' lives is equated with provider output* or the quantity of services consumed; and the common failure to stabilize people in community settings is reduced to predictive diagnostic labels such as "treatment resistent" or "young adult chronic."

Common practice ties providers' services to conventional and facile reimbursement formulas or restrictions, with little incentive to cross agency boundaries to pursue clients' needs or to produce continuity of care even between inpatient and outpatient units of the same large institution. These typical practices represent the cooptation of the Turner–TenHoor CSP agenda. They also create a basic theme—cooptation—that must be carefully examined throughout this section.

Client-driven case management, in contrast, does not begin with treatment plans or service plans controlled by service providers or shaped by their funding formulas. It begins with a set of principles formulated to emphasize clients' potential; their dignity; their capacity to grow and develop when provided with adequate material resources (safe, affordable housing, income, jobs where appropriate, etc.); appropriate supports and assistance to focus on living stable, positive lives; and validation communicated through an ongoing commitment to empowerment. Clients' strengths, goals, or desired life directions take precedence over formal service provider resources as the point of orientation for case managers. Tasks include defining directions or goals; using them as the basis for needs delineation; trying to develop community resources to replace formal provider relationships; strengthening informal support networks that clients' feel *are* supportive; and documenting resource deficits and system dysfunctions that impede clients' development. The dual focus concentrates concurrent attention on the person along with his or her family, and on the system. Providers' resources appropriate to clients' goals are utilized, specifically targeted to identified and carefully elaborated purposes consistent with individual client's direction plans.

In the articles which appear in this section, there will be a thorough examination of case management roles, tasks, functions, and responsibilities. Remember that the critical influence in shaping how these functions are operationalized in practice is the underlying paradigm or problem-defining framework.

Additional factors also require close scrutiny. How are the two dimensions of the dual focus articulated? Do they receive equal attention? How will the two dimensions be integrated? How is advocacy treated? Does advocacy appear as a high priority function necessitated by system deficits and dysfunctions that impede clients' lives? What organizational resources and structural ingredients exist to support workers in their advocacy activities and in the trying, more frustrating aspects of their work?

How is the client perceived—as a whole human being or as a passive, functional or dysfunctional service consumer? Where does autonomy, self-determination, or empowerment fit into various case management models? And how are the entire array of human needs seen—are concrete needs reduced in their validity when compared with subjective needs more amenable to desk-bound psychotherapy? These questions pervade case management practice in mental health. They exist as issues for examination in the four practice models in this section and in Part VI.

Mainstream thinking in mental health policy and case management program development has a provider bias expressed most prominently in the design and use of discharge plans or treatment plans. Typical parameters for clients are confined to mental health services and office-bound practice. It is not accidental that these services are retrospectively financed on a fee-for-service basis so that the more consumption by clients, the greater the income generated by providers to offset or supplement funding contracts. That Medicaid is a primary financing source in public mental health care and functions as a medicalizing constraint on practice sustains typical provider-driven mental health models. It does not excuse them, however, for their frequent inability to assist people to live stable, positive lives in community settings. Nor does it excuse them from perceiving clients simply as consumers of service, with needs prioritized around services that are made available. These issues require careful reflection as we turn to four practice models created by social workers or strongly influenced by social work input.

Libassi sees the connection between social work and case management deriving from the growing use of an "ecological perspective" in social work training. In this view, both people and environments are parts of a unitary system, thus honoring the dual focus of practice concern. Parallels are drawn to the philosophy of psychosocial rehabilitation and its optimistic belief that people can grow and learn when provided with appropriate and sufficient supports to do so. Libassi's work appears to be client-driven, yet little is said about the interorganizational context for delivery of services. Because she addresses a practice arena focused on the mental health system's client population, and not specifically case management, we are unable to learn from her directly how she views advocacy and its implications for interorganizational conflict.

Harris and Bergman describe a model of clinical case management in which aspects of the case management process itself are seen as the primary benefit. They describe integrative, rational and pro-active aspects of the process as therapeutic: "Emphasis is shifted from the material functions onto those aspects of the process which make case management a potential vehicle for intrapsychic growth." (1987, p. 296). What they do not discuss is the context for this frame of reference—the Community Connections program they created in Washington, D.C. This capitation-financed program provides a wide range of services that most mental health case managers must spend the bulk of their time trying to acquire (see Harris & Bergman, 1988). This clinical model requires graduate level staff and is the most psychotherapy-oriented of the four approaches presented here. Advocacy, as a central component of case management practice, is seen as a therapeutic activity.

Witheridge has developed a model of assertive outreach for working with populations that have been the most resistent to typical discharge plans and after-care service providers. The workers function exclusively in teams, work entirely "in vivo" or where clients experience everyday life, and stay with clients even when they are rehospitalized. Individualized packages of community supports (which extend beyond formal service providers to informal networks) are tailored to meet each client's particular situation.

Similar to the Kisthardt–Rapp approach and the advocacy/empowerment design, case managers develop community resources in response to clients' needs. Advocacy is addressed, but again is not linked to its interorganizational implications or the common circumstances when providers' services are not appropriate to clients' needs. Witheridge directly discusses the case managers' task of taking ultimate professional responsibility for clients' well-being. How does this function relate to the empowerment factor discussed earlier? Can there ever be a situation where a program's intense commitment to avoiding hospitalization is antagonistic to clients' self-determination?

Kisthardt and Rapp present a fourth approach—the strengths model. This concept, developed by Rapp and his associates at the School of Social Welfare at the University of Kansas, emphasizes explicit practice principles which it applies across several case management functions. The strengths model, like the assertive outreach model and the advocacy/empowerment design, demonstrates client-driven values and commitments. Caring about clients as people rather than as consumers or agency-bound role players, the strengths model asserts the primacy of clients' individuality. Clients' wants for themselves precede or guide the delineation of needs and serve as the basis for linking clients to resources. The implementation is designed by both client and case manager through use of a personal plan and strengths assessment protocol which appear at the end of the chapter.

The objective of supporting clients to create a life based on community stability appears in case managers' commitment to the identification and acquisition of community resources not tied to or dependent on formal providers. While advocacy is clearly necessary wherever indicated by the clients' wants or needs, there is no explicit framework for examining the implications of advocacy activities for interorganizational relations. Thus, the question arises about where this type of case management could be practiced since it requires organizational supports and commitment. The strengths model is used by the State of Ohio in its case management effort, indicating the degree of validation seen for this model and the extent to which it has been legitimated.

Finally, the Kanter article reintroduces many questions raised in the beginning. Kanter clearly sees the necessity for training and skills beyond simple brokering of services. Clinical interaction and environmental interventions are seen as both necessary and desirable. These, according to Kanter, require additional training and justify graduate level social work participation. Is there any inevitable correlation between professional level staffing and provider-driven or client-driven models?

The emerging context, especially with Public Law 99-660 mandating statewide case management systems, will confront social work with an opportunity of great magnitude. In this window of potential leadership, how will the profession react?

CHAPTER 5

The Chronically Mentally Ill

A Practice Approach

Mary Frances Libassi

Persons with chronic psychiatric disabilities have received increasing attention in the past few years. As a result of deinstitutionalization, community services have expanded in many areas of the country, and the chronically mentally ill are a growing part of the service population in mental health agencies. However, many professionals are resistant to work with this group of clients, and community services are often inadequate (Gerhart, 1985).

The present article presents a conceptual framework for practice with this population that was tested by a group of graduate social work students who found it useful and effective. The approach is illustrated through practice examples of work with clients with chronic psychiatric disabilities. The article provides suggestions and guidelines for practice that may influence attitudes and values of mental health professionals toward persons with psychiatric disabilities and that may stimulate their interest in this underserved population.

The chronically mentally ill have been referred to as an "abandoned population" (Abandoned, 1986). A major public policy initiative for the past twenty years has been that of the deinstitutionalization of the chronically mentally ill and increased attention is being paid to their plight. Although the original motivation for deinstitutionalization was well-intentioned and humane, its consequences have at times been unexpected and even harmful (Bachrach, 1984). For many clients with a psychiatric disability, deinstitutionalization has been a brutal hoax (Abandoned, 1986). Professionals are increasingly asking what went wrong.

THE CHRONICALLY MENTALLY ILL: AN UNDERSERVED GROUP

Various factors are associated with the plight of the chronically mentally ill. First, the development of community programs has not kept pace with the level of deinstitutionalization. Although community programs are now being developed, spurred on by planning and service dollars from the federal government (Turner & Tenhoor, 1978) as well as increased funding by some state governments, systems of care that meet the complex needs of this group of clients are still the exception rather than the rule.

In addition, mental health professionals, including social workers, have not fully accepted responsibility for service to this client population. Nancy Atwood documented a professional prejudice toward psychotic clients in social workers as well as other professionals (Atwood, 1982). Others have discussed the resistance of practitioners toward this client group and have provided detailed reasons for this resistance (Gerhart, 1985; Rubin, 1985). For example, practitioners dislike working with the chronically mentally ill, because psychotherapy or high status work is usually not appropriate; progress is slow and frequently minimal; and practice, especially case management, requires assertive outreach and environmental intervention. Similarly, a study conducted by Peter Johnson and Allen Rubin on the direct-practice interests of student's enrolled in a master's degree program in social work revealed not only a lack of interest in case management interventions, but also a disinclination for work with the chronically mentally disabled. In fact, out of sixteen client groups that the students were asked to rank in terms of preference, the least appealing was the chronically mentally disabled (Johnson & Rubin, 1983). Thus a host of factors result in a lack of motivation on the part of professionals to accept service responsibility for this important and needy segment of our population.

CONCEPTUAL FRAMEWORK

Practice with persons who have a chronic psychiatric disability requires a conceptual framework that fully accounts for the complexities of human beings, the environments in which they live, and their transactions with these environments. The ecological perspective is a basic component of such a conceptual framework.

A central feature of the ecological perspective is its view of people and environments as parts of a unitary system in which each continually shapes the other (Germain, 1979). The person and the environment are understood to be complementary, interdependent parts of a whole—whether one is looking at a person and the family, a patient and the ward, roommates in a residential facility, or any type of community support program within its neighborhood. The development and survival of both the person and the environment depend upon the nature of their transactions or interchanges. The ecological perspective is particularly useful in lifting the environment out of its customary background position and placing it, along with the person, in the foreground. Research on effective practice with persons with psychiatric disabilities increasingly documents the critical importance of an appropriate level of environmental stimulation as well as environmental resources and supports in maintaining clients in the community and in preventing a return to the hospital (Linn et al., 1979, 1980; Hogarty, 1979; Crotty & Kulys, 1985). The ecological perspective enables practitioners to understand the impact of environment, both social and physical, on a client's mental health, and more important, to use the environment to support the coping and adaptive efforts of individual clients and groups of clients in dealing with the stress of daily living.

Flowing from the ecological perspective are ideas about *stress* and *coping* that are congruent with emerging theoretical notions regarding chronic psychiatric disability. For example, the concept of *stress* refers to upsets that occur in the characteristic adaptive balance between person and environment (Germain, 1979). Some stress is zestful and challenging, contributing to growth and development; other stress is problematic and unmanageable, because it exceeds the usual coping limits or because the person perceives a discrepancy between the coping demands and his or her coping capacity. What is defined as stress and how it is defined or experienced varies from person to person and is affected by such factors as vulnerability, previous experience, culture, and so forth. Although it may arise from the environment, it may also arise from internal processes, both physical and psychological. In his discussion of schizophrenia, Gerard Hogarty reports on the "stress–diathesis" model (Hogarty, 1984). The "diathesis" side of the equation refers to a constitutional "vulnerability" or disposition to severe mental disorders related to altered neurotransmission processes in the brain. The midbrain systems are uniquely involved in processing information about both the internal and external world, in regulating emotion and cognition, and in facilitating adaptive behavior. Environmental stress is implicated, interactively, in the tendency toward recurrent episodes or sustained social dysfunctioning, or both (Hogarty, 1984).

In ecological terms, environmental stress in transaction with a vulnerable individual is experienced as unmanageable and responses to that stress become dysfunctional. Interventions must necessarily address the vulnerability of the individual as well as the environmental stress. Research studies on effective treatment have borne out the importance of a combination of both types of interventions for effective social adjustment of the chronic psychiatric client (Hogarty, 1980; Anderson, Hogarty, & Reiss, 1980; Anderson, Reiss, & Hogarty, 1986). Clients who received combined treatments of drugs and sociotherapy adjusted better than did those who received drugs or sociotherapy exclusively. In fact, sociotherapy appeared ineffective, even toxic, without the drug therapy. The enriched cognitive field and the increased expectations for responsibility and productive of some sociotherapy programs were found to be overly stressful for some vulnerable individuals who did not have the benefits of drug therapy as well (Hogarty, 1984). The ecological perspective is a theoretical orientation that helps practitioners appreciate more fully this dual attention to person and environment.

APPROACHES TO PRACTICE

From the ecological perspective emerge approaches to practice that are useful in work with clients with psychiatric disabilities. These approaches include the life model (Germain & Gitterman, 1980) and competence-oriented social work practice (Maluccio, 1981). The life model of practice assumes that the social worker's intervention into a client's situation is patterned after life itself: the approach provides concepts and principles based on life processes that are designed to strengthen coping patterns by changing transactions among people and their environments. In competence-oriented practice, the promotion of competence in the transactions is viewed as a special goal of social work intervention. For persons with chronic psychiatric problems whose competence may be low, social work practice that focuses on the rebuilding of competent functioning to the greatest degree possible is particularly appropriate. These approaches to practice have much in common with developing frameworks for psychiatric rehabilitation treatment (Anthony, Cohen, & Farkas, 1982).

Several guidelines that are especially valuable in effective practice with clients with psychiatric disabilities can be gleaned from the approaches mentioned above.

Humanistic Perspective

Humans are active and purposeful beings who are capable of achieving their potential when necessary environmental resources are made available. In working with clients with psychiatric disabilities, this humanistic orientation leads the practitioner to acknowledge but deemphasize the disability and to emphasize strengths, assets, and potentialities. The focus of intervention is not on treatment or cure of the illness but on supporting or releasing the client's adaptive potential so that he or she can cope with the disability as well as improve his or her social functioning in the environment. This practice guideline suggests that success, that is, effectiveness with clients, should be measured by improvement in the person's competence and functioning in the environment, not by cure of illness. This guideline is especially useful in work with persons with chronic psychiatric disabilities, because much of social work practice activity is focused on enhancing living conditions and promoting competent role performance. As Allen Rubin (1985) reflects, "In a hospital setting, social workers are not expected to cure physical disabilities; their job is to help individuals and families cope with them. Cannot the same be said for mental disabilities?"

Problem Definition and Assessment

A second guideline flows logically from the first and relates to the way in which problems are viewed. In contrast to the emphasis on pathology in more traditional practice approaches, this approach suggests that problems occur when there is not a good match between the person's needs and skills and the demands and resources in the environment (Germain & Gitterman, 1980). Accordingly, problems do not represent weaknesses in the person but rather are outcomes of the transaction of the person with the environment (Maluccio, 1981). The units of attention for both assessment and intervention include the person, the environment, and the transactions between them.

For example, in competence-oriented practice, assessment is redefined as competence clarification—the process of identifying and understanding the person's capacity to deal with environmental challenges at any one time (Maluccio & Libassi, 1984). Through this technique, the competence of the client system is assessed together with the characteristics of the impinging environment that influence the client's coping and adaptive patterns. The purpose of competence clarification is to determine where to intervene in order to enhance the person–environment transactions and thus improve social functioning. Interventions into the person system, the environment, or both are equally important.

Psychiatric rehabilitation programs utilize similar techniques by assessing a client's strengths and deficits in relation to the demands of the particular environment in which the client wants or needs to function (Anthony, Cohen, & Farkas, 1982). In addition, such programs assess environments to ensure that proper resources and supports are available to facilitate the client's success within them. As in competence-oriented practice, interventions may relate to teaching new skills to clients or to modifying environments. Utilizing such sophisticated skills of assessment as guides for intervention is another way to ensure success for both clients and practitioners.

Emphasis on Environmental Work

The emphasis on environment is a natural outgrowth of the ecological perspective and its dual focus on person and environment. This guideline for practice is congruent with the emphasis on the importance of environmental resources and support in much of the literature on services for persons with chronic psychiatric disabilities. These environmental resources "include significant others (e.g., family, other practitioners), services (e.g., transportation), and things (e.g., money)" (Anthony, Cohen, & Farkas, 1982). For example, practitioners working with clients who are schizophrenic speak of the "nitty gritty stuff": intervention with housing and money management issues, advocacy to secure appropriate benefits, and helping clients to find employment and be successful on the job (Dincin, 1985).

Case management is widely regarded as an essential component for pulling together these environmental resources. The psychiatrically disabled have multiple needs. The principle underlying the case management approach is that one worker—the case manager—will link the client to the complex service delivery system and be responsible for ensuring that the client receives appropriate services in a timely fashion (Johnson & Rubin, 1983). James Intagliata describes various functions that are required of case managers, including outreach, client assessment, case planning, referral to service providers, advocacy for clients, direct casework, developing natural support systems, reassessment, advocacy for resource development, monitoring quality, public education, and crisis intervention (Intagliata, 1982). Leonard Stein and Mary Ann Test describe the work of case managers in developing support systems to motivate and encourage patients, educating community residents involved with patients, and assertively persevering in outreach and continued contact with clients (Stein & Test, 1980). These case management activities are examples of the kinds of environmental interventions that are necessary in work with clients with psychiatric disabilities. Evaluation of programs that provide case management have consistently shown that these programs are effective in creating and modifying environments and in promoting the client's effective social functioning.

Johnson and Rubin make an excellent argument in support of implementation of the broad interventions of case management in social work (Johnson & Rubin, 1983). The focus on the person–environment transaction and commitment to enhanced quality of life, social responsibility, and relatedness are compelling arguments for social work activity in the broad area of environmental modification. When these values and ideals are combined with positive results with regard to enhanced client competence, social workers may indeed begin to "take pride in providing (environmental) resources" for this client group (Johnson & Rubin, 1983).

Redefinition of Client and Practitioner Roles

A fourth guideline relates to the role of clients and workers in the helping process. In both the life model of practice and the competence-oriented approach, clients are viewed as resources and as partners in the process. They are encouraged to play active roles in the helping process and to meaningfully participate in such areas as assessment, goal formulation, and selection of interventive strategies (Maluccio, 1981). Practitioners currently working with the chronically mentally ill propose similar roles. For example, Charles Rapp suggests that workers form a helping relationship whereby the client is the principal director of the efforts (Rapp, 1985). Courtenay Harding, a noted researcher on effective practice with persons with prolonged psychiatric disorders, suggests asking clients themselves what they need and what works for them.[1] William Anthony and co-workers state that client involvement in assessment and intervention is an essential ingredient in a psychiatric rehabilitation program (Anthony, Cohen, & Farkas, 1982).

This redefinition of client and worker roles has implications for the therapeutic relationship. Qualities such as mutuality, authenticity, reduction of social distance, honesty, and "human caring" are emphasized (Germain & Gitterman, 1980). Walter Deitchman has captured what this might mean for work with clients with a chronic disability:

> The chronic client in the community needs a traveling companion, not a travel agent. The travel agent's only function is to make the client's reservation. The client has to get ready, get to the airport, and traverse foreign terrain by himself. The traveling companion, on the other hand, celebrates the fact that his friend was able to get seats on the plane, talks about his fear of flying, and then goes on the trip with him, sharing the joys and sorrows that occur during the venture (Deitchman, 1980).

Focus on Life Processes and Experiences

Effective practice with clients with psychiatric disabilities requires the use of natural (real) life experiences and events as instruments for change. Life experiences, events, and processes can and should be used to promote personal growth, learning of new social skills, and the promotion of competence (Maluccio, 1981).

Community support programs, particularly psychosocial rehabilitation programs, often utilize this approach in trying to facilitate successful experiences for their members. Members need rebuilding exercises that slowly increase their level of confidence (Dincin, 1985). Behavioral techniques such as shaping (breaking skills into smaller increments), the use of positive reinforcement, modeling, and role playing are often used to improve competence and social functioning in real-life situations (Rapp, 1985).

A corollary of this focus on life processes and experiences is the emphasis on practice within the environments of clients. Teaching social skills and improving social functioning is best done in *in-vivo* situations rather than in contrived environments. Bruce Hall and John Valano suggest that "life space social work uses the immediate experiences of the client system to pursue developmental goals, maintaining a sense of proportion and optimism for clients' encounters with obstacles to achievement" (Hall & Valvano, 1985). Effective practice with clients with psychiatric disabilities requires that workers move out of their offices into the places where clients live and congregate.

---

[1] This suggestion was made by Dr. Courtenay Harding in an address to the State Board of Mental Health, Wallingford, Connecticut, March 1986.

The Family, A Critical Focus for Practice

From an ecological perspective, the family is a major "environment" that affects the functioning of individual clients. Studies on community-based alternatives to institutional care for those with chronic psychiatric problems support the crucial role that families can and do play in preventing rehospitalization and maintaining a client in the community (Langsley, Flomenhaft, & Mochotra, 1970; Rittenhouse, 1970). In some programs, a psychoeducational approach to family intervention is used. Families are encouraged to discuss their anxieties, are provided with information to increase their understanding of the patient's illness, and are taught skills of crisis management that enable them to better cope with schizophrenic symptomatology (Anderson, Hogarty, Reiss, 1980). Agnes Hatfield has been an advocate and a leader for this approach. Her monograph discusses such topics as understanding chronic mental illness, the treatment of mental illness, creating a low-stress environment, managing disturbing behavior, and promoting growth and rehabilitation (Hatfield, 1982).

The emphasis on family education and intervention is yet another guideline that flows from the conceptual framework and the approaches to practice described herein. As noted above, it is also congruent with theoretical approaches currently utilized by those who work with clients with a chronic psychiatric disability.

PRACTICE ILLUSTRATIONS

The conceptual framework and the practice approaches presented above were tested by a group of graduate social work students placed in a community mental health training unit (Libassi & Maluccio, 1982). The value of the practice guidelines is illustrated through the following examples, which draw from the work of the students who worked in agencies, both institutional and community, that served clients with chronic psychiatric disabilities.[2] The students found that it was essential to reframe their practice along the lines of the conceptual approaches discussed above.

MSG Group

A student placed in a psychosocial rehabilitation center was asked by staff to develop an educational group that would focus on the development of employment skills to facilitate the reentry of psychiatric clients into the job market. Despite his efforts and staff efforts, the group was not successful. Membership was small and attendance poor. In evaluating the group intervention, the

---

[2] These practice examples were contributed by Richard Forleo, Christine Nicols, and Kathy Little, former students at the University of Connecticut School of Social Work.

student solicited input from client group members and discovered several important reasons for the failure of this group. First, the focus of the group was on problems and deficits; the members felt that enough attention was already directed to their weaknesses. Second, the group met in the rehabilitation center, which intensified the feeling among members that the group was a problem-focused group. Finally, the comments of the clients suggested that much of the difficulty in obtaining employment stemmed from systems or environmental problems. The opportunities for employment for an ex-psychiatric client were almost nonexistent. The problems experienced in obtaining employment were just as much an outgrowth of systems and environmental issues as they were of personal deficits. By zeroing in on personal problems only, the group fed the low self-esteem of the clients.

With this evaluation in mind, the student began to reframe his work with the group utilizing the guidelines presented here. First, he made a conscious effort to start with the clients' definitions of their problems. In addition, he changed his focus to client strengths and competencies. The goal became to foster the social competencies that each group member already possessed as well as the competencies of the group as a whole. The group was described to potential members as a social group that would explore any activities *they* wished to pursue in the community. Instead of focusing on problems in self (internal problems), the group focused on the interests, knowledge, and strengths that members already possessed. No restrictions were placed on membership. Anyone who wished to be a part of the group was welcome. The student saw his role as facilitator and encouraged group interaction rather than leader–participant interaction.

Student process notes highlight many of the practice guidelines delineated above.

> T, a group member, volunteered to hold a television-viewing party at his house after the group had elected that activity as the program for the next meeting. T's fears about being a host surfaced, and he started to back down. Group members offered their support, and one member volunteered to help him prepare for the coming meeting.
>
> On the day of the meeting, I drove to the party with some of the group members. They mentioned how scared T must be and how hard it would be for any of them to host the meeting. When we arrived, we were all amazed at the snacks that T had prepared. People quickly prepared their plates and sat down. Little, if any, conversation followed. At first I defined the silence as a symptom of the ex-psychiatric clients' deep-seated problems and became anxious to intervene. However, I quickly recognized that I was falling back into my old deficit mind set and began to reframe what was happening. I recognized that silence can occur in any group and began to relax. T was also upset and suggested to the group that he was a poor host. I responded that the best of hosts had silent parties at times and that it wasn't the host's responsibility to *make* the party work. This comment seemed to break the

> ice for everyone. It served to "normalize" the experience. T and the others began to talk. When the meeting was over, they all felt good at how well it had gone and another member volunteered to use her house for a potluck supper at the next group meeting.

This group, which was initiated five years ago, was the first of its type in the rehabilitation center. It still exists today; it has become the prototype for several other similar groups, all of which enhance the life of the participants. Social competencies are enhanced in natural situations. Self-esteem has grown, and clients with psychiatric disabilities have been helped to move from the role of patient to that of person.

A Resistant Client

A student placed in a psychiatric hospital setting was assigned to work with J, a patient who had attempted suicide. The client had a history of hospitalizations and of long periods of therapy. She was described as hostile, manipulative, resistant, and unmotivated. The student's first task was to complete a psychosocial history. Although J had been hospitalized a number of times, her history was incomplete. There was no clear agreement on what kind of person J was, what had caused her psychosis, or how she perceived herself and her world.

The student's process notes highlight her approach to engagement and her determination to reframe her work with J along the general guidelines presented in this article.

> Before I met J, I was determined to circumvent resistance and fill in the blanks in her history. I felt pressure by the hospital requirement to prepare an interim history for the treatment meeting. However, I decided that I should not allow my sense of unmet responsibility to the hospital procedures to interfere with my work with J.
>
> I approached J with the intent to convey my respect for her choice of utilizing my services rather than to obtain information from her. I hoped to establish a relationship with her by agreeing to work on discharge plans. When I knocked on her door, she asked me to leave her alone. I did, but left her a note explaining my role as her social worker and stating that I'd be back the next day. When I returned, she was reading in her room. "What do you want?" she asked, without looking up. I introduced myself. There were no chairs, so I sat on the floor. "You don't want to be here?" I asked. She responded with a chaotic outburst directed toward the people who ran the transitional living facility where J had been and the psychiatrist on her ward. I was frightened, less by the language than by the intense energy behind the language. I couldn't think of anything to say. I asked J if she minded if I had a cigarette and offered her one. We sat in silence, smoking. She seemed to forget that I was there. She appeared to be listening to something. She shook her head and shoulders rapidly. "Were you hearing voices?" I asked

her. "Get out of here," she replied. "You think I'm loony, too." I said, "I think you are angry and sad and that you don't want to be here. I don't know whether that's loony or not. You know where you are and why you are here. What do you think?"

I sat with her for almost two hours, saying very little. When she spoke, I had difficulty following her train of thought, references to people, and references to politics. I was fascinated by the images she used to illustrate her despondency with the world.

When I left, she asked if I planned to write up her "loose associations" in her chart. I told her that even though they didn't help us deal with her present issues, they helped me to get an idea of what she cared about and how she thought. I told her that I would write that she exhibited an imaginative use of language and that she attributed her depression to external things. She agreed to another meeting, and we shook hands.

I saw J twice a week for almost three months. At first our meetings were erratic in that she continued to refuse to talk to me at times. We met in different places—my office, the ward, and so forth. I realized she was most hostile when we met in my office and commented on this. She said that being there made our talks feel like therapy, which she had no use for. We agreed to have coffee together in the mornings, then talk in the visitors' lounge. It was here that an emotional connection occurred; a working contract was developed that eventually led to discharge and acceptance to a transitional living program.

This humanistic approach to the helping relationship showed respect for the client as a person, allowing the student to give direction to the process and practice effectively with a client who had always been viewed as resistant, unmotivated, and unlikely to succeed in any environment other than an institutional setting.

Life Space Intervention

A public health nurse referred M to a student placed in a community mental health multiservice agency. M had a history of multiple hospitalizations but had been living in the community for about six months. The public health nurse felt M needed support and direction in achieving his goal of obtaining his graduate equivalency diploma (GED). M's goal was to make something of himself and to support himself like other young men his age. He was concerned about the stigma associated with his mental illness and wished to be viewed as one who not only had a mental illness but also had much in common with "normal" young adults his age. The student assured M that she would attempt to view him as a young man working to achieve his potential, not just as an ex-psychiatric patient.

To assess M and his life space, the student used ecomapping (Hartman & Laird, 1983). As she and M developed the ecomap, activities for intervention became clear. For example, M's first goal was to become employable. Therefore, his work on the GED was a primary activity. The student assumed the role of tutor, assigning specific chapters in the GED manual for work, assessing M's capacity in each area, and working with him on specific deficits. For leisure activities, M was encouraged to pursue his interest in basketball in a program offered by a local church. This activity not only helped him structure his leisure time, but also allowed him to meet young men his own age who were not ex-psychiatric clients. To ensure success in this endeavor, the student and M role-played early encounters with members of the new group and also made sure M had adequate directions to get to the church where the program was held. In addition, the student offered to meet the priest with M so that the experience would be less stressful.

Reading was chosen as an area for intervention. The student helped M acclimate himself to the local library, learn how to get there by bus, how to find books he enjoyed, how to solicit aid from the librarian, and so forth. When M found the branch library in the neighborhood inadequate, the student helped him learn how to use the main library.

M's family history indicated overinvolvement by his mother and neglect by his father and brothers. The student helped educate the family about M's potential. In addition, she helped them identify the type of support that would benefit him most.

The practice approach proved effective; two years later M had obtained his GED, was employed, had rented his own apartment, had learned to drive, and was a leader in a social support group at the local social club. He did not require any additional hospitalizations. Currently, M is on the Board of Directors of the social club.

CONCLUSION

The ecological perspective and practice approaches such as the life model and competence-oriented perspective allow comprehensive assessment of problem situations and multiple approaches to interventive activities. Together, they form a rich conceptual framework that enriches practice with those who have a chronic psychiatric disability. The conceptual framework here provides an alternative to the disease or medical models and is congruent with a psychosocial rehabilitation focus. It emphasizes the practitioner's responsibility to identify, mobilize, and ally him- or herself with the potential of the client. It focuses on the interface between the person and the environment, on the practitioner's role in facilitating the person's life and goals, and on matching the client's needs with environmental supports. It emphasizes the need for the availability of services in the person's environment and stresses the importance of the family as a major part of that environment.

These guidelines have been tested by a group of graduate social work students. The response of clients to such practice approaches has been most encouraging and suggests that the practice guidelines may be applicable to work with clients with chronic psychiatric disabilities. The ecological perspective and the approaches to practice from which these guidelines flow are receiving wide acceptance and attention in the field of social work. Explicating services to the chronically mentally ill in conceptual and practice terms that are widely accepted in the field is one way to increase workers' motivation to practice with this underserved population.

REFERENCES

Abandoned. 1986. *Newsweek*. Jan. 6.

Anderson, C. M., Hogarty, G. E., & Reiss, D. J. 1980. Family treatment of adult schizophrenic patients: A psycho-educational approach. *Schizophrenia Bulletin*. 6(3):490–502.

Anderson, C. M., Reiss, D. J., & Hogarty, G. E. 1986. *Schizophrenia and the Family*. New York: Guilford Press.

Anthony, W. A., Cohen, M., & Farkas, M. 1982. A psychiatric rehabilitation treatment program: Can I recognize one if I see one? *Community Mental Health Journal*. 18(2):83–96.

Atwood, N. 1982. Professional prejudice and the psychotic client. *Social Work*. 27(2): 172–177.

Bachrach, L. L. 1984. Asylum and chronically ill psychiatric patients. *American Journal of Psychiatry*. 141:975–978.

Crotty, P., & Kulys, R. 1985. Social support networks: The views of schizophrenic clients and their significant others. *Social Work*. 30(4):301–309.

Deitchman, W. S. 1980. How many case managers does it take to screw in a light bulb? *Hospital and Community Psychiatry*. 31:789.

Dincin, J. 1985. Psychiatric rehabilitation today. In J. P. Bowker (Ed.), *Education for Practice with the Chronically Mentally Ill: What Works?* Washington, DC: Council on Social Work Education, pp. 18–31.

Gerhart, U. C. 1985. Teaching social workers to work with the chronically mentally ill. In J. P. Bowker (Ed.), *Education for Practice with the Chronically Mentally Ill: What Works?* Washington, DC: Council on Social Work Education, pp. 50–66.

Germain, C. B. 1979. Ecology and social work. In C. B. Germain (Ed.), *Social Work Practice: People and Environments*. New York: Columbia University Press, pp. 1–22.

Germain, C. B., & Gitterman, A. 1980. *The Life Model of Social Work Practice*. New York: Columbia University Press.

Hall, B., & Valvano, J. 1985. Life space social work: A new level of practice. *Social Casework*. 66:515–524.

Hartman, A., & Laird, J. 1983. *Family-Centered Social Work Practice*. New York: Free Press, pp. 157–186.

Hatfield, A. 1982. *Coping with Mental Illness in the Family: A Family Guide*. Washington, DC: National Alliance of the Mentally Ill.

Hogarty, G. E. 1979. Aftercare treatment of schizophrenia: Current status and future direction. In H. M. Pragg (Ed.), *Management of Schizophrenia*. Assen, Netherlands: Van Gorcum, pp. 19–36.

Hogarty, G. E. 1984. Curricula and administrative issues addressed to the needs of the (chronic) mentally ill. Paper prensented at the NIMH Division of Human Resources' Workshop, July. Rockville, MD.

Intagliata, J. 1982. Improving the quality of community care for the chronically mentally disabled: The role of case management. *Schizophrenia Bulletin.* 8(4):655–674.

Johnson, P. J., & Rubin, A. 1983. Case management in mental health: A social work domain? *Social Work.* 28(1):49–55.

Langsley, D. G., Flomenhaft, K., & Mochotra, P. 1969. Follow-up evaluation of family crisis therapy. *American Journal of Orthopsychiatry.* 39(5):753–759.

Libassi, M. F., & Maluccio, A. N. Teaching the use of the ecological perspective in community mental health. *Journal of Education for Social Work.* 18(3):94–100.

Linn, M., et al. 1979. Day treatment and psychotropic drugs in the aftercare of schizophrenic patients. *Archives of General Psychiatry.* 36(10):1055–1066.

Linn, M., et al. 1980. Foster home characteristics and psychiatric patient outcome. *Archives of General Psychiatry.* 37:129–132.

Maluccio, A. N. 1981. Competence-oriented social work practice: An ecological approach. In A. Maluccio (Ed.), *Promoting Competence in Clients: A New/Old Approach to Social Work Practice.* New York: Free Press, pp. 1–26.

Maluccio, A. N., & Libassi, M. F. 1984. Competence clarification in social work practice. *Social Thought.* 10(2):51–58.

Rapp, C. A. 1985. Research on the chronically mentally ill: Curriculum implication. In J. P. Bowker (Ed.), *Education for Practice with the Chronically Mentally Ill.* pp. 32–49.

Rittenhouse, J. D. 1970. *Without Hospitalization: An Experimental Study of Psychiatric Care in the Home.* Denver: Swallow Press.

Rubin, A. 1985. Effective community-based care of chronic mental illness: Experimental findings. In J. P. Bowker (Ed.), *Education for Practice with the Chronically Mentally Ill,* pp. 1–17.

Stein, L. I., & Test, M. A. 1980. Alternative to mental hospital treatment: Conceptual model, treatment program, clinical evaluation. *Archives of General Psychiatry.* 37: 392–397.

Turner, J. C., & Tenhoor, W. J. 1978. The NIMH Community Support Program: Pilot approach to a needed social reform. *Schizophrenia Bulletin.* 4(4):319–348.

CHAPTER 6

Case Management with the Chronically Mentally Ill

A Clinical Perspective

Maxine Harris
Helen C. Bergman

With increasing numbers of chronically mentally ill adults being treated in community-based facilities, many program planners are viewing case management as the mechanism whereby patients will be assured of receiving the treatment they need (Bachrach, 1983; District of Columbia Department of Human Services, 1986). Practitioners and planners have viewed case management as incorporating varying degrees of aggressiveness and clinical involvement (Lamb, 1980; Levine & Fleming, 1984; Stein & Test, 1980). Nevertheless, the role of a case manager is generally seen as one of coordinating and overseeing a patient's overall treatment (Schwartz, Goldman, & Churgin, 1982; Sullivan, 1981; Test, 1979). In this sense, case management, while integrally related to it, is a set of functions independent of the treatment itself.

Our hypothesis is that, for many chronically mentally ill patients, case management not only provides coordination of care but is actually a mode of therapy in itself and as such constitutes treatment independent of any other treatments with which the patient is involved. Generally, psychiatric treatments are thought to result in either the remediation or the stabilization of some pathological condition or in an increased capacity on the patient's part to cope and to manage stressful circumstances. Case management, in contradistinction, is usually seen as affecting only the patient's external world without necessarily facilitating any growth or internal change on the part of the patient. We are suggesting that the process of effective case management can enhance patients' own capacities to cope and function in the world. This occurs when patients internalize, as they might in more traditional psychotherapy relationships, the activities of the case management process itself. The emphasis is thus shifted from the managerial functions onto those aspects of the process which make case management a potential vehicle for intrapsychic growth.

We will begin by describing those aspects of the case management process that offer potential identification by the patient. Why these particular process variables are especially suited to the deficits of the chronically mentally ill will then be highlighted. Finally, we will discuss how a process of internalization can occur via the case management relationship and result in patients acquiring new skills and capacities with which they can function independently.

CASE MANAGEMENT PROCESS

The process whereby a case manager accomplishes the various tasks on a client's behalf—from advocating benefits to monitoring outpatient visits—embodies certain principles which transcend any particular activity. Case management, over and above its specific functions, is integrative, rational, proactive, and individualized; it is these process variables which become available to patients for potential modeling and identification.

Integrative

Bachrach (1983), among others, has stressed the primacy of the integrative function in case management. Integration occurs in two ways. First the case manager coordinates and brings together the various aspects of the individual's treatment. By understanding the requirements and expectations in diverse parts of the treatment system, the case manager averts conflicts and disruptions. For example, knowing that entitlement benefits are tied to earnings, the case manager coordinates the patient's earnings at a sheltered workshop so that needed benefits are not curtailed. An overview of all parts of the treatment system enables the case manager to avert the fragmentation that occurs when several clinicians operate independently.

In addition to coordination at the systems level, the case manager also maintains a coordinated view of the patient. In a system without case management, professional personnel often hold only partial views: the vocational counselor knows the patient as a potential worker while the psychiatrist may be aware only of the patient's responses to medication. The case manager, in contrast, collects data from a variety of sources to arrive at a view of the whole person (Cutler, Terwilliger, & Faulkner, 1983). Moreover, by knowing what is going on in several aspects of the individual's life, the case manager can better plan interventions. Thus the process of case management not only embodies the diverse aspects of an individual's treatment but also develops a holistic, integrated view of the individual.

Rational

In addition to being integrative, case management also operates rationally. Planning is generally listed as one of its functions and the very act of planning implies that things are done in an orderly way that makes sense. The case manager uses assessment data to plan treatment so that interventions will follow from a clear sense of who the person is. One does not, for example, apply for an apartment program merely because a bed is available or because it is the first of the month; the application is based on a reasonable assessment of the patient's skills, goals, and readiness for such a move. Not only does the patient come to see the rationale behind particular plans but, more critically, that there *is* a rationale, that is, that events occur for identifiable reasons.

Planning also implies an orderly sequence of events leading to particular outcomes. When applying for benefits, for example, the case manager's instrumental knowledge not only gets things done but also, indirectly, demonstrates to the patient that events can be understood and anticipated.

Thus, being rational and orderly, the case management process implies a logical view of the world. Events are linked to one another either through temporal sequence or through cause-and-effect. This approach may well contrast with the patient's own unpredictable and often frightening view of events.

Proactive

Case managers must be prepared to deal with crises, but rather than waiting for things to happen, they attempt to control and direct external events. Case management provides a model for operating in the world as a capable individual, secure in the ability to influence external events. This contrasts with the experience of many clinicians engaged in working with chronically mentally ill individuals who feel powerless to have an impact on the treatment system (Stern & Minkoff, 1979). Regrettably, this sense of powerlessness frequently parallels the patient's own feeling of inadequacy in managing his or her life. Ideally, when a mental health system decides to incorporate a case management component, it empowers its case managers to have an impact on the system. Thus the patient is presented with a model of a powerful adult, with whom the patient can initially ally and eventually emulate.

Individualized

Finally, the process of case management is individualized (Cutler, Terwilliger, & Faulkner, 1983). Through careful assessment, the case manager creates the profile of a particular patient. A plan is constructed to fit that patient's needs, goals, and skills, and it is put into operation in a language that has meaning for the patient. For example, while the objective for many chronic patients may be to increase social skills, for one patient that may mean calling a friend to go to the movies while for another it may entail spending an hour a day with other people.

In mental health systems, where many patients have to be treated with limited resources, the treatment is apt to become mass produced. All patients may receive group therapy because that is the only modality available in a given program rather than because it meets specific patients' needs. Ideally, case managers should have flexibility and authority to match patients to a range of treatments. In this way the patient comes to appreciate his or her importance as an individual.

To recapitulate, case management may be described in terms of its characteristic processes: integration, rationality, proaction, and individuality. We shall demonstrate that, while such an approach holds the potential of being therapeutic for most patients, it is particularly responsive to the deficits of chronically mentally ill patients who typically experience life in a fragmented, irrational, passive, and global manner.

CHRONIC MENTAL ILLNESS

Both program planners and researchers have tackled the difficult task of defining and delineating the population of chronic mental patients (District of Columbia Department of Human Services, 1986; Talbott, 1984). From an epidemiological perspective (Freud, 1940), variables such as diagnosis, extent of disability, and duration of illness have served to identify the population. This discussion will focus on the psychological variables that contribute to the subjective experience of being a chronically mentally ill person.

First and foremost is the chronically mentally ill individual's lack of stable identity and secure sense of self (Blatt, Schimek, & Brenneis, 1980; Will, 1980). As one young man put it, "I don't think I have a self and I'm not sure I want one." This lack of cohesive identity outside of one's delusional system contributes to the sense of dread and panic that many patients experience (Will, 1980). It also makes any realistic plans for treatment difficult (Harris & Bergman, 1984). If the patient's core identity is in jeopardy, he or she can only play at goal planning. Issues of survival and just making it to the next day are too overwhelming to permit plans for next month or beyond.

Related to this deficit in the development of a stable identity is the patient's experience of being scattered, disorganized, and easily distracted. Pepper and Ryglewicz (1984), among others, have highlighted the intrapsychic fragmentation and disorganization characteristic of young adult chronic patients. Regardless of whether this experience is the result of underlying cognitive deficits, intrapsychic defenses, or organic damage secondary to substance abuse, the experience for the chronically mentally ill person is frequently one of confusion and befuddlement. Unfortunately, the profile of a patient who leaves home in the morning bound for a clinic appointment and is found several hours later wandering through a distant part of town without any idea of how or why he or she managed to get there is not an atypical one.

Perhaps as the result of these deficits, chronically mentally ill persons often find themselves easily overwhelmed by changes in external events or contingencies (Neligh & Kinzie, 1983). Research has focused not only on the special vulnerabilities of schizophrenic patients to stressful events but also on the increase in stressful life events that goes with being a chronic mental patient (Zubin & Spring, 1977). These factors contribute to the patient's sense that he or she lacks the capacity to cope with even minor changes. Some patients will seem almost as overwhelmed by a change in appointment times or bus routes as by a major move or disruption in their life circumstances.

All of these difficulties are exacerbated by the fact that chronic patients often lack even rudimentary problem-solving skills (Liberman et al., 1980). When confronted with a situation that demands a solution, the chronic patient is often unable to deal with it rationally. One young man at the Community Connections program in Washington, D.C. (Harris, Bergman, & Greenwood, 1982), when faced with not having enough money to pay his rent, decided to solicit donations from wealthy and famous people. His strategy failed and not only was his instrumental need unmet, but he also experienced himself as unable to manage his own affairs.

Other patients do not even conceptualize any strategies, however impracticable. For them, the task of solving a problem is completely unmanageable and they find themselves passively dependent when confronted with the need to devise a plan of action or solve a problem.

Given a patient with this particular constellation of vulnerabilities (lack of stable identity, tendency toward disorganized thinking, vulnerability to stress, and inability to solve problems) case management emerges as an effective means of stabilizing the individual in the community; it provides an integrative, rational and stable approach to community living. Beyond this accommodative function, however, case management can also serve as a model for potential internalization by the chronic patient and in that way facilitate growth.

Internalization

The internalization process is usually cited by analytic writers (Freud, 1940; Kohut, 1984; Meissner, 1981; Schafer, 1968) as the mechanism whereby an individual absorbs some aspect of the external world and makes it his or her own. In his original discussion of superego formation, Freud (1940) asserted that functions initially performed by significant others in the external world come to be internalized and subsequently performed by the individual. Schafer (1968) extended the concept by proposing that both real and imagined regulatory actions and characteristics of the environment are available for potential internalization. The process may start as mimicry (Meissner, 1981) but eventually identification occurs and the behavior comes to belong to the mime.

Clinicians (Blatt, Schimek, & Brenneis, 1980) have discussed the role of internalization in the psychotherapy of chronically mentally ill individuals, but not in connection with the case management relationship. Because case management is generally seen as a managerial, oversight function, its clinical aspects tend to be ignored. A notable exception is Lamb's (1980) work on the therapist–case manager, although he approaches the dual role from the perspective of the therapist who also performs case management functions rather than the case manager whose work is therapeutic.

Because case management entails the development of a close working relationship between manager and patient, it affords the opportunity for identification in much the same way as a psychotherapy relationship. At first the patient may use the case manager as an auxiliary ego, in the performance of certain functions (Pepper, Ryglewicz, & Kirshner, 1982). This dependency may be replaced by a phase of imitation in which the patient merely repeats or copies behaviors of the manager. This can be superseded by a period in which the patient undertakes the case manager's mode of reasoning. One young woman at Community Connections, for example, would approach problems by asking herself, "Now how would [her case manager] handle this?" She would then approach the problem in what she saw as the case manager's manner and at their next meeting would present her reasoning for feedback. In the final stage of identification the activity is summoned as the patient's own, without reference to the case manager.

By this process the patient can come to identify with the dynamic aspects of case management, its integrative, rational, and proactive stance, in the context of an individualized relationship. While the patient may also come to learn such discrete behaviors as riding the bus or monitoring medication, the internalization of case management functions will ultimately provide a greater flexibility and capacity to cope with a variety of situations.

Integration and Sense of Self. With access to data about the patient from a variety of sources, the case manager is able to develop a reliable and integrated view of the patient and often discerns certain aspects of the patient's identity before the patient does. Thus, the case manager can label behavior and deduce general traits for the patient. In the Community Connections program, one young man with a history of intellectual accomplishments did not see himself as intelligent; he seemed unable to step back from his academic successes and identify in himself the endowment which allowed them. The case manager, aware of the patient's history, saw him as a smart young man and reflected this back to the patient. Because he identified with the case manager's image of him, the patient came to know himself as intelligent.

This evolution of a personal identity is akin to what Winnicott (1965) and others describe as part of healthy child development. Bach (1985) suggests that a child's theory of self is developed in relationship with another person. If development proceeds normally, a child internalizes an accurate and stable sense of identity.

A chronically mentally ill person has failed to form this stable sense of identity and the mental health system, with its multiple care-givers and often fragmented service delivery (Bachrach, 1979), does not usually reflect a stable identity back to the patient in the present. The case manager, however, as coordinator, is able to form a stable sense of the patient and reflect it back in the treatment planning process.

Rationality and Ego Functions. It is frequently remarked that clinicians may need to function as auxiliary egos for chronic patients (Pepper, Ryglewicz, & Kirshner, 1982). The full import of this statement can best be appreciated by examining what is entailed in ego functioning. Hartmann (1951) identified several dimensions of the ego, including those related to problem-solving and to overall coordination and synthetic function.

In its role as problem-solver, the ego tests reality, anticipates events, sets goals, makes plans for the future, remembers past events and brings them to bear on present and future behaviors, and imposes thought on impulsive actions. Since these are many of the functions that the case manager performs for the chronic patient, it is apparent why the former is likened to an auxiliary ego.

By the same token, the case manager also provides a model of healthy functioning with which the patient can identify. Initially the patient may repeat the case manager's problem-solving approach in a rote manner; some patients even appreciate a written "how-to" version and this can function as a transitional object for the patient (Winnicott, 1958). Eventually, however, with no explicit instruction, patients can internalize a problem-solving approach and are able to use it independently of the case manager.

In its coordinating function for the personality, the ego serves as the center of the personality, regulating and synthesizing various personality functions. The case manager in coordinating all aspects of the treatment system, temporarily becomes the center of the patient's world. Thus, in practical terms the patient has a single consultant for a variety of concerns. On a more symbolic level, the case manager becomes a model of a centered universe to counter the patient's hitherto fragmented one. In the internalization of this integrative function, the coordinating capacity of the patient's ego is enhanced.

Proaction and a Sense of Power. At the beginning of the case, the case manager may need to provide the patient with a respite from stressful external events. By directly intervening to gain control over a family or work situation that appears overwhelming to the patient, the case manager brings the patient real relief and at the same time demonstrates that one can have power over external events.

The patient initially experiences this control and power through alliance with the case manager. As one patient said about confronting his (borderline) wife, "You [the case manager] do it this time, and I'll watch." This process seems to parallel the pleasure and security of a young child in sharing parental power.

With the acquisition of a more stable sense of self and more consistent ego controls, the patient begins to experience a more competent self. Identification with a competent case manager as well as a growing belief that mastery of external events is possible may help develop a more positive sense of self in the patient. Such development can contribute to the amelioration of poor self-esteem, so often a problem among chronic patients (Pepper & Ryglewicz, 1984).

DISCUSSION

Emphasis has so far been on the positive therapeutic aspects of a case management approach, focusing on the ways in which chronic patients may come to identify with the stable, integrative, and problem-solving aspects of the process. A word of moderation is needed, however. Clearly, for some percentage of the chronically mentally ill the capacity for internalization is impaired as a result of biological illness. For these individuals, the need for the auxiliary ego functions of the case manager may persist. However, for many others, perhaps even the majority, the capacity for some intrapsychic growth remains and the initially dependent relationship with the case manager can be transformed (Anthony, Cohen, & Cohen, 1984).

Interventions with the chronically mentally ill can focus on growth or on maintenance (Kanter, 1985). Generally, while psychotherapy and psychosocial rehabilitation are seen as growth promoting interventions, case management is usually listed with the maintenance strategies. By emphasizing the potential for internalization of stable and integrative functioning in the case management process, practitioners can come to consider case management as an intervention with real psychological growth as a possible outcome.

REFERENCES

Anthony, W., Cohen, M. & Cohen, B. 1984. Psychiatric rehabilitation. In J. Talbott (Ed.), *The Chronic Mental Patient: Five Years Later.* Orlando, FL: Grune and Stratton.

Bach, S. 1985. *Narcissistic States and the Therapeutic Process.* New York: Jason Aronson.

Bachrach, L. 1979. Planning mental health services for chronic patients. *Hospital Community Psychiatry.* 30:387–392.

Bachrach, L. 1983. An overview of deinstitutionalization. *New Directions for Mental Health Services.* 17:5–14.

Blatt, S., Schimek, J. & Brenneis, B. 1980. The nature of the psychotic experience and its implications for the therapeutic process. In J. Strauss et al. (Eds.), *The Psychotherapy of Schizophrenia.* New York: Plenum.

Brown, G. & Birley, J. 1968. Crisis and life changes and the onset of schizophrenia. *Journal of Health and Social Behavior.* 9:203–214.

Cutler, D., Terwilliger, W. & Faulkner, L. 1983. Integrating an aftercare plan for the chronic patient. *New Directions for Mental Health Services.* 19:95–104.

District of Columbia Department of Human Services. 1986. Final Mental Health System Implementation Plan, Washington, DC.

Freud, S. 1940. An outline of psychoanalysis. In *Standard Edition.* London: Hogarth Press.

Harris, M., & Bergman, H. 1984. Reassessing the revolving door: A developmental perspective on the young adult chronic patient. *American Journal of Orthopsychiatry.* 54:281–289.

Harris, M., Bergman, H., & Greenwood, V. 1982. Integrating hospital and community systems for treating revolving door patients. *Hospital and Community Psychiatry.* 33:225–227.

Hartmann, H. 1951. Ego psychology and the problem of adaptation. In D. Rapaport (Ed.), *Organization and Pathology of Thought.* New York: Columbia University Press.

Kanter, J. 1985. Clinical issues in treating the chronic mentally ill. *New Directions for Mental Health Services.* 27.

Kohut, H. 1984. *How Does Analysis Cure?* Chicago: University of Chicago Press.

Lamb, H. 1980. Therapist-case managers: More than brokers of services. *Hospital and Community Psychiatry.* 31:762–764.

Levine, I., & Fleming, M. 1984. *Human Resource Development: Issues in Case Management.* University of Maryland: Center for Rehabilitation and Manpower Services.

Liberman, R. et al. 1980. Social and family factors in the course of schizophrenia: Toward an interpersonal problem-solving therapy for schizophrenics and their families. In J. Strauss et al. (Eds.), *The Psychotherapy of Schizophrenia.* New York: Plenum.

Meissner, W. 1981. *Internalization in Psychoanalysis.* New York: International Universities Press.

Neligh, G., & Kinzie, J. 1983. Therapeutic relationships with the chronic patient. *New Directions for Mental Health Services.* 19:73–83.

Pepper, B., & Ryglewicz, H. 1984. Treating the young adult chronic patient: An update. *New Directions for Mental Health Services.* 21:5–16.

Pepper, B., Ryglewicz, H., & Kirshner, M. 1982. The uninstitutionalized generation: A new breed of psychiatric patient. *New Directions for Mental Health Services.* 14:3–13.

Schafer, R. 1968. *Aspects of Internalization.* New York: International Universities Press.

Schwartz, S., Goldman, H., & Churgin, S. 1982. Case management for the chronic mentally ill: Models and dimensions. *Hospital and Community Psychiatry.* 33:1006–1009.

Stein, L., & Test, M. 1980. Alternative to mental hospital treatment. I. Conceptual model, treatment program, and clinical evaluation. *Archives of General Psychiatry.* 37:392–397.

Stern, R., & Minkoff, K. 1979. Paradoxes in programming for chronic patients in a community clinic. *Hospital and Community Psychiatry.* 30:613–617.

Sullivan, J. 1981. Case management. In J. Talbott (Ed.), *The Chronically Mentally Ill.* New York: Human Sciences Press.

Talbott, J. (Ed.). 1984. *The Chronic Mental Patient: Five Years Later.* Orlando, FL: Grune & Stratton.

Test, M. 1979. Continuity of care in community treatment. *New Directions for Mental Health Services.* 2:15–23.

Will, O. 1980. Comments on the 'elements' of schizophrenia, psychotherapy, and the schizophrenic person. In J. Strauss et al. (Eds.), *Psychotherapy of Schizophrenia.* New York: Plenum.

Winnicott, D. 1958. Transitional objects and transitional phenomena. In *Collected Papers.* London: Tavistock.

Winnicott, D. 1965. *The Maturational Processes and the Facilitating Environment.* New York: International Universities Press.

Zubin, J., & Spring, B. 1977. Vulnerability: A new view of schizophrenia. *Journal of Abnormal Psychology.* 86:103–126.

CHAPTER 7

The Assertive Community Treatment Worker

An Emerging Role and Its Implications for Professional Training

Thomas F. Witheridge

In recent years, a new treatment approach for long-term mental health consumers has grown in acceptance and sophistication. Known by a variety of names—including assertive community treatment, assertive outreach, and assertive or intensive case management—this approach can be traced to the work of Pasamanick and associates (1967), Hetrick (1969), and other pioneers. It was further developed and refined during the 1970s by Stein and Test in Madison, Wisconsin (1980, 1985, 1976). Their exceedingly robust model has proven adaptable to diverse geographical and agency settings, consumer subgroups, and treatment applications.

In 1978 the model was adapted to the realities of an inner-city mental health system by the Thresholds Bridge Program in Chicago (Significant achievement awards, 1981; Witheridge, 1987; Witheridge & Dincin, 1985; Witheridge, Dincin, & Appleby, 1982). Although that program is eclectic in origin, it owes particularly heavy debts to the Madison model and to the psychosocial rehabilitation methods employed at its own parent agency, Thresholds (Dincin, 1975, 1981; Dincin, Selleck, & Carter, 1980; Dincin & Witheridge, 1982). Related concepts and methods can be found throughout the literature on the community treatment of long-term mental health consumers (Kanter, 1985; Lamb, 1982; Stein, 1979; Talbott, 1978, 1981).

As it will be described here, assertive community treatment includes several characteristic features: a virtually exclusive reliance on home visiting and other "in vivo" intervention methods; a focus on the highest-priority service recipients, however they might be defined in a given treatment situation; an explicit mission to reduce psychiatric hospital use by improving the quality of the participants' everyday lives; a favorable ratio of staff to participants, generally 1 to 10 or better; a heavy emphasis on staff teamwork; a willingness to assume ultimate professional responsibility for the participants' well-being, no matter how they might become involved with the service delivery system; tenacious advocacy across myriad system boundaries; the anticipation and prevention of crises; a rapid response when crises unavoidably occur; and a commitment to working with participants as long as their needs persist, whether or not they can demonstrate "growth" or "progress."

Because of its limited scope, this paper does not enter into the increasingly lively debate among the proponents (Baker & Weiss, 1984; Harrod, 1986; Intagliata, 1982; Lamb, 1980) and critics (Franklin, 1988) of case management in its many forms. Nor does it seek to synthesize the various offshoots of the Madison model that are currently evolving in the United States (Bond et al. 1988; Mulder, 1988) and abroad (Hoult et al., 1983). Instead, it pursues the more modest aim of clarifying the role of the assertive community treatment worker, using the Thresholds Bridge Program as a case in point. The first section describes the activities conducted by members of the core services team (Test, 1979) at each of several inner-city locations. The second section identifies some of the implications of that work for professional training programs in the major mental health disciplines.

FUNCTIONS OF THE ASSERTIVE COMMUNITY TREATMENT WORKER

It is difficult to write a job description for the assertive community treatment worker, because the tasks performed vary tremendously from consumer to consumer and from day to day. Even so, experience suggests that possible activities include all of the following, among others.

Identifying Members of the Target Population

The assertive community treatment team maintains cordial working relationships with its major referral sources, such as hospitals and community mental health centers. The goal is to identify those individuals who are in the greatest need of attention from a core services team of assertive community treatment workers. Thus, the outreach worker ensures that prospective participants (whether they are called members, clients, ex-patients, or patients) meet the team's relatively strict eligibility criteria.

In the Thresholds Bridge Program, for example, prospective members ordinarily present with at least five prior psychiatric admissions or with a longstanding pattern of homelessness. The typical candidate has been hospitalized upwards of 20 times; however, some of the most appropriate candidates have managed to avoid frequent institutional confinement.

Engaging New Participants

The outreach worker initiates the engagement process very carefully, recognizing full well that the new participant may have rejected or overwhelmed professional helpers in the past. Ideally, the worker begins by assisting the consumer with a concrete task—for instance, leaving the hospital and moving into affordable housing—to demonstrate the advantages of participation right from the outset.

With the consumer's permission, the worker explains the team's assertive approach to family members and collaterals, obtaining in return as much pertinent information as possible. Then the worker introduces the new participant to the rest of the outreach staff, one worker at a time, so that a whole team of helping personalities can be enlisted in the community support and rehabilitation efforts to come.

Conducting Assessments and Planning Interventions

The members of the core services team perform an initial assessment of the person's strengths, difficulties, existing resources, and remaining needs (Kanter, 1985). Then they look for novel ways to interrupt the chain of events that previously led to the person's distress in the community and subsequent rehospitalization or homelessness. In consultation with the consumer and his or her family, the team members develop an intervention strategy, intervene as planned, observe the consumer's response, and modify the strategy accordingly. The goal is to get a handle on the constellation of factors responsible for the person's inability to thrive in the community.

Assuming Ultimate Professional Responsibility

The core services team assumes ultimate professional responsibility for the consumers' well-being, helping them to assemble coherent, individually tailored packages of community supports (Talbott, 1978, 1980). Many of these supports can be provided directly by the team; others must be farmed out. Moreover, in most assertive community treatment programs, individuals may participate on a long-term basis—even if they are rehospitalized repeatedly or terminated by other agencies. Consequently, the staff must show unusual tolerance for "unresponsive" or "difficult" behavior.

Home Visiting

The outreach worker meets with people on their own turf, where the problems arise and the solutions must be found (Test & Stein, 1976; Test, 1979). Typically, this may mean starting a a person's home and proceeding to a nearby restaurant for coffee and light conversation. But the worker soon becomes intimately familiar with a variety of locations that are seldom (if ever) visited by the conventional practitioner: low-rent hotels, boarding houses, and apartment buildings; welfare offices; police lockups; public shelters; unsavory street corners; and the like. In general, the friendly visit takes place where the consumer happens to be, wants to be, or needs to be, not necessarily where the worker would prefer to be.

Attending to the Concrete Details of Everyday Life

The assertive community treatment worker focuses on improving the quality of the participants' everyday lives so that the community can become a satisfactory alternative to the total institution (Test & Stein, 1976; Test, 1979). This means, in practice, that the worker pays close attention to such basic, largely concrete matters as entitlement funding, money management, food, clothing, shelter, and medical care. After all, it is the seemingly "trivial" activities of daily living that produce some of the most stubborn and critical problems for people with psychiatric disabilities (Davis, 1988).

Providing in Vivo Assistance and Training

The outreach worker provides on-the-spot help with a wide range of independent living tasks, from the most elemental (for example, operating a space heater) to the more complex (for example, leasing an apartment). The worker experiments with psychosocial rehabilitation and other practical, behaviorally grounded techniques for helping consumers to pursue higher-level goals, such as residential independence and gainful employment (Dincin, 1975, 1981; Dincin, Selleck, & Carter, 1980; Dincin & Witheridge, 1982; Anthony, Cohen, & Cohen, 1984). In order to minimize any problems associated with the transfer of training, this help is generally provided in a natural or naturalistic setting (Test & Stein, 1976; Stein, 1988). The worker encourages the consumers' involvement with social, recreational, and self-help programs, where interpersonal skills can be learned, practiced, and consolidated.

Thus the worker helps the participants to develop greater self-confidence and to execute more sophisticated behaviors whenever possible, gradually reducing the participants' reliance on external support as they gradually internalize the functions of the team (Harris & Bergman, 1987). If this strategy fails, however, the worker continues to provide hands-on support, accepting the participants' dependency and looking for ways to make life in the community more comfortable, dignified, and satisfying than life in the hospital (Lamb, 1982).

Arranging for Psychiatric and Other Medical Services

The assertive community treatment worker is willing to take an active role in the consumer's quest for high-quality medical services. If necessary, for example, the worker may actually take the person to the mental health clinic, accompany the person into the room for the psychiatric interview, and take the person back home—perhaps via the nearest drive-through restaurant for a refreshing and reinforcing snack. In other cases, the worker plays a more subtle and indirect role in the process, helping the person to arrange his or her own medical services and monitoring to make sure that all goes well. In general, the worker strives to make the participant's use of these services a less intimidating experience than it might otherwise become.

Providing Interagency Resource Brokering and Advocacy

The outreach worker functions as an all-purpose resource broker, facilitating efforts by the many private and governmental agencies on which people with psychiatric disabilities routinely depend (Test & Stein, 1976; Test, 1979). The worker spends a great deal of time and energy serving as an advocate on the consumers' behalf in their confrontations with the complex, impersonal, and often irrational bureaucracies to which they must turn for help, especially in big cities like Chicago.

Whatever the bureaucracy, the worker rapidly gains a worm's-eye view of its customs and peculiarities. In the course of a year, the worker contacts a bewildering variety of agencies, learns their idiosyncratic policies and procedures, and goes over dozens of heads to dozens of supervisors—and to their supervisors, if necessary—in a calculated but sincere effort to systematize the service delivery "nonsystem" (Talbott, 1980).

Developing Community Resources

The worker often finds it necessary to search for hidden resources (for example, an especially tolerant apartment house) or to develop nonexistent resources from scratch (for example, a foster family with sign-language skills). This step is especially important for the consumer whose psychiatric disability is complicated by another disability or medical problem, such as mental retardation, epilepsy, deafness, chemical dependency, or AIDS. Some communities and neighborhoods have a paucity of existing resources, and the worker in such settings must be creative or even entrepreneurial to get the job done.

Facilitating Necessary Readmissions and Working with the Inpatient Staff

As the mental health workers who know their program participants best—more intimately, in most cases, than they are known by any other professionals in town—members of the core services team are generally in a position to recognize prodromal symptoms, signs of distress, and crisis situations first. Occasionally, the tide of breakdown simply cannot be reversed, and the outreach worker must make the inescapable decision to initiate a rehospitalization.

At such times, the worker must exercise sound clinical judgment, often on the spur of the moment, and often with little or no useful support from others on the scene. The logistics can be incredibly complicated: dealing with confused or hostile bystanders; reviewing the options with concerned family members; if necessary, calling the police and persuading them to cooperate; presenting the facts at the hospital emergency room; arranging for the interim care of pets and plants and the storage of personal belongings; and so forth.

Once the individual has been safely hospitalized, the core services team turn their attention to the inpatient staff, helping them to understand the new patient and his or her predicament, as well as to devise a practical discharge plan. The goals at this stage are to streamline the inpatient process and to put together a package of community supports that will enable the person to leave the hospital just as soon as his or her mental status permits.

In theory, this interagency collaboration should be more or less automatic. In practice, it breaks down with frustrating regularity so that the outreach worker must become an active transport mechanism, as it were, across a seemingly impermeable inpatient–outpatient barrier. The worker must find ways to become insinuated into the inpatient world, using all of the diplomacy and resourcefulness at his or her command. In other words, the worker must act as if the core services team and their inpatient counterpart constituted a single, continuous, planfully integrated system, even though they seldom do (Frances & Goldfinger, 1986; Torrey, 1986).

Working in Partnership with Families

The outreach worker recognizes that living with severe mental illness is an exquisitely painful experience for everyone concerned: not only for the primary consumers themselves, but also for the family members who care about them. Therefore, the worker is quite willing to expand the advocacy role to include activities on behalf of entire families. It is axiomatic, moreover, that the worker treats family members as partners, not as adversaries, in the community support and rehabilitation efforts (Kanter, 1985; Dincin, Selleck, & Streiker, 1978; Bernheim & Lehman, 1985; Hatfield, 1979).

IMPLICATIONS FOR PROFESSIONAL TRAINING

What are the implications of this emerging practice role for professional training programs in the major mental health disciplines? The preceding comments suggest one conclusion so obvious that it almost goes without saying: certain aspects of the assertive community treatment worker's role cannot readily be taught. Because of their aptitudes, their interests, and even their temperaments, certain individuals are unquestionably cut out for the job; others are not. Furthermore, the correlation between suitability and prior professional training is weaker than one might expect it to be.

At this writing, the largest number of Thresholds Bridge staff workers hold bachelor's degrees in such fields as social work and psychology. A smaller but growing number hold master's degrees in social work, counseling, and related fields. The director and of course the consulting psychiatrists hold doctorates. However, the program's hiring supervisors have learned over the years to focus on the person, not the degree. More precisely, while recognizing that the degree does convey important information about the applicant, they generally consider personality factors first, and credentials second, in the hiring process (Dincin, 1975).

Even so, academic and professional programs could certainly do more than they have done thus far to meet the training needs of the assertive community treatment field (Bowker, 1985). If one were to design a curriculum at the undergraduate or graduate level to prepare students for the work described in the previous section, that curriculum would pay special attention to the following key areas.

Professional Attitudes, Values, and Beliefs

The prospective outreach worker should be given repeated opportunities to explore, clarify, question, and modify his or her preexisting attitudes, values, and beliefs. Assertive community treatment requires a genuine concern for people with seriously disabling psychiatric problems, most of whom are living below (or just above) the poverty line. It requires an ability to put the consumers' needs ahead of the worker's desire for the trappings of professional success.

It requires a clear understanding that the rights, the self-determination, and the empowerment of consumers are at the very center of ethical practice. At the same time, it requires a willingness to accept the protracted dependency exhibited by some program participants. It requires a truly nonjudgmental attitude toward the participants and their families. Finally, it requires an openness to the veritable revolution in beliefs about the etiology and course of severe mental illness currently taking place within the medical and behavioral sciences and the human service disciplines.

Biological, Psychological, and Sociological Foundations

The prospective outreach worker should be given a thorough introduction to the relevant foundation areas. For example, assertive community treatment requires an especially solid familiarity with recent developments in biological psychiatry, psychopharmacology, rehabilitation theory, and psychodiagnostics. It requires basic familiarity and comfort with selected topics in sociology and anthropology, including social systems, race, ethnicity, class, and culture. It may not require, but it benefits greatly from, familiarity with the most commonly used evaluation research strategies.

Historical Foundations

The prospective outreach worker should be given a hearty welcome to the mainstream of the mental health professions, through a systematic orientation to their venerable traditions of service to individuals and groups in the greatest of need. Assertive community treatment becomes less burdensome and more meaningful with the awareness that we are not alone; that we are following the examples of pioneers like Dorothea Dix, Jane Addams, Julia Lathrop, Clifford Beers, Adolf Meyer, and so many others; that the friendly visit preceded the 50-minute hour by decades; and that the alleviation of suffering among those who are poor, powerless, and disabled is a fundamental and noble mission of the professions, not just something we do to make ends meet until the private practice is off and running. In addition, this work entails at least a survey-course familiarity with the recent history of social welfare, mental health law, and related topics.

Methods of Intervention

Both in the classroom and in the field, the prospective outreach worker should be exposed to a variety of approaches that have shown particular promise in the treatment of long-term consumers. These approaches include psychosocial rehabilitation; home visiting and other out-of-the-office methods; resource brokering and service coordination; consultation with families, professionals, and community representatives; crisis residential services; consumer- and family-run alternatives; and supportive counseling and group work.

If possible, a significant portion of the practical training should take place within an assertive community treatment program. The team approach used in these programs makes them well suited for the training of apprentices. The student can be eased into progressively greater responsibility for the team's shared caseload, and every member of the team can serve as a de facto auxiliary field instructor (Urbanowski & Dwyer, 1988). In this fashion, the

Thresholds Bridge Program has trained numerous social work and nursing students over the years, several of whom have been invited to join the staff.

CONCLUSIONS

Assertive community treatment places heavy demands on the frontline workers who carry it out. This paper has addressed their increasingly important role within the service delivery system and has identified some of the implications of that role for professional training programs.

In general, assertive community treatment requires a willingness to abandon narrow ideology, to step outside the traditional schools and guilds of mental health practice, and to experiment with innovative techniques whose merit has yet to be conclusively demonstrated. Above all, this work requires a willingness to fit the service to the members of the target population. If those persons cannot, will not, or simply do not use the service, it can hardly be construed as therapeutic.

REFERENCES

Anthony, W., Cohen, M., & Cohen, B. 1984. Psychiatric rehabilitation. In J. A. Talbott (Ed.), *The Chronic Mental Patient: Five Years Later.* Orlando: FL: Grune & Stratton.

Baker, F., & Weiss, R. S. 1984. The nature of case manager support. *Hospital and Community Psychiatry.* 35:925–928.

Bernheim, K. F., & Lehman, A. F. 1985. *Working with Families of the Mentally Ill.* New York: Norton.

Bond, G. R., et al: 1988. Assertive case management in three CMHCs: A controlled study. *Hospital and Community Psychiatry.* 39:411–418.

Bowker, J. P. (Ed.) 1985. *Education for Practice with the Chronically Mentally Ill: What Works?* Washington, DC: Council on Social Work Education.

Davis, S. 1988. "Soft" versus "hard" social work. *Social Work.* 33:373–374.

Dincin, J. 1975. Psychiatric rehabilitation. *Schizophrenia Bulletin.* 13:131–147.

Dincin, J. 1981. A community agency model. In J. A. Talbott (Ed.), *The Chronic Mentally Ill: Treatment, Programs, Systems.* New York: Human Sciences.

Dincin, J., Selleck, V., & Carter, S. 1980. Implementing the rehabilitation approach in a community residential setting. *Rehabilitation Counseling Bulletin.* 24:72–83.

Dincin, J., Selleck, V., & Streicker, S. 1978. Restructuring parental attitudes: Working with parents of the adult mentally ill. *Schizophrenia Bulletin.* 4:597–608.

Dincin, J., & Witheridge, T. F. 1982. Psychiatric rehabilitation as a deterrent to recidivism. *Hospital and Community Psychiatry.* 33:645–650.

Frances, A., & Goldfinger, S. M. 1986. "Treating" a homeless mentally ill patient who cannot be managed in the shelter system. *Hospital and Community Psychiatry.* 37:577–579.

Franklin, J. L. 1988. Case management: A dissenting view. *Hospital and Community Psychiatry.* 39:921.
Harris, M., & Bergman, H. C. 1987. Case management with the chronically mentally ill: A clinical perspective. *American Journal of Orthopsychiatry.* 57:296–302.
Harrod, J. B. 1986. Defining case management in community support systems. *Psychosocial Rehabilitation Journal.* 9:56–61.
Hatfield, A. B. 1979. The family as partner in the treatment of mental illness. *Hospital and Community Psychiatry.* 30:338–340.
Hetrick, 1969. Psychiatry gets off the couch and hits the streets. *Life.* Aug 8: 48–51.
Hoult, J., et al. 1983. Psychiatric hospital versus community treatment: The results of a randomised trial. *Australian and New Zealand Journal of Psychiatry.* 17:160–167.
Intagliata, J. 1982. Improving the quality of community care for the chronically mentally disabled: The role of case management. *Schizophrenia Bulletin.* 8:655–674.
Kanter, J. S., (Ed.) 1985. Clinical issues in treating the chronic mentally ill. *New Directions for Mental Health Services.* 27.
Lamb, H. R. 1980. Therapist-case managers: More than brokers of services. *Hospital and Community Psychiatry.* 31:762–764.
Lamb, H. R. 1982. *Treating the Long-Term Mentally Ill.* San Francisco: Jossey-Bass.
Mulder, R. 1988. Evaluation of the Harbinger program, 1982–1985. Lansing: Michigan Department of Mental Health.
Pasamanick, B., Scarpitti, F. R., & Dinitz, S. 1967. *Schizophrenics in the Community: An Experimental Study in the Prevention of Hospitalization.* New York: Appleton-Century-Crofts.
Significant achievement awards for 1981: Visiting programs for recidivists. 1981. *Hospital and Community Psychiatry.* 32:723–725.
Stein, L. I. (Ed.). 1979. Community support systems for the long-term patient. *New Directions for Mental Health Services.* 2.
Stein, L. I. 1988. "It's the focus, not the locus." Hocus-pocus! *Hospital and Community Psychiatry.* 39:1029.
Stein, L. I., & Test, M. A. 1980. An alternative to mental hospital treatment, I: Conceptual model, treatment program, and clinical evaluation. *Archives of General Psychiatry.* 37:392–397.
Stein, L. I., & Test, M. A. (Eds.). 1985. The training in community living model: A decade of experience. *New Directions for Mental Health Services.* 26.
Talbott, J. A. (Ed.) 1978. *The Chronic Mental Patient: Problems, Solutions, and Recommendations for a Public Policy.* Washington, DC: American Psychiatric Association.
Talbott, J. A. 1980. Toward a public policy on the chronic mentally ill patient. *American Journal of Orthopsychiatry.* 50:43–53.
Talbott, J. A. (Ed.) 1981. *The Chronic Mentally Ill: Treatment, Programs, Systems.* New York: Human Sciences.
Test, M. A. 1979. Continuity of care in community treatment. *New Directions for Mental Health Services.* 2:15–23.
Test, M. A., & Stein, L. I. 1976. Practical guidelines for the community treatment of markedly impaired patients. *Community Mental Health Journal.* 12:72–82.
Torrey, E. F. 1986. Continuous treatment teams in the care of the chronic mentally ill. *Hospital and Community Psychiatry.* 37:1243–1247.
Witheridge, T. F. 1987. The effectiveness of an assertive home-visiting intervention for

frequent psychiatric recidivists. Unpublished doctoral dissertation. Evanston, IL: Northwestern University.

Witheridge, T. F., & Dincin, J. 1985. The Bridge: An assertive outreach program in an urban setting. *New Directions for Mental Health Services*. 26:65–76.

Witheridge, T. F., Dincin, J., & Appleby, L. 1982. Working with the most frequent recidivists: A total team approach to assertive resource management. *Psychosocial Rehabilitation Journal*. 5:9–11.

Urbanowski, M. L., & Dwyer, M. M. 1988. *Learning Through Field Instruction: A Guide for Teachers and Students*. Milwaukee: Family Service America.

CHAPTER 8

Bridging the Gap between Principles and Practice

Implementing a Strengths Perspective in Case Management

Walter E. Kisthardt
Charles A. Rapp

Since the inception of the Community Support Program (CSP) in 1978, no service has received the attention devoted to case management. State and local officials, practitioners, researchers, educators, and consumer groups have engaged in an effort to develop and enhance case management services through policy, practice, and training. This level of activity, instead of waning after a decade, promises to increase with the passage of P.L. 99-660, requiring states to assure case management services are provided to people suffering from severe and persistent mental illness.

The strengths model of case management has been the subject of eight years of development and testing. The research and evaluation have produced consistent results for consumers in terms of increased community tenure, high levels of individual goal attainment, improved vocational and independent living status, and high levels of consumer satisfaction (Rapp & Chamberlain, 1985; Modrcin, Rapp, & Poertner, 1988; Rapp & Wintersteen, 1989).

The strengths model is based on six principles which guide the intervention process (Modrcin, Rapp, & Chamberlain, 1985):

1. Persons with severe and persistent mental illness possess the inherent capacity to learn, grow, and change.
2. The focus is on individual strengths, not deficits or pathology.
3. The helping process is guided by a rigorous standard of consumer self-determination.
4. The consumer–case manager relationship is primary and essential.

5. The community is viewed as an oasis of resources, not as an obstacle or target for blame.
6. Community integration is fostered by assertive outreach.

These principles are interrelated; the expression of one serves to replenish attention to the others. The six functions in the strengths-oriented case management helping process are directly influenced and buttressed by these six principles. This chapter provides a description of how the six principles become observable activities within the functions required by the strengths model.

For purpose of clarity, the six functions will be discussed separately. In actual practice, however, we have found that as changing consumer wants and needs dictate, each function may be implemented in a spontaneous manner. Recognizing the nonlinear dynamics of the helping process, the functions to be described include engagement, strengths assessment, planning and implementation, collective and continuous collaboration, advocacy, and graduated disengagement.

ENGAGEMENT: THE FIRST STEPS IN THE HELPING JOURNEY

In the strengths model, engagement is viewed as a distinct function. It constitutes the initial steps of relationship building so vital to any helping effort. In implementing this function, the case manager's primary goals are threefold. First, the case manager must plainly and simply reeducate the consumer regarding the unique nature of the case management process. This exchange, referred to as "role induction," is one where clients are encouraged to question the case manager. Second, the effort is made to describe how involvement in this process may help consumers realize their own unique wants and needs. Believing in and being able to clearly articulate the unique role of case management become two prerequisites for effective engagement. Third, an atmosphere is created where case manager and consumer may get to know each other as people. At these initial meetings, forms are not necessarily introduced and inquiries regarding psychiatric history are not the primary focus. Case managers must be secure and comfortable in sharing personal information (which they feel is appropriate) in a manner similar to what they will be asking consumers to do.

In the strengths perspective, reluctance and a modicum of suspicion on the part of the consumer are not understood as symptoms of paranoia. These responses are expected as a normal reaction to an uncertain and somewhat invasive interpersonal situation. Most people experience some misgivings and doubt when asked to become involved in an endeavor that is new or which has not turned out well for them in the past. Most people are somewhat guarded and distrusting when being persuaded to become involved in a relationship that is unclear. We need to give that same consideration to clients as we reach out to them, without resorting to familiar labels that place this normal reaction in the context of paranoid ideations or other symptoms.

Engagement is fostered by the principle of assertive outreach. Meeting with clients for the first time wherever *they* are most comfortable constitutes a new way of doing mental health business. Allowing clients the power to determine when and where this initial meeting will take place sends a clear signal early in the relationship that the client will play a major role in directing the helping process.

The engagement process is facilitated by establishing a nonthreatening and enjoyable atmosphere for communication. Discussing topics that are of interest to consumers helps to develop such an atmosphere. Here again, a primary focus on those aspects of clients' lives that are viewed as strengths rather than problems or deficits may serve to catalyze their desire to become involved in the case management process.

Each initial meeting with clients is unique. Some of our clients who have been involved with the strengths model over the years begin immediately with a list of things that they would like to do. Others may take several weeks before they feel comfortable meeting with the case manager face to face. We have found that maintaining regular indirect contact during the initial stages of engagement, such as telephoning, writing letters, and leaving brief notes when stopping by a client's home or apartment, is effective in the trust-building process. First, and foremost, we must demonstrate to clients that we truly care about them as people; conveying this concern breathes life into each of the helping functions that will occur during the course of the relationship.

As the initial meetings with consumers take place, a picture of who they are in terms of their unique situation and personal desires begins to emerge. As each consumer begins to understand the process, this information begins to be documented in the strengths assessment (see Tables 8–1 and 8–2).

STRENGTHS ASSESSMENT: REDISCOVERING PERSONAL AND ENVIRONMENTAL POTENTIALS

In the most general sense, assessment refers to the process whereby a professional, on hearing the specifics of the client's initial problem, calls on a particular theoretical base to render a judgment, conclusion, or determination as to possible causes or correlates. This assessment then legitimates a particular course of helping designed to ameliorate the problem.

Within a strengths perspective, however, the assessment is produced by both the client and the case manager. Information is generated relative to the uniqueness and capabilities of each client. Case managers may possess neces-

TABLE 8–1. CASE MANAGEMENT: CONSUMER STRENGTHS ASSESSMENT

Case Manager's Name ____________ **Consumer's Name** ____________

Date ____________

Current Status: What's going on today? What's available now?	Individual's Desires/ Aspirations: What do I want?	Resources, Personal/ Social: What have I used in the past?
	Life domain Daily living situation	
	Financial/insurance	
	Vocational/educational	
	Social supports	
	Health	
	Leisure/recreational supports	

What are my priorities?

1.

2.

3.

4.

Case Manager's Comments:	Consumer's Comments:
Case Manager's Signature Date	Consumer's Signature Date

TABLE 8–2. CASE MANAGEMENT PERSONAL PLAN

For: ____________ Case Manager: ____________ Date: ________

Planned Frequency of Contact: ____________

Life Domain
Focused Upon:

______ Daily Living Situation
______ Social Supports
______ Financial/Insurance
______ Vocational/Educational
______ Leisure/Recreational Supports
______ Health

Consumer's Long-Term Goal

Measurable Short-Term Goals Toward Achievement	Responsibility	Date To Be Accomplished	Date Accomplished	Comments:

______________________ Consumer's Signature ____________ Date

______________________ Case Manager's Signature ____________ Date

______________________ Psychiatrist's Signature ____________ Date

______________________ Collateral Signature ____________ Date

sary knowledge and understanding of the nature of mental illness symptomatology and may be well versed in the principles of psychiatric rehabilitation. However, they cannot be expected to know the special qualities, the hopes, the dreams, and the aspirations of the person they are charged to help by focusing on the generic deficiencies that are so frequently associated with mental illness.

The goal of the strengths assessment is to generate a holistic portrait of the client. Information is gathered across six "life domains." These life domains include, residential, financial, vocational, health, leisure time, and social supports (see Tables 8–1 and 8–2). Identifying information within each life domain will serve to direct and support short-term goals that develop during the planning and implementation stage. For example, if the client sets a goal to get out of the apartment more on weekends, the people or places that are listed in the social supports domain may be a valuable resource in becoming involved in the client's plan for a weekend activity. Recognizing these natural helpers as potential collaborators provides opportunities for case managers to replace themselves in specific activities and thereby reduce dependence and increase the client's supportive network.

Each individual's behavior is influenced by the confluence of their own personal history, their present social context, and their visions of what they would like to achieve. Consequently, the strengths assessment focuses on gaining as detailed a description as possible of each client's present status, his or her desires for the future, and historical information of a specific kind within each life domain. Historical data are gathered relating what each client has accomplished. Specific descriptions in terms of what each client has done in an effort to satisfy wants and needs in each life domain serve to more fully inform efforts that will be undertaken during the course of the helping process. As Bertha Reynolds, a renowned social work teacher and theorist once said, "Our first question to the client should not be 'What problem brings you here today,' but rather, 'You have lived life thus far, how have you done it?' "

The strengths assessment is not designed to generate a list of client "needs" as seen by the case manager. Rather, it is designed to generate a clear statement of "wants" as perceived by the client. Once a client has stated, for example, that he or she wants his or her own apartment, needs such as learning to manage money or remaining compliant with medication regimen may be discussed in relation to something that holds meaning for that individual. We have found that beginning with what clients have said they wanted, and then tailoring each plan to support these wishes, elicits problem areas such as poor personal hygiene or lack of motivation without ever having to focus on them as the target of the intervention.

The strengths assessment is a component of the helping process that consistently demands the attention of case managers. Information regarding potential support people, leisure time interests, and other possibly long-overlooked skills is regularly gathered. This information frequently becomes known to the case manager after a trusting relationship has been developed. Not surprisingly, much of this important information is obtained while riding together to an appointment or having coffee together and not in the context of a formal interview at the mental health center.

Case managers who become well versed in the strengths assessment process use this interaction consciously as an indicator of opportunities for immediate, tangible helping efforts. The client whose supplemental security income payment has been discontinued after a lengthy hospitalization may request assistance in reactivating it. If the client wishes to begin the initial steps necessary to accomplish this goal, the focus of the interaction may shift at that point into the mutual goal planning and implementation phase of work. Case managers, working within the strengths model, do not feel constrained by the belief that intervention cannot take place until they have completed the assessment. In actual practice, the strengths assessment is never completed; it is viewed as an ongoing, formative process.

PERSONAL PLANNING AND IMPLEMENTATION: ACCOMPANYING CLIENTS ON THEIR JOURNEY

Planning, as a general case management function, has been recognized since the inception of the CSP concept of case management. The actual form of this process, however, varies widely between and within the context of particular treatment programs.

Planning, within the strengths model, is best understood in conjunction with implementation (see Tables 8–1 and 8–2). From the outset of the helping relationship, the message to the client is that "we are in this together." Consequently, as plans are developed in terms of short-term goals, the case manager assumes an active role in assisting the client in implementing these goals. This might entail accompanying clients to the social security office or assisting them with their grocery shopping.

These shared activities are not viewed as trivial or as singularly isolated events. Rather, they are viewed as an opportunity for teaching, counseling, and modeling functional behaviors in the natural environment. The objective becomes to provide each client with a sense of mastery and personal empowerment from which future independent behaviors may emerge. Needless to say, case managers who are asked to respond to the wants and needs of 60 or 70 clients are forced by pragmatics to assume brokerage functions rather than a mutual implementation function.

In developing a client's personal plan, the case manager is guided by the following hierarchy of questions that influence the "level of accompaniment." First, is the goal something the client can do by himself or herself? Spending time discussing both the client's personal level of comfort as well as capabilities is an important safeguard against proceeding too quickly with the assumption that he or she is able to complete the task alone. Additionally, helping clients to break down a goal into smaller, incremental tasks often produces areas where they can do certain tasks by themselves. Exploring the resources in the environment, such as transportation, helps to guide the planning process in terms of additional supports that may bear on successful completion of the goal.

This process frequently leads to the consideration of a second question; is there someone in the client's support network who can assist him or her in implementing the goal? At this stage, the case manager may review the information that has been collected in the strengths assessment in an effort to identify these potential collateral helpers. The clients plays a key role in this review process, and collaterals are not approached unless the client agrees that this strategy is a desirable one.

The final two questions in the planning process relate directly to the mutual helping relationship. Case managers explore whether this goal is one that they can attain *with* clients; and finally, whether it would be desirable for them to attain this goal *for* clients. Asking these questions during the planning process and discussing alternative approaches with the client helps to ensure an individualized approach. Additionally, it incorporates the client in the decision-making process in an active manner. Finally, this process attempts to build in the involvement of a wide range of natural helpers at the planning and implementation stage.

The goal planning process is guided by the belief that people grow by building on successful endeavors in areas of their life that hold meaning *for them*. For many clients, being successful has been defined as conforming to the expectations of the mental health center. Most of our clients did not grow up with the aspiration of being "a compliant patient." Frequently, what they want to do is viewed as "inappropriate" or "contraindicated" by professionals who purport to know better than they what is "best" for them. For some professionals, the notion of returning responsibility for the direction of the helping effort back to the client is one which may be viewed as "setting the client up to fail." Some may even see it as unethical.

Practice guided by a philosophy of empowerment, however, supports nothing less than attempting to maximize client self-direction. In every life, success may not be permanent, but by the same token, neither is failure. By moving with clients in directions chosen by them, where they feel most competent, capable, and willing, small successes may lead to renewed involvement and personal achievement.

The principle of normalization directly affects the personal planning stage of the helping process. As case managers and clients discuss alternatives for how to go about achieving a particular goal, the case manager is careful to avoid mental health myopia. Mental health myopia refers to the all too common, ritualistic response that often accompanies an identified client need. A client's desire for her or his own apartment becomes converted into the "need" for transitional living; a desire for a job becomes a "need" to complete a prevocational training program.

Every client does not need, nor for that matter want, to become involved in activities that have been deemed by the treatment team to be necessary. From the strengths perspective, individuality must be considered before the "appropriate linkage" is effected. Planning and implementation, as perceived from the strengths model, constitute a qualitatively different way of understanding the concept of "linkage."

We have learned that initial and ongoing linkage with community resources constitutes much more than a referral. The initial, and possibly the most critical, "linkage" appears to be the strength of the case manager–client relationship. In our work to date, this variable is emerging as an important factor with clients who have achieved a level of tenure in the community. This may be due, in part, to the consistent attention to and familiarity with each client's current circumstances, which has generally been discussed as the monitoring function.

SUSTAINING CLIENT GAINS: IMPLEMENTING THE THREE C'S

We believe that the monitoring function of case management constitutes an intensive and multidimensional process. Typically, "monitoring" has become synonymous with "checking on a regular basis to see how things are going"; it fails to capture the range of activities necessary to assist clients in sustaining gains made during their involvement in case management. In its place, we see monitoring as incorporating the three C's: *c*ollective and *c*ontinuous *c*ollaboration. In an effort to clarify the activities inherent in this function, we will examine each component more closely.

To assist clients in sustaining gains they have made, a collective of supports and supporters needs to be developed. In the development of this collective there is a recognition that the case manager cannot hope to be the exclusive guarantor of the client's success. Family members, friends, employers, landlords, law enforcement officials, Alcoholics Anonymous sponsors, nurses, therapists, psychiatrists, and others with whom the client comes into contact may have a profound impact on sustaining present levels and continuing growth on the part of the client.

The efforts of this collective of caregivers are continuous. Once a client has achieved a desired end, such as beginning a volunteer job, the case manager takes the position that much of the work is yet to be done. Continuous contact is maintained with the client, family, job supervisor, and any other key person in the collective of caring. The case manager seeks to identify strategies such as altering the work schedule or building in reinforcers with the job supervisor, which are designed to assist the client in his or her quest for mastery in the particular context. The focus of this continuous involvement attends to the desires and needs of the client as well as the desires and needs of the individuals composing the collective.

Collaboration represents the third side of the triangle in the process of assisting clients to sustain gains they have achieved. Case manager, client, and the caring collective interact as collaborators, each partner recognizing the value of his or her unique input, as well as the benefits of making the helping journey a mutually advantageous effort.

Inextricably entwined within the function of sustaining client gains is the case management function of advocacy. Advocacy within the case management relationship is a complex, demanding, and at times frustrating endeavor. It represents a function that requires creativity, persistence, skills in influencing resource gatekeepers, and knowledge of entitlements and legislative sanctions that promote equal opportunity and seek to inhibit discrimination. Advocacy is a function that may be expressed on several levels, which we classified as the four A's.

AAAADVOCACY: IMPLEMENTING THE FOUR A'S

In a general sense, advocacy is understood as an effort to influence the social welfare, educational, legal, correctional, and mental health systems to be more responsive to the unmet needs of clients. Most frequently, these unmet needs are found in four areas: ***a***vailability, ***a***dequacy, ***a***ccessibility, and ***a***ccommodation.

Consider the client who enjoys working on cars and would like to become a mechanic. As an advocate, the case manager begins with the availability issue. Are there continuing education courses at local high schools or junior colleges that provide such training? Are there mechanics in the community who would be willing to have the client help out at the service station in return for some hands-on training? Are there junkcar businesses that would provide an opportunity for the client to become familiar with car engines by stripping parts for resale? Identifying the availability of opportunities constitutes the first step in the advocacy process.

Accessibility becomes the next important area for consideration. Identifying obstacles, such as lack of transportation, or expectations of the service system, such as attending a prevocational group at the center five days a week, may functionally render this resource inaccessible to the client. In such cases, efforts of the case manager may involve initially transporting the client to the resource site or arranging for a family member, friend, or other collateral to meet this need. Additionally, efforts may need to be made within the CSP to be more responsive and supportive of the client's plan.

Once issues of availability and accessibility have been addressed, the case manager must consider how accommodating the resource will be. This refers to the nature of interaction and communication the client will experience in any given resource context, be it the garage or the social security office.

Case managers who work with people with mental illness know that clients who have been treated in an abusive or less-than-compassionate manner in a given context in the past will be reluctant to involve themselves in a similar situation. Consequently, addressing this area of accommodation frequently involves initial work in educating and supporting the potential resource person, such as the employer or landlord. Explaining any special needs the client may have may help set the stage for a more successful advocacy effort. For example, a case manager was working with a particular client who wanted to have a permanent wave put in her hair, but was extremely fearful of going in the shop to have it done. With her approval, the case manager went in to talk with the woman who ran the shop to explain the client's wishes and her particular situation. As it turned out, the beautician had experienced mental illness in her family and was receptive to accommodating the needs of the client. She scheduled a time at the end of the day when there would be no one else in the shop, gave the client permission to smoke if she needed to, and was reassuring and friendly in her approach. The client got her hair "permed," which made her feel wonderful, and the beautician gained a regular customer.

A final consideration in the advocacy effort is that of adequacy. This issue relates to the extent which the resource meets the needs of each particular client. Is the connection giving the client a sense of personal fulfillment and satisfaction? Does the living situation meet minimal standards for decency and safety, such as adequate heat, cooling, and freedom from infestation? Do the clients' vocational or volunteer involvements allow them to use their own unique talents and abilities, or are clients involved exclusively in what the program has to offer?

As we have traveled from Alaska to Delaware providing training and consultation for case managers, we have observed direct evidence that attention to these principles yields results. From the case manager in Alaska who arranged for a plane to fly her to clients in "the bush," to the case manager in Kentucky who arranged for a retired school teacher to help her clients learn to read, we have seen the strengths perspective in action.

The specifics of how each case manager acquires these resources may vary, but they all seem to share seven common characteristics:

1. They view their efforts as a worthwhile challenge.
2. They believe in a desire of human beings to help others.
3. They know their clients extremely well in terms of what skills and abilities they possess that could benefit the resource person.
4. They enjoy talking to people about the type of work they do.
5. They are not satisfied with the status quo.
6. They view their work with collaterals as a parallel process.
7. They devote the same caring and nurturing of their relationship with collaterals as they do with their clients.

GRADUATED DISENGAGEMENT: EMPOWERMENT EXPRESSED

Graduated disengagement represents a case management function that attempts to guide the later stages of the helping relationship. As clients secure entitlements, achieve a level of stability in their residential circumstances, and become involved on a regular basis with vocational or volunteer activities, the level of intensity of the case management relationship may begin to want. The function of graduated disengagement suggests that although contacts with clients may become less frequent, they need the reassurance of continued support and also may require tangible assistance as circumstances change.

Implementing graduated disengagement means that case managers must convey to the clients that their relationships are not ending. This represents an alternative to the notion of termination as the final stage of the helping relationship. For some clients, who truly value the case management relationship, termination as a consequence of doing well may create a negative incentive to "get well." In the spirit of such current concepts as "lifetime case management" and "zero-reject policies," the notion of graduated disengagement is one that provides for clients' growth and independence, while maintaining a personal connection that may be essential for clients to maintain a reasonably high quality of community life.

The concept of graduated disengagement as a case management function attempts to apply the principle of normalization to the helping relationship. As with any social relationship in which there is an actor who is identified as the "helper" and another identified as the "receiver of help," there will come a time when the actual helping will change in terms of form and function. This change must be recognized and even anticipated by case managers; for in this awareness, the process may be used as a learning and growing experience for both parties.

There are two indicators that might suggest that the case management helping process warrants the graduated disengagement function. First, the activities during helping meetings may become routine. At these times, the case manager may begin to question the necessity or even the level of professionalism of their involvement. These feelings should be used to fuel efforts to integrate a friend or family member to become more actively engaged in these activities with the client, while the case manager gradually disengages. Second, the client may begin to appear less and less available for regular meeting times. Growing client interests or involvements may make meeting with the case manager, merely for the sake of meeting, appear to be more of a chore and less of a beneficial activity.

The process of empowerment represents a paradoxical relationship where the overarching purpose of engagement is designed to foster and promote disengagement. The function of graduated disengagement, given this premise, is one that becomes intertwined within each of the other functions. During initial engagement the case manager states that the primary purpose of his or her help will be to empower the client; to assist and support him or her in making decisions and engaging in behaviors that hold meaning and relevance. Data collected during the strengths assessment are purposively designed to generate potential windows of opportunity for case managers to identify others who may replace them as they gradually disengage with clients. During the planning and implementation stage, collaterals are considered and may become an active resource in graduated disengagement. Finally, efforts that are made in the advocacy function may yield ongoing supports which may remain in place long after the case manager has ceased to be an active part of the client's life.

CASE MANAGEMENT IN THE NINETIES: A CLIENT-DRIVEN APPROACH

This chapter has described the manner in which principles of a strengths ideology are translated into concrete functions of helping. From the initial efforts of attempting to engage clients in the process, to the advocacy efforts involved in securing a section eight apartment, the tangible forms of help are legitimated and supported by the six principles that lie at the heart of the helping effort. Consequently, the nature of the relationship between mental health professionals and those they seek to help has changed and will probably continue to change dramatically.

Case managers in the 1990s will become more like case management consultants. This ongoing consultation will be provided from the actual case managers, who, in reality, become the clients themselves. Consultants listen to what their clients want to achieve and then help them to recognize how their strengths may be used to support these desires, as well as how their weaknesses should be considered in their planning and implementation. Consultants recognize that they should not try to coerce their clients into accepting advice that is incompatible with their own visions.

The strengths perspective mirrors these consulting protocols. Throughout, the theme of consumer empowerment and self-determination pervades the process and generates activities that are consonant with this belief. The functions described in this chapter become the bridge that spans the abstract shore of ideology to the empirical shore of daily living.

REFERENCES

Kisthardt, W. E. in press. A strengths model of case management: The principles and functions of a helping partnership with persons with persistent mental illness. In D. Saleebey, (Ed.), *Power in the People: A Strengths Perspective in Social Work Practice,* White Plains, NY: Longman.

Modrcin, M., Rapp, C. A., & Chamberlain, R. 1985. *Case Management with Psychiatrically Disabled Individuals: Curriculum and Training Guide.* Lawrence, KS: The University of Kansas School of Social Welfare.

Modrcin, M., Rapp, C. A., & Poertner, J. 1988. The evaluation of case management services with the chronically mentally ill. *Journal of Evaluation and Program Planning.* 11(4).

Rapp, C. A., & Chamberlain, R. 1985. Case management services for the chronically mentally ill. *Social Work.* 30:417–422.

Rapp, C. A., & Wintersteen, W. T. 1989. The strengths model of case management: The results of twelve demonstrations. *Journal of Psycho-Social Rehabilitation.* 13(1):23–32.

CHAPTER 9

Mental Health Case Management

A Professional Domain?

Joel S. Kanter

As the importance of case management in caring for the long-term mentally ill increasingly becomes recognized, many authors have questioned the value of using professional staff to provide these services (Johnson & Rubin, 1983; Intagliata, 1982; Levine & Fleming, 1984). The social work profession itself is divided on this question. Although some social work leaders argue that case management is a demanding modality that is enhanced by professional skills (Harris, 1987), others advocate a model of nonprofessional case management to replace allegedly costly and ineffective professional interventions (Rapp & Chamberlain, 1985). Because the controversy will influence policy decisions regarding mental health staffing, practicing case managers must participate in a dialogue that has been dominated by administrators and policymakers.

Professional case management services are, in fact, both effective and practical. A careful examination of case management practice and recent empirical research supports the value of professional interventions that effectively integrate clinical and environmental approaches.

Case managers are confronted daily with situations that require knowledge, professional skill, and personal commitment. For example, a case manager receives a call from a client who shows signs of a prodromal psychotic state. What have these signs meant in the past? How can the managerial relationship be handled to avoid eliciting further anxiety from a client with persecutory fears? Should the case manager contact family members or others to share information and coordinate efforts? How can the client be persuaded to take medication if the client believes that the case manager and family are conspiring to poison him or her? At what point should a decompensating client be hospitalized to relieve community caregivers? Regardless of their program's stated objectives, all case managers frequently encounter situations that call for expert clinical skills and a willingness to intervene directly.

Case managers practicing in diverse settings increasingly have recognized that their work involves more than brokering services or chauffering their clients to community resources. The work of case managers involves maintaining clients' physical and social environments to facilitate their physical survival, personal growth, community participation, and recovery from or adaptation to mental illness. This task is complicated by the often unpredictable course of chronic mental illness and the tendency of these disorders to impair human relationships severely.

Effective case management necessitates that case managers should maintain continuity of care, titrate support and structure, tailor managerial interventions to address diverse client needs for outreach and frequent contact, and recognize and facilitate client resourcefulness. Each aspect of case management practice is enhanced by professional skills and training.

Continuity of care involves more than developing elegant discharge plans or maintaining attractive records. Competent case managers, sensitive to their clients' fears of intimacy and control, gradually develop relationships of increasing trust with clients, families, and other caregivers (Lamb, 1980; Kanter, 1985a). In the context of these relationships, case managers develop a longitudinal view of their clients' illnesses, functioning, and resources (both psychological and environmental) that enables them to intervene effectively over a period of years, preventing crises when clinical status or external resources change (Strauss, 1985; Kanter, 1985b; Harding et al., 1987a).

It is unlikely that low-paid, nonprofessional case managers will be motivated both to develop the requisite skills and to remain in this stressful work for an extended time. Indeed, many community support programs have serious problems with personnel turnover, as staff burnout, return to school for professional training, or seek more remunerative employment. Models of case management that rely on student staff maintain enthusiasm while disrupting the continuity of care.[1]

Effective case managers also titrate the environmental support and structure each clients needs (Kanter, 1985a; Harris & Bergman, 1987). This task requires ongoing assessment of each client's changing clinical status, level of functioning, motivation, and external resources. Advocates of nonprofessional case management often view this work simplistically as centering on

---

[1] While arguing that case management should be delivered by nonprofessionals, some programs rely on graduate social work interns to provide all direct service. It is unclear how the proponents of this model justify using a professional internship to train social workers in a modality that allegedly does not require professional skills. *See* Rapp and Chamberlain, 1985.

service provision. They frequently overlook the necessity of intermittently withholding support to elicit further growth. For example, although arranging for transportation to a community agency might be necessary after hospital discharge, case managers must consider carefully when clients are able to use public transportation. Case managers make similar judgments when they decide where (agency or community) or how often to meet with clients. Familiar with the longitudinal studies that demonstrate the adaptive capabilities of most chronic mentally ill persons (Bleuler, 1978; Harding et al., 1987b), these staff develop clinical skills that enable them to recognize and facilitate client resourcefulness in managing their own lives and utilizing informal support networks (Strauss et al., 1987).

With such capabilities, professional case managers can function more efficiently while supporting clients in their strivings to manage their own lives. Skilled case managers can handle a caseload of 30 to 40 mentally ill clients, some of whom they see frequently and some of whom they see only occasionally. Case managers intermittently become more actively involved with the latter group when clients encounter the death or illness of a relative, eviction, loss of benefits, or other stressful life changes. However, even when more intensive support is necessary, these staff effectively mobilize natural support systems and other community resources to provide needed assistance (Anderson, Reiss, & Hogarty, 1986; Harris & Bergman, 1985).

With such caseloads, case management by capable professionals can hardly be viewed as excessively expensive. If such services incorporate a collaborative approach to discharge planning and family psychoeducation, cost savings in the form of decreased recidivism can be empirically demonstrated (Altman, 1982; Hogarty et al., 1986). Nonprofessional staff, however, lack the skills and knowledge to offer these interventions. Even when case managers have a caseload of fewer than ten high-risk clients, careful studies have demonstrated the cost-effectiveness of such intensive programs (Weisbrod, Test, & Stein, 1980; Witheridge, Dincin, & Appleby, 1982).

Finally, the argument that social work professionals are unwilling to move beyond a psychotherapeutic model deserves more careful scrutiny. Although some authors have cited studies from the 1970s that found that social workers in mental health were uninterested in case management (Johnson & Rubin, 1983), a new generation of professionals in this rapidly expanding field is incorporating a more responsive value system. Stern and Minkoff presented useful guidelines for reorienting staff to address effectively the complex needs of the mentally ill (Stern & Minkoff, 1979; Minkoff & Stern, 1985). Whereas they stress the necessity of realistic goals and recognition of the professional challenges involved, others continue to devalue this work by insisting that it is best done by low-paid nonprofessionals.

Establishing a nonprofessional cadre of case managers, often working apart from other members of the client's mental health treatment team, risks unnecessary duplication at best and destructive fragmentation at worst (Deitchman, 1980; Schwartz et al., 1983). As social workers who have worked in the relatively cohesive structure of hospitals recognize, staff conflicts are a common source of difficulty in treatment. Integrating clinical and managerial functions within an interdisciplinary mental health team encourages a creative dialogue between psychiatrists and case managers who share a common language and knowledge base.

Thus, it is essential that case management of the mentally ill be delivered by skilled mental health professionals who can implement the complicated tasks of this practice modality. Although social work institutions have paid little attention to the mentally ill in recent years, our social casework tradition, integrating psychological and environmental interventions, has much to contribute to the field of case management (Johnson & Rubin, 1983).

REFERENCES

Altman, H. 1982. Collaborative discharge planning for the deinstitutionalized. *Social Work*. 27:422–427.

Anderson, C., Reiss, D., & Hogarty, G. 1986. *Schizophrenia and the Family: A Practitioner's Guide to Psychoeducation and Management.* New York: Guilford Press.

Bleuler, M. 1978. *The Schizophrenic Disorders: Long-Term Patient and Family Studies.* New Haven, CT: Yale University Press.

Deitchman, W. S. 1980. How many case managers does it take to screw in a light bulb? *Hospital and Community Psychiatry.* 31:788–789.

Harding, C., et al. 1987a. Chronicity in schizophrenia: Fact, partial fact or artifact? *Hospital and Community Psychiatry.* 38:477–486.

Harding, C., et al.: 1987b. The Vermont longitudinal study of persons with severe mental illness. *American Journal of Psychiatry.* 144:718–735.

Harris, D. V. 1987. From the president: Case management is gaining popularity in the public sector. *National Association of Social Workers News.* 32:2.

Harris, M., & Bergman, H. 1985. Networking with young adult chronic patients. *Psychosocial Rehabilitation Journal.* 8:28–35.

Harris, M., & Bergman H. 1987. Differential treatment planning for young adult patients. *Hospital and Community Psychiatry.* 38:638–643.

Hogarty, G., et al. 1986. Family psychoeducation, social skills training, and maintainance chemotherapy in the aftercare treatment of schizophrenia. *Archives of General Psychiatry.* 43:633–642.

Intagliata, J. 1982. Improving the quality of community care for the chronically mentally disabled: The role of case management. *Schizophrenia Bulletin.* 8:655–674.

Johnson, P., & Rubin, A. 1983. Case management in mental health: A social work domain? *Social Work.* 28:49–55.

Kanter, J. S. 1985a. *Clinical Issues in Treating the Chronic Mentally Ill.* San Francisco, CA: Jossey-Bass.

Kanter, J. S. 1985b. The process of change in the chronic mentally ill: A naturalistic perspective. *Psychosocial Rehabilitation Journal.* 9:55–69.

Lamb, H. R. 1980. Therapist-case managers: More than brokers of services. *Hospital and Community Psychiatry.* 31:762–764.

Levine, I. S., & Fleming, M. 1984. *Human Resource Development: Issues in Case Management.* Baltimore, MD: Maryland Mental Health Administration.

Minkoff, K., & Stern, R. 1985. Paradoxes faced by residents being trained in the psychosocial treatment of people with chronic schizophrenia. *Hospital and Community Psychiatry.* 36:859–864.

Rapp, C. A., & Chamberlain, R. 1985. Case management services for the chronically mentally ill. *Social Work.* 30:417–422.

Schwartz, S. R., et al: 1983. The young adult chronic patient and the care system: Fragmentation prototypes. In D. L. Cutler (Ed.), *Effective Aftercare for the 1980s.* San Francisco, CA: Jossey-Bass.

Stern, R., & Minkoff, K. 1979. Paradoxes in programming for chronic patients in a community clinic. *Hospital and Community Psychiatry.* 30:613–617.

Strauss, J., et al. 1985. The course of psychiatric disorder: III. Longitudinal principles. *American Journal of Psychiatry.* 142:289–296.

Strauss, J., et al. 1987. The role of the patient in recovery from psychosis. In J. Strauss, W. Boker, & H. Brenner (Eds.), *Psychosocial Treatment of Schizophrenia.* Toronto, Canada: Hans Huber.

Weisbrod, B. A., Test, M. A., & Stein, L. I. 1980. Alternative to mental hospital treatment II: Economic benefit-cost analysis. *Archives of General Psychiatry.* 37:400–405.

Witheridge, T. F., Dincin, J., & Appleby, L. 1982. Working with the most frequent recidivists: A total team approach to assertive resource management. *Psychosocial Rehabilitation Journal.* 5:9–11.

PART III

Case Management in Health Care

Contextual Factors and Their Influence on Social Work and Case Management

Cost containment issues saturate health care literature. Articles discussing case management in the field begin with its central tasks unquestioned: containing costs and rationalizing care. Some debate exists about the relative emphasis given to these two tasks. In some cases, particularly in private sector case management, client contact has been replaced by rationing care, by reducing allowable costs. More often, case management in health care involves cost containment through rationalizing care: trying to produce continuity of care between major inpatient services; coordinating inpatient and outpatient sectors; or arranging appropriate home care services through discharge planning and implementation. Thus, case management becomes a service rationalizing function, orchestrating the most effective and efficient coordination of services, both within hospitals and after discharge.

Case management in health care consists of quite complicated tasks and functions. Primarily, the complexity occurs because the patients most likely to be referred are those with chronic conditions that often require extended attention, those patients with severe illness or injury. The medical complications are compounded by social policy intrusion: How care will be paid for and what will be made available as treatment are uncertain, in part because they interact with payment mechanisms.

In Chapter 10, Reamer discusses the larger historical policy context for case management in health care. He vividly reminds us that case management in this sector emerges as a reaction to system dysfunction. In the prospective payment system known as diagnostic related groups (DRGs), Reamer identifies the tasks of making care coherent within hospitals as well as trying to coordinate it with discharge planning and implementation. The chapter by the American Hospital Association (AHA) supports this view, but from the perspective of the provider.

Case management that facilitates patients' compliance with hospital policy and practice rationalizes care and contributes to containing costs, while presumably contributing to improvement in the patients' quality of life. As a trade association, we could expect no less from the AHA. But the position they take, applied to health care and long term care, can indicate a convergence of clients' and providers' interests that differs from other service sectors where the relation of the service to the reality of life is more tenuous.

Case management in health care often appears as "managed care." This refers to the attempt to coordinate services among disparate units in complex medical settings, particularly when serious illness or injury require input from numerous services. Reamer's article highlights the case manager's need to know contextual factors shaping client outcomes. Included are DRG policies and practices; potential incursions into self-determination of patients and families created by funding limitations; possible reluctance to use all available resources because of funding controls; potential refusal to accept high risk patients or patients with diagnoses that do not commonly correspond to the DRG allotment of payment for inpatient days; and projected discrimination against the most vulnerable populations.

Reamer also raises a very important question for social workers in the health care arena—the impact of DRGs on our domain. Psychosocial assessment and support, long the terrain of professional social work, have been reduced by DRGs and replaced by heavy emphasis on discharge planning. Because discharge planning and follow-up require medical certification and prescription for home health care, more medicalized intrusions into psychosocial assessment and care have brought nursing more actively into the domain. In many instances, the two professions are now competing for control over discharge planning, with structural incentives favoring nursing. These incentives, in addition to those mentioned, include the inherent medicalized bias in the funding-streams underwriting postdischarge care (still paid for by insurance mechanisms, retrospectively) and the fact that most hospital care ends at the hospital's walls. Thus, the social work functions of developing, orchestrating, and monitoring community resources are often designated as irrelevant, especially because they cannot be easily paid for within hospital settings. Yet, when hospital practices end at the walls of the building, hospitals inadvertently may be turning control over readmissions to unreliable, frequently for-profit organizations in the community. Social work, as the only health care profession with roots in both areas, may want to reexamine its reluctance to aggressively develop this linkage through case management services.

Reamer also discusses another central point, one that appears in all of the other articles in this section. It is the ultimate provider-driven forms of care that exist in health care case management. Among the authors, Reamer seems the most troubled by the intrusion into patients' capacity for self-determination under DRGs. The AHA, as the membership organization of providers, must be expected to hold a provider-oriented view. Examine its position on advocacy; when mentioned at all, its purpose is restricted to making the funding stream function more efficiently. While Loomis reminds us that appropriate services and available services to specific patients are not necessarily the same, he presents no advocacy strategies to consider when patients could be harmed by the outcome. However, he does alert case managers to examine the decision-making processes in hospitals to ascertain whether patients' interests or hospitals' cost estimates are the data base for outcomes in delivery of care.

Henderson and Collard believe that case management in health care has three functions. It begins with the task of locating the lowest cost of high quality care or the most effective care outside hospital walls. Case managers also must coordinate care among family members and providers. And, finally, case managers have to optimize the use of patients' benefit plans to cover needed services. Opportunity exists to explore how these tasks might be done in a client-driven case management model. None of the tasks appear to be inherently provider-driven. But, as with the other authors after Reamer, the issue seems ephemeral. When Henderson and Collard study how case managers in health settings spend their time, or how they allocate and prioritize their time among a variety of activities, client or family contact is not even mentioned. Certainly, given this finding, neither is there any mention of empowerment, self-determination, or client-centered focus on participation in treatment or service plans.

Given the complexities of the health care system, can there be a client-driven form of case management? Must people's autonomy dwindle or evaporate when they enter the health care system? Or is autonomy, like resources, a matter of inequity? Where does self-determination enter, and can it be reconciled with an ever more technological form of medical care? What role do social workers have in supporting clients and families? Can a significant difference be made when case managers have some authority over resource allocation?

Hopefully, these questions will occur as the health care articles are read. Can social work develop models in the health arena that correspond to those created for mental health? Clearly, the functions of social work in health care have been substantially rearranged. Its very existence in hospital settings has already been called into question by the Health Care Financing Administration. How can the profession generate support for its role and for the validity of its participation in comprehensive health care? The practice paradigms that guided its work may no longer apply to the political and economic context reflected in DRGs.

Perhaps case management can be a new beginning for social work involvement. However, it seems apparent that a case management model that accepts the hospital walls as boundaries and providers' definitions of need as exhaustive, will fall to nursing. Experience in the health maintenance organizations may provide some alternative, but this is unlikely because they too are funded through restrictive medicalized arrangements. The flexibility of full prospective payment may open a window of opportunity for social work and client-driven models of case management, but that will require assertive leadership and system impact methods of evaluation in order for system reform in health care to be stimulated.

As we turn to the articles in this section, the focus or the key issues include self-determination and autonomy; provider-driven impacts framed by financing issues; the complexities of integrating high medical technology with empowerment; and the role for social work advocacy within the health care arena.

CHAPTER 10

Facing Up to the Challenge of Diagnosis Related Groups

Frederic G. Reamer

The staggering cost of health care ranks high on the list of major national and international problems. In recent years in this country, scores of blue-ribbon commissions, congressional subcommittees, panels, and symposia have convened with a determination to tame a health care system that, in the eyes of many, has gone berserk. Insurance premiums, per diem rates, and the costs of outpatient care and other ancillary services have increased exponentially. As the price of today's impressive health care technology slips beyond society's grasp, a sense of panic is growing in many health care circles.

To place a lid on skyrocketing costs, a wide variety of cost-containment measures has been introduced in both the public and private sectors, including the Certificate of Need program (P.L. 93-641) to review purchases of hospital equipment and the development of new facilities; utilization review committees to monitor hospital admissions, lengths of stay, and priorities; and Professional Standards Review Organizations (PSROs) to monitor the cost, utilization, and quality of care provided under the Medicaid, Medicare, and maternal and child health programs (McClure, 1981; McCarthy, 1981; Mechanic, 1979; Phillip & Hai, 1976). These developments have provided some relief, but it is widely acknowledged that they have not evolved into the panaceas most hoped they would be.

The shortcomings of these programs are complex and, some argue, intractable. The litany of criticisms is familiar. Certificate of Need committees have not found ways to relieve the ever-present pressures on hospitals to upgrade their technology and facilities (Cohen & Cohodes, 1982). Utilization review committees have carried out their work inconsistently, and the mechanisms they use are neither well understood nor well documented (Wilson & Neuhauser, 1982). There is little evidence that PSROs have effectively slowed the escalation of health care costs, and the design of these organizations has proved cumbersome (Fulchiero et al., 1978; Goran, 1979). The negative commentary goes on and on.

A point on which many critics have agreed is that hospitals and their staffs must have stronger incentives to limit the cost of services billed to third parties. Because third-party payers are billed for the cost of care per patient, there is little incentive for health care providers to shorten lengths of stay, cut back on laboratory tests, or pare ancillary services. It is no surprise, then, that the most recent developments in health care financing have focused on the revision of the traditional practice of retrospective reimbursement for services.

DIAGNOSIS RELATED GROUPS

The introduction of diagnosis related groups (DRGs) represents the most recent major attempt to stall the rise of health care costs in the United States. Directed primarily at hospitals, the DRG approach is designed both to streamline the administration of health care and to introduce incentives to reduce the cost of care per patient. Instead of reimbursing hospitals retrospectively for the total cost of care per patient, DRG policy institutes a prospective payment system. It categorizes illnesses according to nearly 500 DRGs and attaches specific payment rates to each of them; the rates are arrived at by considering a large number of factors, including the nature of the illness, accepted treatment procedures, whether the hospital is a teaching facility, local wage scales, and the hospital's location. Although DRG policy permits allowances for special circumstances, such as for patients with unusually long or costly lengths of stay—the so-called outliers—the key assumption is that the cost of delivering care for particular illnesses can be standardized and that, with some exceptions, the actual cost of care should not vary considerably from hospital to hospital (U.S. Department of Health and Human Services, 1984).

The DRG approach was first introduced at the Yale–New Haven Hospital in 1975; this was followed by a widely publicized pilot program in New Jersey beginning in 1976. As reported in rules and regulations pertaining to the Medicare program issued by the Health Care Financing Administration (HCFA) of the U.S. Department of Health and Human Services, DRGs were formally introduced on a national level in October 1983 (U.S. Department of Health and Human Services, 1984). This nationwide DRG application is designed to reduce the wide variations in the cost of Medicare services existing since the program began in 1965.

Although DRGs currently apply on a national scale only to Medicare patients, some states have instituted similar guidelines for other patients as well. In New Jersey, for example, all payers, including Medicare, Medicaid, Blue Cross, commercial insurance companies, and uninsured patients, reimburse hospitals based on preestablished rates. The rates for each DRG are established prior to the beginning of each year so that hospitals know in advance how much they will be reimbursed for treating patients in each category. Rates are based on the hospital's actual cost of providing care to these categories of patients and on a statewide standard cost—the average of all hospitals' costs, calculated separately for teaching and nonteaching hospitals (Wasserman et al., 1983).

Under the DRG system, hospitals retain the difference between the reimbursement rate and the actual cost of providing a patient's care if the discrepancy is in the hospital's favor; if the cost of care exceeds the reimbursement, the hospitals absorb the loss. This gives hospitals a substantial economic incentive to reduce the costs involved in treating each patient. If they are not reimbursed directly for each laboratory test, X ray, medical procedure, and day an inpatient bed is occupied, hospital staff presumably will be considerably more restrained in the costs they run up for each patient.

This, briefly, is how DRGs are designed to work, in principle. If all goes well, straightforward laws of economics should bring about a healthier health care system. However, as members of a profession with nearly a century of experience in hospital settings, social workers know that policies designed for apparently noble and sound purposes often have unintended consequences that jeopardize the welfare of their clients. Our job as conscientious professionals whose primary mission is to attend to the psychological, social, and, in turn, physical well-being of patients is to anticipate as best we can what these consequences may be.

EFFECTS ON HOSPITAL POLICY

The potential risks DRGs pose for hospital social workers and their clients affect several key areas of hospital policy: admission criteria, inpatient care, discharge planning, and personnel standards. As already indicated, under DRG policy, hospitals absorb the loss if the cost of care for any given patient exceeds the reimbursement permitted for the relevant diagnostic category. Therefore, hospitals may be unenthusiastic about admitting patients whose conditions fall into DRGs that tend, in the long run, to produce a net cost to the hospital. Because hospitals have relatively little experience thus far with DRGs and only limited track records for the many diagnostic groupings, it may take time for this phenomenon to unfold. In due time, however, hospitals may be faced with disincentives for treating patients whose care is too costly or not sufficiently profitable. This problem may be particularly acute in profit-seeking hospitals.

This is a special concern for social workers because of social work's long-standing commitment to protecting and enhancing the welfare of those who are most vulnerable and least advantaged. It is well known that lower-income people, as a group, experience far greater health care problems than upper-income people and often develop many medical complications once hospitalized (Kosa, Antonovsky, & Zola, 1969; Antonovsky, 1967; Pond, 1961; Stockwell, 1962; National Center for Health Statistics, 1979). Over time, it may turn out that low-income and minority groups with histories of poorer physical health fall disproportionately into those DRGs that hospitals are less motivated to treat. As a consequence, many of the profession's clients may have difficulty gaining admission to the hospital of their choice and may be referred with regularity to the proverbial county hospital of last resort. This, in turn, may exacerbate the pressures already felt by publicly financed hospitals that provide more than their share of care for low-income patients.

Although DRG policy is too new for anyone to predict with confidence the extent to which such selective admissions may occur, precedents exist in other social work arenas that may foreshadow what is to come in health care. In the field of juvenile justice, for instance, a similar problem can be seen regarding youths who have substantial court records and histories of offenses, difficult placement histories, or certain psychiatric symptoms. It is well known and well documented that because of the inordinate costs and trouble it takes to care for such youths adequately, many private community-based programs decline admission to them when contracted with a state agency to provide service based on prospective payment (Reamer, 1983a). Youths who require extensive services are often referred elsewhere. In Utah, this problem of "skimming" or "creaming" was considered so substantial that the state juvenile corrections agency instituted a provision in its contracts stipulating that each private community-based program be willing to accept a specified percentage of hard-to-place youths (Billings, Pace, & Vickrey, 1981). Similar problems have been found in programs for the elderly and mentally ill when the programs have had incentives to discourage admission of clients whose problems stand to be exceptionally complex or costly to solve (Frankfather, 1976; Milofsky, 1976; Protta's, 1976; Wiseman, 1970; Blau, 1963).

The use of DRGs also has implications for the quality of care provided to patients once they are admitted to a hospital. As noted earlier, the prospective reimbursement plan creates financial incentives for hospitals to reduce the number of medical procedures and related services they provide. Although social workers are not, as a rule, in a position to render authoritative judgments about the necessity of specific medical procedures, they are trained to offer informed opinions about a wide variety of patient needs and the services that may be required to respond to them. Workers may begin to notice that pressure, subtle or otherwise, is brought to bear on hospital staff to reduce the number of referrals to such specialists as occupational and physical therapists, speech pathologists, and social workers themselves because of the costs that are associated with their services.

DISCHARGE PLANNING

A serious risk to which patients may be subjected as a result of DRGs concerns the handling of discharges from the hospital. As is evident from the program's design, DRG policy provides incentives to discharge patients as early as possible. A startling and well-publicized incident that took place in Milwaukee shortly after DRGs were introduced may portend the frightening consequences of this policy. In December 1983 a Medicare patient in her seventies was discharged from the hospital and sent to a nursing home even though she still showed symptoms of congestive heart failure and pneumonia. She died shortly thereafter, before she could be readmitted to the hospital. According to nursing home personnel, the woman was one of at least six Medicare patients who had been "dumped" there by hospitals because DRG reimbursement had run out (Curry, 1984).

Although the vast majority of hospital staff do their best to ensure that patients are not discharged prematurely, it is likely that in occasional instances pressures exist to discharge a patient before it is medically appropriate. This may occur more frequently in cases where a patient's illness falls into a DRG involving less profitable or more costly treatment. Only time will tell whether this is so. Nevertheless, the implication of the DRG policy seems so straightforward in this respect that social workers will need to be especially vigilant to avoid any pressures to arrange premature discharges. Davidson noted the pressures that can be brought to bear on social workers in this regard:

> The urgent need of hospitals to comply with regulatory agencies and to meet constraints in order to obtain reimbursement makes pressure for early discharge high. This furthers the notion of discharge planning as a role in service of the institution rather than of the individual client. In order to make the discharge role acceptable to professional values of client self-determination and rights to quality health care, the social worker must redefine the "administrative" role of discharge planner so as to be in the best interest of the client and not to serve the institution at the expense of the client's well-being. (Davidson, 1978)

A related by-product of a policy such as the DRG approach concerns the pressure it can bring on the social work profession to alter its mission in hospital settings. In recent decades, hospital social workers have made major strides in their efforts to expand their role beyond that of discharge planning. Social workers have introduced an impressive number of innovations related to psychotherapy and group work with a wide variety of patients, including general hospital patients, substance abusers, oncology patients, burn victims, adolescent mothers, dialysis patients, the terminally ill, and the families of patients. It would be tragic if reimbursement policies turned back the professional clock of hospital social work and led to a preoccupation with discharge planning.

This is not to say that social workers cannot use the introduction of DRGs as an opportunity to effect appropriate and well-planned discharges. It is necessary, however, to guard against discharge for reasons of financial expedience. Kane noted this as a possible consequence of DRGs:

> Prospects seem mixed. On the one hand, if social workers can demonstrate an ability to facilitate timely discharges, their place in the hospital may even be strengthened. Early discharge obviously lowers the hospital's cost per admission. On the other hand, the pressures to make hasty nursing-home placements will be greater than ever. This will be particularly true as more and more hospitals come to own the nursing home down the street, another trend worth watching. (Kane, 1983; *see also* Davidson, 1983; Abramson, 1981)

ETHICAL CONCERNS

Social workers in hospitals governed by DRG guidelines thus face an imposing set of responsibilities to ensure that these regulations do not jeopardize the quality of care available to patients. At the foundation of these responsibilities are values and ethical principles concerning the patient's right to self-determination, the allocation of scarce or limited health care resources, whistle blowing, and participation on institutional ethics committees.

The patient's right to self-determination—among the sturdiest of values in social work—is at risk as a result of DRGs. The obligation to help clients pursue goals that are personally meaningful to them is paramount in social work, and it is incumbent on hospital social workers to ensure that the implementation of DRGs does not interfere with patients' autonomy and wishes about care necessary to their well-being (Biestek, 1975; Bernstein, 1960; Keith-Lucas, 1963; Perlman, 1965; Soyer, 1963).

A serious possibility is that social workers may be expected to explain to patients a hospital policy or decision conflicting with the right to self-determination. This would place the social worker's genuine concern for patients' wishes and welfare in conflict with the duty to comply with hospital policy. Unfortunately, such instances of divided professional loyalties are all too common in social work. A special danger in these situations involves the temptation to justify the hospital's policy as one that is "in the patient's best interest" when it may not be. Although it is sometimes appropriate to interfere with patients' right to self-determination to protect them from serious harm—true paternalism—it is pseudopaternalism if patients are led to believe that a policy is in their best interest when it is not. This must be avoided at all costs, lest social workers jeopardize the trust that patients traditionally place in them (Dworkin, 1971; Carter, 1977; Gert & Culver, 1976; Buchanan, 1978; Reamer, 1983b).

Threats to patients' right to self-determination under the DRG system result in large part from measures adopted to cope with limited or scarce resources. Controversy related to distributive justice is chronic in health care, however, and it often relates to both microallocation and macroallocation. With respect to microallocation, or the distribution of limited resources in individual hospitals, social workers must pay close attention to the criteria used to allocate beds and services that are likely to be more scarce as a result of DRGs. Do patients receive care on the basis of medical need or their ability to pay for care once DRG limits are reached? The risks involved here are illustrated by a recent investigation conducted by the American Medical Peer Review Association. The association found physicians' notes on medical records stating that patients must leave acute-care facilities "since the DRG reimbursement had run out" and other sources of funds were not available (Curry, 1984).

Sober questions of distributive justice also arise at the macro level, that is, concerning the nationwide allocation of health care resources. Today the Medicare program is two decades old and represents a most impressive success of the Great Society era, when social workers lobbied for subsidized health care that would be provided as a right to which Americans over 65 are entitled, rather than as a charity or a privilege. However, the development of DRGs stems from shortfalls in the Medicare Trust Fund, which the Congressional Budget Office predicted would be bankrupt by 1987 unless drastic cost-saving and revenue-enhancing measures were adopted (Bayer, 1984). As such, DRGs represent a fundamental threat to Medicare as an institutional form of welfare, similar to a public utility or entitlement, rather than a residual form of welfare, under which assistance is considered temporary and restricted (Kahn, 1979). This potential danger is especially striking in light of the results of a recent survey of public opinion conducted by Yankelovich, Skelly, and White for the Health Insurance Association. The study indicated that 54 percent of those surveyed favored a limitation on Medicare "so that only those who need financial help would actually get it" (Bayer, 1984).

Thus, a program that many have hoped would serve as a precursor to comprehensive national health insurance may ultimately further the narrowing of the range of entitlements available in the United States. As Bayer noted in his discussion of the significance of DRGs and other cost-cutting measures,

> Rather than a first step toward comprehensive insurance coverage for all Americans, Medicare now appears to many an unwarranted and over-

> generous public program for those whose needs seem to dictate no such special attention. Rather than serving as a model for all Americans, the universal social insurance foundations of Medicare have taken on the features of a benefit for a privileged special interest. (Bayer, 1984)

The scramble for scarce health care resources that may be occasioned by DRGs may be difficult for many health care professionals, but it is likely to place an especially heavy burden on social workers, who are expected to advocate for patients whose needs are not adequately met. At times social workers may find themselves in particularly awkward and uncomfortable positions in relation to other hospital staff, especially when they have evidence that colleagues are compromising the quality of care to reduce costs. For example, evidence gathered by the American Medical Peer Review Association documents instances of multiple admissions and readmissions, which provide hospitals with larger DRG reimbursement but which represent "grave compromises in quality" and a threat to patients' health. In one instance, a patient was hospitalized for malnutrition, developed a second ailment, and was discharged to a nursing home. One half-hour later, the patient was readmitted to the hospital with the second "new" diagnosis, thus providing the hospital with a second reimbursement (Curry, 1984).

Another disturbing illustration of a suspicious medical practice comes from a New Jersey hospital, where a staff physician apparently was pressured to consider performing cesarean sections in cases where vaginal deliveries seemed justifiable. The reason for this was that cesareans tended to be reimbursed at a favorable rate, whereras vaginal deliveries often resulted in a net cost to the hospital (Wasserman et al., 1983). Although the vast majority of physicians are too conscientious and principled to engage in such unconscionable practices, social workers who become privy to such disconcerting information need to think carefully about their conflicting obligations to their employers, colleagues, patients, and themselves. Nobler instincts may push the worker to blow the whistle without hesitation, but it is also necessary to reflect on the propriety and likely efficacy of less drastic measures (Glazer, 1983; Westin, 1981; Stuart, 1980; Nader, Petkas, & Blackwell, 1972). Social workers who reach the conclusion that a patient is not receiving the care he or she needs must be exceedingly deft at reconciling conflicting duties and negotiating differences of opinion and priority that may prevail among staff. Full-scale whistle blowing may be necessary in rare instances, but it is incumbent on social workers to rehearse and plan for less provocative ways of ensuring that patients receive adequate care.

Thoughtful planning and policy development by hospital staff can usually prevent the egregious incidents that call for whistle blowing, and social workers should do what they can to encourage such foresight. A specific mechanism that has been effective in a large number of hospitals is the use of institutional ethics committees (IECs) to help draft guidelines to prevent abuses under DRG regulations. IECs counsel hospital staff on ethical matters ranging from individual case decisions about the withdrawal of life-support systems to hospital policies concerning discharge criteria. They tend to be interdisciplinary in membership and to include physicians, nurses, clergy, attorneys, hospital administrators, and social workers. Workers would do well to encourage their hospitals' IECs to draft guidelines pertaining to the implementation of DRGs, organize IECs in hospitals where they do not exist, and strive to ensure that social workers are represented on them (Levine, 1984; Randal, 1983; Joseph, 1983).

TRADEOFFS AND POTENTIAL THREATS

Forceful policies are needed to control rising health care costs in the United States. Because the problem transcends local boundaries and is a function in large part of nationwide economic trends, these policies must be national in scope. The rate of inflation, wage scales, rate of unemployment, investment trends, interest rates, and a wide array of similar economic phenomena interact to influence the cost of caring for citizens' health.

DRGs represent a brave attempt to place controls on a health care system growing increasingly unwieldy. Although DRG policy is currently restricted to the Medicare program and the few states that have implemented it for other groups of patients, the initial DRG applications are likely to be models for more comprehensive reimbursement plans to come. The logic behind the DRG plan—the use of prospective rather than retrospective reimbursement—lays the foundation for a trend in health care that is likely to be more than a passing fad.

The DRG approach rests on a classic law of economics. This law holds that a cost-conscious organization will respond to economic incentives and disincentives affecting its ability to deliver a service or put forth a product without incurring a net loss. It may be that this fundamental principle of economics governing so much of the commercial world will bring about greater efficiency and quality in health care as well. However, it is important for social workers to be mindful that the tradeoffs we tend to tolerate in commerce (what economists refer to as externalities or external diseconomies) may not be acceptable in health care settings. No one objects too strenuously when the laws of the marketplace drive a mediocre restaurant or clothing store out of business or cause the price of red roses to increase around Valentine's Day. But the stakes are considerably higher when health care is involved, and social workers have a special duty to ensure that health care administrators—many of whom have received their training in traditional business schools concerned primarily with the private, for-profit sector—are sensitive to the risks that policies such as the DRG plan pose for the profession's clients. Seiden has made a similar point cogently:

> The mission of hospitals is determined by the unique demands society makes regarding health care. An individual who appears at an automotive showroom without a dime to his name and asks to be given a new car will be shown to the door, no matter how valid his reasons for needing private transportation. There are very few who will argue for any other outcome. However, an individual who appears at a hospital without a dime to his name and asks to be given care that is worth the price of many multiples of a new car can expect to be shown to an inpatient bed. A majority of society will still argue that this is not merely the best possibility, but that it is the only possible outcome. (Seiden, 1983)[1]

The need for social workers to monitor the implementation of DRGs is particularly important considering the ironic fact that HCFA, the agency introducing DRGs, has also authored a controversial regulation that would eliminate current federal standards for social work departments in hospitals participating in the Medicare and Medicaid programs. This policy would affect nearly 1500 hospitals that are not certified by the Joint Commission on Accreditation of Hospitals or the American Osteopathic Association. The current federal regulations, which were instituted in 1966, specify organizational and staffing standards for hospital social work departments where such departments exist. In their place, HCFA would require only that "hospitals provide services to meet the social, psychological, and educational needs of patients" and would permit these facilities to decide themselves how best to meet these needs (Latest Hospital Rules, 1984). Thus, the implementation of DRGs occurs at approximately the same time that HCFA is retreating in its enforcement of standards in hospital departments of social work. This could translate into a systematic retrenchment among hospital social workers and place responsibility for monitoring the quality of care delivered to patients under DRG guidelines in the hands of less qualified social service workers. The recent comments of Henry Aaron, senior fellow at the Brookings Institution, concerning the implications of DRGs and related measures for the profession of social work are especially sobering:

> As cost pressures begin to make themselves felt you're going to see pressures on items that the medical establishment regards as frills, extras—as things that are not really important to the medical cure of the patient. And one leading candidate for beheading in that, I think, will be the medical social worker. . . . I think the main implication is that we should mourn what is likely to be the outcome for medical social work of cost limitation, but I don't think we should fool ourselves about the likelihood of its

---

[1] It must be anticipated that hospitals beginning to experience losses as a result of DRGs will begin to shift costs to other payers, including patients. This stands to be a particular problem for the medically indigent, who constitute a substantial portion of hospital social workers' clients. See Paul L. Grimaldi, "Calculating DRG-based Payment Rates," *Hospital Progress,* 64 (October 1983), p. 80.

> coming along. (Latest Hospital Rules, 1984; *see also* Grossman, Harrell, & Melamed, 1979)

Policing the impact of DRGs may thus become more than a matter of safeguarding the care of clients for disinterested reasons—it may become a matter of survival for social workers in health care.

LEADERSHIP OPPORTUNITY

The introduction of DRGs may do much to enhance the efficiency and equity of the nation's health care system, but this remains to be seen. In the meantime, social workers cannot afford to be shortsighted about DRGs. Like all policies, this one undoubtedly will produce some unintended consequences—some trivial and some profound—and we would be remiss if we did not try to anticipate them. A utilitarian calculus that designs policies producing the greatest good for the greatest number may be appealing in principle, but measures resulting in the greatest aggregate good may trample on the rights of a minority along the way (Smart & Williams, 1973; Gorovitz, 1971; Reamer, 1982; Frankena, 1973). Social workers must be especially careful to serve as watchdogs when large-scale policies with widespread popular appeal presents risks for clients. To the extent possible, workers should promote the development of hospital-based procedures that will monitor carefully the effects of DRGs on admission criteria, inpatient care, discharge planning, and personnel standards.

It would be naive to argue that hospitals are in a position to care for everyone who arrives on their doorsteps, regardless of ailment or financial solvency. The world does not work this way, and hospital administrators have an obligation to maintain fiscal soundness so that their institutions can fulfill their mission (Vladeck, 1984). However, it is also important to make sure that the measures engaged in to protect a hospital's fiscal integrity do not compromise its moral integrity. In the final analysis, the responsibility is to deliver the best care possible at the most efficient cost, in a way that balances the right of the individual patient to high-quality health care with the rights of the public that is asked to subsidize this care.

If social workers are to succeed in their efforts to monitor the implementation of DRGs and similar measures, they cannot afford to be shy about their capacity to exercise influence and bring about change in the social welfare arena. The profession has developed an impressive track record during its less-than-century-long history, and some of its most noteworthy achievements have been related to health care. Social workers were instrumental in introducing social services in health care settings in the early part of this century and in lobbying for Medicare, Medicaid, and maternal and child health programs. Workers also played key roles in advocating for home-based services for the elderly, regulation of nursing homes, and quality control in hospital social service departments. Although there have been significant obstacles and frustrations along the way, social workers can point with confidence to a proud history of achievements. The inauguration of DRGs represents yet another opportunity for the profession to spearhead efforts to assess and affect the implementation of a major social welfare reform.

REFERENCES

Abramson, M. 1981. Ethical dilemmas for social workers in discharge planning. *Social Work in Health Care.* 6:33–42.

Antonovsky, A. 1967. Social class and illness. *Sociological Inquiry.* 37:311–322.

Bayer, R. 1984. Will the first Medicare generation be the last? *Hastings Center Report.* 14:17.

Bernstein, S. 1960. Self-determination: King or citizen in the realm of values? *Social Work.* 5:3–8.

Biestek, F. P. 1975. Client self-determination. In F. E. McDermott (Ed.). *Self-Determination in Social Work.* London, England: Routledge & Kegan Paul, pp. 17–32.

Billings, J., Pace, S. E., & Vickrey, W. C. 1981. Management issues and the deinstitutionalization of juvenile offenders. (Unpublished report prepared for the National Center for the Assessment of Alternatives to Juvenile Justice Processing, University of Chicago), pp. 48–49.

Blau, P. 1963. *The Dynamics of Bureaucracy.* Chicago: University of Chicago.

Buchanan, A. 1978. Medical paternalism. *Philosophy and Public Affairs.* 7:370–390.

Carter, R. 1977. Justifying paternalism. *Canadian Journal of Philosophy.* 7:133–145.

Cohen, A. B., & Cohodes, D. R. 1982. Certificate of need and low capital—cost medical technology. *Milbank Memorial Fund Quarterly/Health and Society.* 60: 307–328.

Curry, B. 1984. Hospitals save, but at a price. *Providence Sunday Journal.* July 8:A-3.

Davidson, K. W. 1978. Evolving social work roles in health care: The case of discharge planning. *Social Work in Health Care.* 4:51–52.

Davidson, S. M. 1983. Current acronyms, National Health Line. *Health and Social Work.* 8:239–243.

Dworkin, G. 1971. Paternalism. In R. A. Wasserstrom (Ed.). *Morality and the Law.* Belmont, CA: Wadsworth. pp. 107–126.

Frankena, W. K. 1973. *Ethics* (2d ed.). Englewood Cliffs, NJ: Prentice-Hall.

Frankfather, D. 1976. *The Aged in the Community: Managing Senility and Deviance.* New York: Praeger.

Fulchiero, A., et al. 1978. Can the PSROs be cost effective? *New England Journal of Medicine.* 299:574.

Gert, B., & Culver, C. M. 1976. Paternalistic behavior. *Philosophy and Public Affairs.* 6:45–57.

Glazer, M. 1983. Ten whistleblowers and how they fared. *Hastings Center Report.* 13:33–41.

Goran, M. J. 1979. The evolution of the PSRO hospital review system. *Medical Care.* 17(5, Supp.).

Gorovitz, S. (Ed.). 1971. *Utilitarianism.* Indianapolis, IN: Bobbs-Merrill Co.

Grossman, L., Harrell, W., & Melamed, M. 1979. Changing hospital practice and social work staffing. *Social Work.* 24:413.

Joseph, M. V. 1983. The ethics of organizations: Shifting values and ethical dilemmas. *Administration in Social Work.* 7:47–57.

Kahn, A. J. 1979. *Social Policy and Social Services* (2d ed.). New York: Random House. pp. 72–76.

Kane, R. A. 1983. Minding our PPOs and DRGs (Editorial). *Health and Social Work.* 8:84.

Keith-Lucas, A. 1963. A critique of the principle of client self-determination. *Social Work.* 8:66–71.

Kosa, J., Antonovsky, A., & Zola, I. K. (Eds.). 1969. *Poverty and Health: A Sociological Analysis.* Cambridge, MA: Harvard University Press.

Latest Hospital Rules Undermine Standards. 1984. *NASW News.* 29:1.

Levine, C. 1984. Questions and (some very tentative) answers about hospital ethics committees. *Hastings Center Report.* 14:9–12.

McCarthy, C. 1981. Financing for health care. In S. Jonas (Ed.), *Health Care Delivery in the United States* (2d ed.). New York: Springer, p. 274.

McClure, W. 1981. Structure and incentive problems in economic regulation of medical care. *Milbank Memorial Fund Quarterly/Health and Society.* 59:107–144.

Mechanic, D. 1979. *Future Issues in Health Care, Social Policy, and the Rationing of Medical Services.* New York: Free Press.

Milofsky, C. 1976. *Special Education: A Sociological Study of California Programs.* New York: Praeger.

Nader, R., Petkas, P. J., & Blackwell, K. (Eds.). 1972. *Whistle Blowing.* New York: Bantam Books.

National Center for Health Statistics. 1978. Annual summary for the United States, 1978: Births, deaths, marriages, and divorces. *Monthly Vital Statistics Report.* 27(13).

No easy answers for rising health costs. *NASW News.* 29:11.

Perlman, H. H. 1965. Self-determination: Reality or illusion? *Social Service Review.* 39:410–421.

Phillip, J. P., & Hai, A. 1976. Hospital costs: An investigation of causality. In R. W. Foster, et al. (Eds.). *The Nature of Hospital Costs: Three Studies.* Chicago: Hospital Research and Educational Trust, pp. 109–197.

Pond, M. A. 1961. Interrelationship of poverty and disease. *Public Health Reports.* 76:967–968.

Prottas, J. M. 1979. *People Processing.* Lexington, MA: Lexington Books.

Randal, J. 1983. Are ethics committees alive and well? *Hastings Center Report.* 13: 10–12.

Reamer, F. G. 1982. *Ethical Dilemmas in Social Service.* New York: Columbia University Press.

Reamer, F. G. 1983a. The concept of paternalism in social work. *Social Service Review.* 57:254–271.

Reamer, F. G. 1983b. Social services in a conservative era. *Social Casework.* 64: 451–458.

Seiden, D. J. 1983. Ethics for hospital administrators. *Hospital and Health Services Administration.* 28:82.

Smart, J. J. C., & Williams, B. 1973. *Utilitarianism: For and Against.* Cambridge, England: Cambridge University Press.

Soyer, D. 1963. The right to fail. *Social Work.* 8:72–78.

Stockwell, E. G. 1962. Infant mortality and socioeconomic status. *Milbank Memorial Fund Quarterly.* 11:101–102.

Stuart, L. P. 1980. 'Whistle blowing' implications for organizational communication. *Journal of Communication.* 30:90–101.

U.S. Department of Health and Human Services, Health Care Financing Administration. 1984. Medicare program: Prospective payment for medicare inpatient hospital services. *Federal Register.* 49.

Vladeck, B. C. 1984. Comment on "hospital reimbursement under medicare." *Milbank Memorial Fund Quarterly/Health and Society.* 62:269–278.

Wasserman, J., et al. 1983. The doctor, the patient, and the DRG. *Hastings Center Report.* 13:23–25.

Westin, A. (Ed.). 1981. *Whistle Blowing? Loyalty and Dissent in the Corporation.* New York: McGraw-Hill.

Wilson, F. A., & Neuhauser, D. 1982. *Health Services in the United States.* (2d ed.). Cambridge, MA: Ballinger.

Wiseman, J. 1970. *Stations of the Lost: The Treatment of Skid Row Alcoholics.* Englewood Cliffs, NJ: Prentice-Hall.

CHAPTER 11

Case Management

An Aid to Quality and Continuity of Care

American Hospital Association

PURPOSE

The purpose of this document is (1) to educate hospital managers to the emergence of case management as an aid to continuity of care, (2) to describe the state of the art, and (3) to recommend and promote appropriate support for a concept that will improve quality of care. Case management is more than a simple discharge planning function. Recipients of case management services can be episodically ill, chronically ill, disabled, or catastrophically ill individuals requiring medical or medical/social services, as well as elderly or rehabilitated populations requiring social and/or vocational services to maintain independence and productivity in society.

OVERVIEW

Of the many changes that have occurred in the health care industry during the last decade, one of the most fundamental has been the greater involvement of parties outside the medical community in the health care process. As medical costs have risen, those who pay the bills—employers, government, insurers, and reinsurance companies—have demanded a greater voice in such matters as which services will be provided, who will provide them, who will receive them, etc. By the year 2000, it is expected that 70 percent of insurance premiums will be paid to some sort of managed care plan as opposed to traditional insurance (McManis & Hopkins, 1987).

One manifestation of the growing relationship between health care providers and those they serve is the rise of case management. Since its emergence, case management has found applications in such diverse areas as episodic illness and injury, catastrophic illness and injury, long-term care of the elderly and chronically ill, and vocational rehabilitation for the disabled. With growing frequency, the treatment planning such cases is determined not solely by a physician but jointly by a consortium of professionals representing a number of interests.

Case management is designed to realize the maximum value from health care expenditures by allocating resources to the most appropriate and effective form of care. (In some social models, health care expenditures play a secondary role to that of providing other nonhealth services to maintain the greatest degree of independence for the client.) In some instances it may actually mean spending *more* in the short term for a particular service or facility to achieve a faster and/or higher level of recovery, which ultimately results in lower costs. Cost effectiveness, not cost reduction, and quality of health care are the goals of case management.

Case management, like competition, is not a new concept created by today's health policy gurus. Case management demonstrations first received public attention in 1971, when it was one of a series of projects funded by the U.S. Department of Health, Education, and Welfare as part of the Services Interaction Target for Opportunities (SITO) program. The goal was to test a variety of mechanisms for integrating social and health services for clients, including information retrieval, patient tracking, and case management. Even before then, case management in its various forms was practiced informally by physicians, social service agencies, and hospitals. What changed recently was that case management is now a more formalized process and in many instances is reimbursable as a direct service (Merrill, 1985). Case management has strong roots in the basic social case work method, which is predicated on assessment of the client and client system, appropriate treatment interventions, and follow up to assure maintenance of the system. Intrinsic to social work are concepts of coordination of services, negotiating and mediating systems, a team approach, viewing patient needs within a social system, and enhancing self-determination.

Acceptance of case management as standard practice in potentially high-cost cases is probable, and medical professionals and facilities are increasingly likely to work with case managers. An understanding of case management fundamentals can promote more cooperative and productive endeavors and thus, better outcomes.

DEFINITION OF CASE MANAGEMENT

It has been said that the term "case management" is misleading because case managers do not manage cases, they manage services. Case management is defined as the process of planning, organizing, coordinating, and monitoring the services and resources needed to respond to an individual's health care needs (AHA, 1986).[1] Case management is sometimes confused with managed care, a term generally associated with direct cost containment measures because some carriers use "case management" and "managed care" interchangeably, or use yet other terms for similar strategies. However, the two concepts are quite different. Managed care techniques are designed to avoid hospitalization when possible and to shorten unavoidable hospital stays—to reduce costs by discouraging the unnecessary use of medical services.

The intent of case management is not to avoid medical care. On the contrary, it is designed to obtain the best and most appropriate treatment for patients whose need for care is beyond question. Instead of discouraging consumption of medical or social services, it encourages the most effective use of health care or social services and dollars.

Case management and managed care also differ in another respect: Managed care techniques are designed to accommodate large numbers of people, such as participants in a group insurance plan. Case management, on the other hand, applies to a relatively small population. It has been estimated that 2 percent of the population consumes about 30 percent of all hospital resources in the United States, and it is this group of high-cost users that medically based case management seeks to address—those with chronic and

---

[1] The *Glossary of Terms and Phrases for Health Care Coalitions* defines specific terms as follows:

Independent Case Management: Comprehensive professional coordination of the health resources necessary to the support of the patient's diagnosis, treatment, and recovery, facilitating the ability of the patient to function with as much independence as possible through the convergence of physical, psychological, social, functional, and personal services. Case management also describes a gatekeeping function which may be assigned to the primary care physician, who controls and directs patient access to specialty care and institutional services; or to the planning, coordinating, and provision of care to a defined population, such as Medicaid, and health maintenance organization or preferred provider organization enrollees. Individual case management is evolving into a distinct, reimbursable service.

Managed Care: Organized program to control access to health services, designed to ensure the medical necessity of the proposed service and the delivery of the service at the most cost effective level of care. A managed care program imposes access and payment requirements upon the traditional fee-for-service system, similar to those found in health maintenance organizations and preferred provider organizations. Managed care programs are usually established by the purchaser or payer. A managed care program may include preadmission certification, second surgical opinions, fee negotiation, treatment protocol review, preadmission testing, continued stay review and discharge planning. Failure to comply with managed care program requirements or decisions usually reduces health benefit coverage for claims. These penalties may affect both the patient and the provider(s).

disabling problems who need assistance in coordinating services to meet their needs. Research reports on employee benefit plan reviews show that 80 percent of benefit dollars are being spent by 20 percent of the population, and 3 percent of those people, who use 40 percent of those benefit dollars, suffer from catastrophic illnesses and injuries, and the other 17 percent are chronic cases.

Case management can be applied to different needs, practiced by different professionals, and initiated by different sources. Five basic models are currently in use.

Medical Case Management. Medical case management is the model that generally applies to catastrophic or high-cost medical situations such as head injury, spinal cord injury, burns, stroke, and high-risk birth. It may be either internal, as when the facility has its own case management staff and program, or external, as when a third-party payer retains an independent manager to handle a case. The objective of medical case management is to help the individual achieve the highest level of function while practicing appropriate preventive measures to avoid unnecessary complications and sustain the individual's best level of health.

Primary Care Case Management. In this model, the primary care physician makes all specialty referrals, preauthorizes all nonemergency ambulatory care, plays a significant role in determining whether admission to a hospital is necessary, and in many cases manages the patient's care in the hospital. Primary care case management has evolved as a means of controlling resource use and, in turn, as a cost cutting strategy. Examples of this function are the gatekeepers in HMOs and recent Medicaid demonstrations. Thus, the focus is on identifying the most economical care alternatives and eliminating unnecessary or duplicative services (Kane, 1984).

Medical/Social Case Management. This model typically applies to a population already at risk, such as elderly or chronically ill persons who have historically been institutionalized for their medical problems. In addition to medical case management, medical/social case management employs alternative measures such as delivered meals, transportation services, emergency communication devices, and adult day care to give persons the greatest possible degree of independence while ensuring that they receive the services they need and have access to all available community resources.

Social Case Management. Social case management is focused on the physically healthy individual living in the community who needs basic supportive services rather than health care. The purpose is to maintain individuals, particularly the elderly, in the community and prevent a need for institutionalization that may result more from their inability to carry out basic activities than from a serious medical problem. This approach is a departure from most current efforts dealing with the elderly that tend to serve that group after they become sick rather than respond to the basic daily living needs of an essentially healthy population. Most elderly persons, even most of those over age 75, do not suffer from a serious disabling illness.

Vocational Case Management. An offshoot of the social model, vocational case management helps disabled persons increase their independence by improving their ability to achieve gainful employment by returning to their previous job, by modifying the position, or by looking at vocational alternatives. It covers a wide variety of services including assessments of job potential and independent living, job skills training, and job placement assistance. Candidates for this type of case management include not only those who have severe disabilities but those who have less debilitating conditions.

Although these models differ in the types of needs they address and solutions they propose, it is important to note that the case management approach is the same for all models. The essence of case management is the organization and sequencing of services no matter what the need or the type of service required. The circumstances may change, but the basic case management process is the same.

The goal of case management, like the technique, is the same for each of these models. Its purpose is to help the individual achieve the optimum outcome while taking appropriate preventative measures to avoid complications and sustain the individual's best level of health. It strives to ensure that the person receives the best possible care, that there is good communication among everyone involved, and that costs are controlled without compromising the quality of care.

THE CASE MANAGEMENT PROCESS

The case management process consists of five basic steps initiated by the person designated by the hospital or company responsible for the case management process:

1. *Identification.* The first step is to identify the need for case management and the appropriate person(s) to be responsible for managing the case (i.e., physician, nurse, social worker, or most appropriate referral source).
2. *Assessment and Planning.* This step assesses the individual's condition to determine what services and resources are necessary and to plan for their most appropriate delivery.

When an individual is identified as a possible candidate for case management, one of the first requirements is to establish effective communication channels among the patient, family, providers, and payers. Case management requires teamwork, and it is most effective when all parties understand the process and their roles in it.

There are various ways of flagging potential cases, including pre-admission certification, diagnostic codes, insurance claims, and personal contact with patients or their families. Whatever the method, speed is crucial. The sooner the case management process can begin, the more beneficial it is likely to be.

The next step is to evaluate certain factors that determine whether case management is appropriate for a given situation. These factors are:

Patient characteristics, including age, demographics, medical history, psychosocial status, diagnosis, and treatment plan

Family dynamics

Current care providers

All available resources that may be applicable to the individual's care and treatment

When this information has been collected and reviewed, there are three possible conclusions. The first is that the necessary services are already in place and no intervention is needed. The second is that immediate attention is not needed, but arrangements should be made with specific providers for later stages of treatment. The third is that the immediate intervention of a case manager could improve the quality and/or cost effectiveness of the treatment plan.

If case management appears to be the best alternative, the case manager should provide a prospective cost/benefit analysis. This information will help confirm the appropriateness of the decision. This process may be less formal for primary care case management and social case management models where the only consideration may be to determine the extent of need.

3. *Coordination and Referral.* The ability to identify and coordinate the many diverse elements of a treatment plan is the core of case management. The case manager should be able to refer the individual to the most appropriate provider and, if necessary, recommend various social, financial, and other services that may be desirable in addition to medical care.
4. *Patient Treatment.* The implementation of the treatment plan is the fourth step in case management. Although case managers do not participate in the treatment, they serve as a focal point for centralized communication and coordination.

5. *Monitoring and Review.* As the case progresses it must be monitored continuously to ensure that services are being provided as prescribed and that they remain appropriate. When necessary, the plan should be reevaluated to respond to any complications or changes in condition that arise.

CASE MANAGER ROLES AND CHARACTERISTICS

Case management services are available from a variety of sources. When the process is initiated by an employer or insurance company, the case manager is frequently an independent individual or organization whose services are retained on a case-by-case basis. However, a few very large employers, especially those that self-insure their health care benefits, and some insurance companies are beginning to employ their own case management specialists. Case managers may be nurses, social workers, physicians, or psychologists depending on the primary purpose of the management model, and they may in some instances participate directly in rendering aspects of treatment. Such decisions, however, would be based on professional availability and are not directly related to the case management role.

Regardless of the source, a case manager's role includes certain standard duties and responsibilities. These are

Patient evaluation
Family evaluation
Provider evaluation
Communication facilitation
Assessment of available resources
Treatment plan coordination
Monitoring patient progress
Ancillary service coordination
Cost/benefit analysis assistance
Patient/family assistance

To provide this array of services, a case manager should have certain characteristics.

The case manager must be technically qualified to understand and evaluate specific diagnoses, which generally requires clinical credentials and experience. A clinical background also enhances the case manager's ability to work cooperatively with the attending physician and other providers. In addition and especially important is the ability to assess psychosocial dynamics and factors that may impede the patient's appropriate use of services as well as an understanding of cultural variables.

Communication skills are another key requirement. Case managers work with many different parties and must be able to speak each one's language. They must be conversant in medical terminology and usage so they can deal with providers; they must be able to explain medical jargon in simple terms for patients and their families; and they must be able to communicate with employers and insurers in a way that is meaningful to them. Good case managers are able to deal assertively and diplomatically with people at all levels.

Good business sense is an indispensable quality. A case manager must be able to assess a situation objectively from all angles to determine when case management is and is not appropriate.

Case managers must have knowledge of the available resources pertaining to a specific injury or illness, and they must be aware of the strengths and weaknesses of various providers and resources. This knowledge enables them to recommend the most appropriate ones for a given case.

While case managers are probably most concerned with the medical aspects of a case, except for social models, they must also be familiar with employee benefits or insurance and be able to address these concerns. An understanding of insurance terms and procedures is advantageous as is the ability to see issues from the payer's point of view.

Case managers must be able to act as advocates for both the patient and the payer in models relying on third-party payment. This means that they are responsible for seeing that the patient receives the best possible treatment while assuring the third-party payer that its funds are being used wisely and effectively.

BENEFITS OF CASE MANAGEMENT

One of the most convincing arguments for case management is that it benefits everyone involved in a case. It provides a win–win situation; no party gains at the expense of the others. Following are the major advantages of case management for the major participants.

For the Patient. Most individuals have little knowledge of health care providers and procedures, and they may find it confusing, intimidating, and overwhelming to deal with complex medical matters. Case management gives patients the best chance for achieving their highest level of function, it improves their ability to sustain that level of health, it assures them that claims dollars are being used appropriately, and it helps them communicate with other parties.

For the Family or Significant Other. The responsibility for overseeing the patient's affairs usually falls to the family or significant other, but family members or loved ones are often unprepared to handle them appropriately. Case management assures them that the patient is receiving the most appropriate form of treatment, it helps them make decisions about the patient's care, it provides psychological support, and it helps them communicate with others who are involved.

For the Providers. A common tendency among providers is to focus on a certain aspect of treatment rather than to view a case from an overall perspective. Case management helps them to coordinate their part of the patient's care with other aspects of the treatment plan and to provide a continuum of care, it helps them to monitor the quality of care they provide and to measure outcomes, it assures them that they will receive payment for the services they provide, it encourages exploration of creative alternatives for care with the payer, and it enhances communication with other parties.

For the Payers. Case management ensures that claims dollars are used appropriately, it improves the insured's satisfaction with the company's services; it helps the payer communicate more effectively with the other participants in the case, and it enhances the company's image as a concerned, responsible organization.

HOSPITAL'S ROLE

Case management offers hospitals a way to provide or ensure the coordination of a full range of necessary health services for their patients in the most appropriate setting and in a manner that respects human dignity.

The hospital's role in case management can assume a variety of forms as a result of the new payment systems and structures of health delivery. For example, capitated, consolidated programs usually include hospitalization as a service in the plan, traditionally seen as a managed care approach in HMO models, while vertical hospital integration, a trend stimulated by DRG reimbursement, requires an internal case manager so that the hospital can use its own inpatient and community resources effectively. Hospitals are managing cases more and more through a variety of established services such as nursing, social work, medical triage, etc., to allocate the array of services offered under hospital auspices. This function is valuable for the patient as well, assuming that the focus is on the patient's needs rather than on maximizing resource use.

Hospital-based case management can also occur apart from a consolidated delivery system where the hospital introduces expanded case finding and posthospital follow-up (Kane, 1984). This approach is used in some physical rehabilitation programs where the case manager enhances the communication mechanism. Case managers should be invited/encouraged to participate in team conferences for rehab cases, have access to baseline information, and be allowed to participate in the decision-making process. In some experimental social model case management systems for elderly persons in the community, case management can forestall unnecessary or premature institutionalization.

Possible hospital-case management relationships can include the following:

> Hospital personnel may perform functional assessments for case management patients in the hospital.
>
> Hospital personnel may perform both hospital assessments and the discharge planning phase of case management.
>
> A person designated by a case management program may be housed in the hospital and participate with the health care team.
>
> Hospital personnel may run a full-fledged case management system (Merrill, 1985) that can be contracted for by payers, families, or community and governmental agencies.

With the potential for a variety of parties to be involved in case management, hospital managers may wish to develop a system to coordinate the various sources of case management sponsored by individual payers or the hospital itself. If the hospital has the case management responsibility, the role can be incorporated or expanded into an existing discharge planning or nurse review function or a new coordination level can be created. If the case manager is employed by an outside agent and that agent requires the presence of a case manager for the hospital to be reimbursed for services, the hospital manager may wish to institute a coordinating or monitoring function to facilitate information requests, reduce unnecessary duplication of effort, etc. Case management goes considerably beyond simple discharge planning or record review functions and should not be confused with these activities. The benefits of case management are great enough to compensate for minor inconveniences and should be supported by hospital managers.

The AHA philosophy supports mechanisms to promote high-quality, efficient care according to the hospital's mission, either through direct involvement in case management or through linkage or affiliation.

Case management makes sense from a health and human perspective. As the health care system becomes increasingly complex, those who must find their way through the system are likely to appreciate the coordination of services provided by case management.

REFERENCES

American Hospital Association. 1986. *Glossary of Terms and Phrases for Health Care Coalitions.* Chicago: AHA Office of Health Coalitions and Private Sector Initiatives.

Kane, R. A. 1984. *Case Management in Long-Term Care: Background Analysis for Hospital Social Work.* Chicago: American Hospital Association.

McManis, G. L., & Hopkins, M. 1987. Managed care plans: CFOs weigh the benefits. *Healthcare Financial Management.* May:52–61.

Merrill, J. C. 1985. Defining case management. *Business and Health.* July–Aug:5–9.

RECOMMENDED READING

American Hospital Association. 1983. *Policy and Statement on Continuity of Care for the Chronically Ill and Disabled.* Chicago: American Hospital Association.

American Hospital Association. 1986. *Glossary of Terms and Phrases for Health Care Coalitions.* Chicago: AHA Office of Health Coalitions and Private Sector Initiatives.

Anderson, R. E. 1987. Case management (Unpublished monograph submitted to AHA Section for Rehabilitation Hospitals and Program). Minneapolis: Northwestern National Life Insurance.

Case management: Going beyond claims payment. 1986. *Employee Benefit Plan Review.* 4(3, December).

Channeling Effects for an Early Sample at 6-Month Follow-Up. 1985. Princeton, NJ: Mathematica Policy Research.

Evashwick, C., Ney, J., & Siemon, J. 1985. *Case Management: Issues for Hospitals.* Chicago: Hospital Research and Educational Trust, pp. 92–95.

Kane, R. A. 1984. *Case Management in Long-Term Care: Background Analysis for Hospital Social Work.* Chicago: American Hospital Association.

McManis, G. L., & Hopkins, M. 1987. Managed care plans: CFOs weigh the benefits. *Healthcare Financial Management.* May: 52–61.

Mazoway, J. M. 1987. Early intervention in high cost care. *Business and Health.* Jan.

Merrill, J. C. 1985. Defining case management. *Business and Health.* July–Aug.:5–9.

Rossen, S. 1985. Diversification sparks concern over continuity of care. *Hospitals.* Nov. 16.

Tate, D. G., Habeck, R. V., & Schwartz, G. 1986. Disability management: A comprehensive framework for prevention and rehabilitation in the workplace. *Rehabilitation Literature.* 47 (9–10, Sept.–Oct.): 230–235.

CHAPTER 12

Case Management in Health Care

James F. Loomis

Case management is in vogue in health care today, but the term *case management* can be confusing because it is used to describe many different activities. Social workers have long been familiar with case management in the fields of mental health and developmental disabilities (Johnson & Rubin, 1983; Kurtz, Bagarozzi, & Pollane, 1984). However, case management in the health care field is a fairly recent phenomenon. The current popularity of the concept is a direct result of the desire to lower or control health care costs, but case management is much more than cost control.

Case management also is not simply preadmission screening or utilization review, although both elements may be part of the process. Instead, according to Merrill (1985), case management focuses on the organization and sequence of services and resources to respond to an individual's health care problem. Kane (1984) asserts that case management is a system of locating, coordinating, and monitoring a defined group of services for a defined group of people.

Case management comprises five essential components: (1) case finding (or entry); (2) assessment; (3) goal setting and service planning; (4) care plan implementation; and (5) monitoring and evaluation (Austin, 1983; Kane, 1984; Merrill, 1985; Newald, 1986; Steinberg & Carter, 1983). The activities of these components vary depending on the particular case management model. *Case finding* is the process of identifying and screening those persons likely to be eligible for case management services. *Assessment* is the formal procedure for determining the client's needs and usually is performed by social workers, registered nurses, or physicians. *Goals setting and service planning* is the formulation of a strategy to meet the client's assessed needs. The case management must be thoroughly familiar with existing resources and may be able to create innovative service arrangements depending on whether he or she can authorize funding and waive normal eligibility criteria and reimbursement restrictions. The *implementation of the care plan* may or may not fall to the case manager. Often, the case manager is a broker who coordinates service provision by other agencies or practitioners. Sometimes, the case manager has authority to direct, authorize, or deny certain services. With or without this authority, the case manager still has the responsibility to make referrals and ensure that services are carried out in the implementation of the care plan. *Monitoring and* evaluation is the process of reviewing services delivered to the individual client and also includes identifying service gaps in the community and collecting and analyzing management information data to evaluate cost-effectiveness of the program.

Case management services can be organized in different ways, depending on certain factors (Austin, 1983; Kane, 1984; Steinberg & Carter, 1983). Factors that influence the organization of the services include the primary purpose for the case management, whether the case management is a part of or separate from the service delivery organization, and the organizational setting of the case management program—for example, a planning agency, such as an area agency on aging; an information and referral agency; an institution, such as a hospital; or a membership association, such as a health maintenance organization (HMO). Other factors that may influence service organization are the authority base of the case management (public law, membership group, or funding authority); the limits of the case management budget; the centralization or decentralization of the case management system; the scope of the case management program (geographic area served, persons targeted for case management, duration of involvement, and type of services to be provided); and the individual or team functioning of the case managers and their professional background.

CASE MANAGEMENT MODELS

Despite the various mix of these factors, any case management program can be categorized in one of three models: (1) social; (2) primary care; or (3) medical-social (Merrill, 1985). Case management in the social model focuses on well individuals who live in the community and whose needs are for basic supportive services rather than health care. An example is the U.S. Department of Housing and Urban Development Congregate Housing Services Program, in which social workers coordinate nonhealth services that are offered to a population of frail elderly people who live in a housing project (Merrill, 1985).

This article focuses on the other two models. Primary care case management is based on the traditional medical model and often is associated with a gatekeeper function (Merrill, 1985; Simenstad, 1985). The major examples of primary care case management are HMOs and the various Medicaid-managed care demonstration programs (Spitz, 1985). Although providing appropriate care in a coordinated fashion is the major goal of primary care case management, controlling the cost of that care is the primary motivation. The physician is the case manager, and he or she controls access to other medical services. Depending on the structure of the program, the primary physician is financially at risk if excessive care is rendered to the patient, and that situation can cause underutilization of needed services (Berenson, 1985; Egdahl, 1986; Merrill, 1985). Berenson (1985) referred to this form of case management as "regulated . . . restricted . . . and rationed care" (p. 22). As antithetical as this concept is to social work values, this form of health care nonetheless is increasing dramatically. Between 1970 and 1986, operational HMOs increased from fewer than 25 to more than 500. In some communities, HMOs serve nearly 50 percent of the population covered by health insurance (Anthony, 1986).

The medical–social model of case management focuses on clients already at risk (Merrill, 1985). Programs in this model frequently are designed to prevent or delay institutionalization of clients; services are rendered to maintain clients in their homes. Often, the case manager or case management agency has access to money from grants or has authority to waive normal client eligibility criteria for needed services. Two major examples of this model are the National Channeling Demonstration Project (which Congress authorized in 1980) and the Medicaid Home and Community-Based Long-Term Care Waiver Program (Section 2176 of the 1981 Omnibus Budget Reconciliation Act) (Austin, 1983; Guy, 1984; Kane, 1984; Omnibus Budget, 1981). Both programs prohibit expenditures in excess of that required for institutional care but provide funds for structuring services that otherwise would not be available.

The effectiveness of case management depends on the methods used to measure outcomes. Certainly, health care services are provided and coordinated, and hospital admissions are decreasing. However, no consistently conclusive data exist to demonstrate that case management saves money. Even in primary care models, in which cost control is of primary importance, the generally healthy nature of the client population introduces a selective bias that makes analysis and long-range prediction of savings difficult (Merrill, 1985; Thorpe, Thorpe, & Barhydt-Wezenaar, 1986). Despite the inconclusive results of case management programs, however, the trend in health care seems to be toward more case management.

ISSUES FOR SOCIAL WORK

The primary issue regarding case management that is important to social workers is whether case management is designed to facilitate client access to needed services or to contain costs. Because these two goals are not necessarily diametrical in actual practice, social workers must understand the fundamental intent of the case management program in question. An intent to contain or control costs could have the effect of providing services that might not otherwise be funded, such as day care for the elderly rather than nursing home care; limiting services that otherwise might have been available; diverting clients from desired services to less expensive services; or determining in what setting and with which health care providers clients will be served. An intent to improve service delivery potentially could allow case managers to coordinate the services of multiple providers for clients' benefit as no single provider or service agency could alone. Understanding the intent of individual case management programs can help social workers to design social services within their setting that best complement the services provided by the programs. Social workers can avoid working at cross purposes to the case management program, which can lead to counterproductive results, poor client care, and professional frustration (Merrill, 1985).

The second issue that is important for social workers is ownership of the case management program. Authorization for case management can come from federal or state government, regional or local agencies, private organizations, or insurance companies. Authority and ownership confer certain powers, such as funding approval and eligibility determination; therefore, the issue is significant. First, ownership affects and is affected by laws and regulations that govern how health care services can be delivered. Second, the ability to integrate and fund social services with health care services may be determined by the authority of the case management program—the premier example is the Social Health Maintenance Organization (Nassif, 1986). Finally, that authority may determine where in the health care system social services will be provided. Since the advent of prospective payment, the focus in hospital social work departments has changed from attention to psychosocial needs to a greater emphasis on discharge planning. The advent of case managers outside of the hospital or other health care setting could shift the responsibility and authority for the coordination of client care from the organization providing service to an external case manager. For example, this could affect profoundly the ability of hospitals to plan and coordinate the discharges of patients and also would influence hospital social work staffing needs.

The third case management issue that concerns social workers is whether case managers should have centralized authority to pay for proposed or delivered services. If the intent of case management is cost containment, case managers likely will have this authority. Some HMOs have high levels of centralized authority, but some independent practice associations have more decentralized controls (Berenson, 1985; Glick & Taylor, 1986; Thorpe, Thorpe, & Barhydt-Wezenaar, 1986). Various insurance companies and Medicare and Medicaid exercise reimbursement authority by denying payment for hospitalization for certain conditions and by requiring certain procedures and surgeries to be performed on an outpatient basis. If case managers control the funds for care provided in all settings, then case managers exert significant influence when service providers decide if clients should be treated in a hospital, a nursing home, or under hospice or home care. Case managers can decide what additional services, and in what amount, are necessary or unnecessary to care adequately for clients. If case managers do not control the funding for services, then they have little authority other than persuasion with which to coordinate services effectively among multiple service providers. Social workers in any health care setting could argue that they already perform this coordination role, but most social workers do not have the ability to follow clients beyond the point where other services performed by the workers' agencies stop (Lindenberg & Coulton, 1980). Hence, case management without authority over funding can be a valuable adjunct to services provided by health care social workers. Case management with funding authority can be restrictive and can hamper the ability of providers or agencies to deliver coordinate appropriate or desirable services, although such case management can be beneficial in that case managers can authorize payment for innovative types and combinations of services that otherwise would not be possible. For example, Title XIX and Title XX funds might be combined and authorized by a case manager to finance various home care services that would not be authorized by either funding source independently. The result of this case management could be a client maintained at home with individualized support services at a lower cost than the traditional nursing home alternative (Lee & Stein, 1980).

A final important issue for social workers is the question of whether the case managers also are service providers. In the primary care case management model, the primary physicians are both service providers and case managers, and have a vested interest in cost control. In the medical–social model, which recognizes the need for case managers to be experienced clinicians, most case managers are professionally trained nurses or social workers. The question is whether case managers or case management agencies should perform the care plan implementation. Although that arrangement contains some inherent conflict of interest, it does use fewer channels of communication and perhaps allows a more direct response to client needs. The conflict of interest becomes more pronounced if case managers also have the power to authorize payment for services, as in the primary care model (Parrish, 1984). A similar issue is the question of who should perform case finding, assessment, goal setting, and service planning. Health care social workers, nurses in home health agencies, and hospital discharge planning departments all would claim that authority and responsibility. In some cases, case managers from outside agencies would accept that and then would oversee care plan implementation, monitoring, and evaluation. In many cases, however, case management agencies or subsequent service providers would want to verify or repeat some of those inital steps; in fact, such verification may be required by law or licensure in some states. Even where it is not, most providers would be inclined to prepare an assessment and care plan of their own before delivering or coordinating services prescribed by others, which poses problems of authority and autonomy for social workers, case managers, and other service providers and attendant problems of sanction, effectiveness, and timeliness of service provision (Austin, 1983; Guy, 1984; Kane, 1984).

TRENDS IN CASE MANAGEMENT

Kane (1984) identified two possible case management trends for the future. The first possibility was continued growth of community-based case management programs, which might have authority over Medicare and Medicaid benefits for long-term care and would require preauthorization for nursing home care. The second possible trend was the growth of capitate models of case management. Both of these predictions appeared likely at the time they were written, but now require some comment.

The growth of community-based case management programs will be slowed significantly by the Gramm-Rudman-Hollings deficit reduction requirements (Balanced Budget, 1985). It is unlikely that substantial new money will be spent on community-based case management, especially of the medical–social type. In particular, the inconclusive results of such case management programs as the National Channeling Demonstration Project will preclude any significant new growth except in isolated areas. However, states that currently do not require Medicaid preauthorization for nursing home care likely will begin to do so.

Capitate models of case management, or primary care case management, are likely to grow substantially. In addition to the HMO forms of managed care, commercial insurance carriers also will begin to use case managers to lower their health care claim costs. A prime example is case management provided to motor vehicle accident victims who need long-term rehabilitation. This service, which the motor vehicle insurance carrier provides, is intended to find the most appropriate level of services that will have the least financial impact on the carrier. Likewise, business and industry executives increasingly will turn to programs of managed care to reduce the growing cost of their health care benefits packages (Hembree, 1985).

SUGGESTED SOCIAL WORK RESPONSE

Social workers in health care need to be active in developing case management policy in their settings and agencies. Such policy should include coordinated services for elderly persons, who make up an increasing number of the clients of the health care system. The advent of Medicare HMO programs will mean that more and more elderly persons will receive case management services. Social workers therefore should seek to collaborate with case management programs, because as financing for existing methods of health care services becomes more scarce, health care social workers will have fewer resources and less time to serve clients in traditional ways. The possible exception is in home health care agencies, where existing funding for social work is limited but could increase with the increased emphasis on home care as an alternative to institutionalization. For the most part, however, social workers will need the assistance of colleagues in case management agencies to meet the needs of their organizations' clients. Social workers in existing health care settings will need to focus their attention on the needs of their clients and seek the most viable ways to meet those needs. Case management will have to be assessed from that perspective, and social workers will need to be careful not to view case management as simply a threat to their own setting, authority, and autonomy. Even though case management may pose such a threat, it also may present a better way to meet the social service and health care needs of an ever-changing client population in a changing national environment (Austin, 1983). For example, a pilot program entitled CARELINK provides case management services to Medicare HMO clients in Kansas City, Missouri (McNulty, 1986). Nurses provide the case management, work with hospital discharge planners on posthospital care plans, and then monitor the provision of service delivered by various social service and health care providers. The Medicare intermediary bears the expenses in an attempt to reduce acute care costs. Hospital social workers can choose to collaborate with such programs or to battle for control of the total discharge planning process. Ideally, social workers would establish and operate such programs in their own communities.

A variety of possible ways exist in which social workers can approach case management programs (Table 12-1). In most settings, medical–social workers would find it advantageous to collaborate with case management programs, especially if the program is community-based, because the program may be able to access and coordinate client services that the social worker cannot access because of the limitations of his or her organizational setting. If an insurance carrier or HMO operates the case management programs or has authority to authorize or deny funding for certain services, the need for collaboration is heightened by the possible financial impact of case management on the social worker's clients and organization. However, social workers also potentially can assist their organization to become designated by that carrier

TABLE 12-1. POSSIBLE SOCIAL WORK RESPONSES TO CASE MANAGEMENT IN HEALTH CARE

	Case Management Model	
Social Work Setting	***Medical–Social***	***Primary Care***
Larger hospital	Collaboration	Collaboration, preferred provider organization, case management provider
Smaller hospital	Collaboration	Collaboration, preferred provider organization, case management provider
Home health agency	Case management provider	Preferred provider organization, case management provider
Hospice	Collaboration	Preferred provider organization
HMO	Collaboration	Case management provider

as a preferred provider organization as they deliver high-quality, cost-effective services to their clients.

Home health care agencies could bid on case management grant opportunities and seek to become the community-based management agency in their areas, which could improve services to their clients and increase the stature and prestige of the agency. Home health care social workers can take a leadership role in such an endeavor. O'Brien has called for home health care agencies to develop case management services to sell to HMOs, predicted cost savings for HMOs and increased business for home health care agencies, and called for nurses to be the case managers (O'Brien, 1986). Certainly, social workers could fill this role as well.

Social workers in HMOs could develop internal case management programs for their own subscribers to improve services and to reduce costs for unnecessary services such as hospitalization. Although most appropriate for social workers, that role is being ignored by those employed in HMOs (Poole & Braja, 1984).

Because large hospitals are more likely to be located in urban areas and have larger social work departments than smaller hospitals, larger hospitals are more likely to be able to coordinate and provide more comprehensive services to their clients. Therefore, collaboration with case management programs becomes increasingly important for social workers as the size of the hospital or social work staff decreases and as the access to multiple services usually found in urban settings diminishes (Kane, 1984).

Many health care organizations, especially hospitals, serve clients from various communities with a variety of services and funding sources, so social workers must be able to respond to different case management programs simultaneously. For example, a hospital-based social worker may collaborate with a community-based case management program, provide case management to clients of a particular insurance company through a preferred provider arrangement, and be viewed as an unnecessary cost by the case manager of a client hospitalized by an HMO. To coordinate services effectively with various case management programs, social workers must understand the available programs, their primary purpose, the target groups they serve, the services they provide, and the financial impact they can have on the social workers' clients and organization.

The social work profession needs to address the issue of the fundamental intent of case management. Although a simple delineation of that intent is either to facilitate client access to services or to reduce costs, many case management programs strive to accomplish both. Case management can be a labor-intensive, highly clinical service, yet cost-effectiveness can be demonstrated when institutionalization is avoided. To play a leadership role in case management programs, social workers, especially social work administrators, must integrate the two goals of improved client services and reduced costs. The challenge lies in finding organizational methods to do so, because the cost of providing case management easily could fall to a different agency than the one that enjoys the cost-benefit. For example, under current reimbursement policy, a hospital would not be inclined to provide post-hospital case management services to Medicare patients to prevent the need for their admission to nursing homes, even though such service might be cost-effective. Medicare prospective payment would not reimburse the hospital for providing that service. Social workers need to develop methods to deal with such constraints. Working examples exist: The American Hospital Association recently reported on four innovative programs that use case management services (Newald, 1986). It is essential that social workers play a leading role in developing cost-effective programs that enhance the delivery of health care and social services.

On the broader scale, social workers should remain apprised of case management developments in federal and state governments. Because case management deals with the delivery of social services and health care services, it is entirely fitting that health care social workers play a role in the development of policy regarding case management. The National Association of Social Workers, the Society for Hospital Social Work Directors, and their state chapters appropriately could provide direction and guidance for implementing case management programs.

By adapting the strategies outlined in this article, social workers can be proactive and influential in the development of better service delivery systems in their own settings, in their communities, and at state and national levels. Such action will benefit social workers as well as their clients in social service and health care systems.

REFERENCES

Anthony, M. F. 1986. Developing a network strategy: Involvement with managed care programs. *Caring*. 5:56–62.

Austin, C. D. 1983. Case management in long-term care: Options and opportunities. *Health and Social Work,* 8:16–30.

Balanced Budget and Emergency Deficit Control Act of 1985. 1985. *U.S. Code,* vol. 2, secs. 901–907, 921–922.

Berenson, R. A. 1985. A physician's perspective on case management. *Business and Health*. 2:22–25.

Egdahl, R. H. 1986. Managed care programs: The danger of undercare. *Hospitals,* 60 (13):136.

Glick, S. K., & Taylor, M. 1986. HMOs and home care: An overview. *Caring*. 5:8–10.

Guy, J. S. 1984. Case management: Issues and directions in Michigan. Report prepared for the Michigan Home Health Assembly (Photocopied). Appendix 1.

Hembree, W. E. 1985. Getting involved: Employers as case managers. *Business and Health*. 2:11–14.

Johnson, P. J., & Rubin, A. 1983. Case management in mental health: A social work domain? *Social Work*. 28:49–55.

Kane, R. A. 1984. *Case Management in Long-Term Care: Background Analysis for Hospital Social Work*. Chicago: American Hospital Association.

Kurtz, L. F., Bagarozzi, D. A., & Pollane, L. P. 1984. Case management in mental health. *Health and Social Work*. 9:201–211.

Lee, J. T., & Stein, M. A. 1980. Eliminating duplication in home health care for the elderly: The Guale project. *Health and Social Work*. 5:29–36.

Lindenberg, R. F., and Coulton, C. 1980. Planning for posthospital care: A follow-up study. *Health and Social Work*. 5:45–50.

McNulty, E. (Ed.). 1986. Missing link in aftercare. *Discharge Planning Update*. 7:8, 11–12.

Merrill, J. C. 1985. Defining case management. *Business and Health*. 2:5–9.

Nassif, J. Z. 1986. The social health maintenance organization. *Caring*. 5:34–36.

Newald, J. 1986. Diversifying? Better think case management. *Hospitals*. 60 (16):84.

O'Brien, M. 1986. HMOs and home care: Cost containment allies. *Caring*. 5:16–20.

Omnibus Budget Reconciliation Act. 1981. *U.S. Code,* vol. 42, sec. 1396n.

Parrish, R. L. 1984. Social HMOs: An innovative response. *Michigan Hospitals*. 20:11–17.

Poole, D. L., & Braja, L. J. 1984. Does social work in HMOs measure up to professional standards? *Health and Social Work*. 9:305–313.

Simenstad, P. O. 1985. Health care delivery in a multispecialty group. *Business and Health*. 2:27–30.

Spitz, B. 1985. Medicaid case management lessons for business. *Business and Health*. 2:16–20.

Steinberg, R. M., & Carter, G. W. 1983. *Case Management and the Elderly: A Handbook for Planning and Administering Programs*. Lexington, MA: D.C. Heath & Co.

Thorpe, K. E., Thorpe, J. L., & Barhydt-Wezenaar, N. 1986. Health maintenance organizations. In S. Jonas (Ed.)., *Health Care Delivery in the United States*. New York: Springer, pp. 166–182.

CHAPTER 13

Measuring Quality in Medical Case Management Programs

Mary G. Henderson
Anne Collard

Medical case management for high-cost illness is designed to contain costs and enhance quality for patients likely to incur higher than average costs. Commonly managed cases include high-risk infants, traumatic head injury patients, spinal cord injury patients, patients with end-stage cancer or acquired immune deficiency syndrome (AIDS), and patients with chronic psychiatric or substance abuse problems. Although most programs began in the 1980s, the historical roots of medical case management can be traced to the rehabilitation-based models of case management that have been used for workers' compensation cases since the 1940s. Furthermore, like the workers' compensation case management programs of the 1940s, today's medical case management was developed by major insurance and health management firms.

Since 1986, Brandeis University's Bigel Institute for Health Policy has been involved in a two-year project, funded by the Robert Wood Johnson Foundation, to evaluate medical case management programs for high-cost illnesses. The project includes a detailed evaluation of one major private insurer's case management program and a survey to gather general information on case management programs offered by 18 private insurers and 6 health management firms (Henderson & Wallack, 1987; Henderson et al., forthcoming; Henderson, Souder, & Bergman, 1987).

The Brandeis survey found that medical case management is offered by virtually every major private insurer in the United States (Henderson & Wallack, 1987). Intracorp, a national health care management firm, is generally credited as being the first to apply case management principles to the medical claims arena. In addition, several large employers, including Ciba-Geigy and Zenith Corporation, offer in-house medical case management through their occupational health or medical department. Increasingly, state Medicaid programs are either contracting with private firms to provide case management or developing their own capabilities to do so.

Health care providers also offer medical case management services. Most Health Maintenance Organizations (HMOs) maintain that they have always performed case management. HMOs offer specialized programs or services geared to costly, complex, or "technologically dependent" patient cases as part of their basic services. Recently, hospitals have also been looking into the possibilities of extending their discharge planning services to managing patients even after they are discharged from the hospital. In Boston, for example, the New England Medical Center is considering the development of a comprehensive case management program for discharged cardiac patients.

DEFINITION OF MEDICAL CASE MANAGEMENT

What is medical case management and how does it work? Medical case management differs from general case management in that it focuses on patients with severe illesses or injuries that require a great deal of intensive care. The basic difference between medical case management and other cost containment mechanisms (such as preadmission review, second surgical opinion programs, and utilization review systems) is its focus on integrating and mobilizing resources to meet individual patient needs. Thus, instead of *rationing* care, medical case management seeks to *rationalize* a care plan by targeting appropriate resources to meet the individual needs of the patient and family.

The processes of most medical case management programs are similar in a number of ways. Patients are usually referred to a program after being screened according to diagnostic as well as other clinical and cost criteria. The case management program then conducts an assessment of referred cases to determine their appropriateness for management. Many times, only a fraction of referred cases (often less than 20%) are chosen for management. Finally, a case management plan is developed and implemented for patients accepted into the program. The case management plan typically covers three aspects of patient care management: how to obtain patient care that is of lower cost but of comparable or superior quality than care in the traditional hospital setting; how to best coordinate the patient's care among the family members and other providers, institutions, and agencies that may be involved; and how the patient's existing benefits plan can be used to cover needed services.

Benefits management may consist of arranging for payment for services not covered under the patient's existing package. Examples of such services may include hospice care, speech and occupational therapy, use of specialized equipment, and respite care. Benefits management also requires the case manager to continuously monitor the patient's remaining amount of total coverage and to begin seeking alternative sources of coverage before the primary insurance benefits are exhausted.

COST CONTROL AND QUALITY ENHANCEMENT

There is little doubt that medical case management was developed in response to payer and employer fears about the rising cost of health insurance. Experts estimate that if the rise in corporate expenses for health care is not checked, health care costs will absorb profits for the average major U.S. corporation (Herzlinger & Schwartz, 1985). Case management focusing on high-cost cases became especially appealing after studies revealed the tremendous proportion of health care costs attributable to only 5 percent to 10 percent of covered individuals (Rosenbloom & Gertman, 1984). Case management has also become popular because of the perception that care for the severely ill or injured is often excessively expensive due to lack of coordination, failure to use lower cost alternatives to hospital care, and duplication and fragmentation of services. The Brandeis survey of 23 medical case management programs (17 programs offered by insurers and 8 offered by health management firms) found that more than half of the programs surveyed reported no difficulty marketing the program to corporate clients; these clients generally believe that high-cost patients were handled efficiently.

Despite medical case management's focus on containing costs, virtually all programs purport that improving the quality of medical care and of patient and family life is as important as saving money. One major insurer interviewed by Brandeis researchers even acknowledged that the program "doesn't save money on every case but does improve quality." In health care there is a well-recognized relationship between costs and quality such that quality of health care (i.e., care that yields the greatest expected improvement in health status) is maximized at a given level of resources. At resource levels either below or above this optimum, quality is lower. Under ideal circumstances, the primary provider would select and implement the strategy of care that maximizes health status without wasting resources (Donabedian, Wheeler, & Wyszewianski, 1982). The raison d'être of case management is that payers and employers perceive a failure on the part of physicians to act as this expert decision-maker. In reality, the problem is not that physicians are irresponsible, but that physicians often lack the resources and knowledge to develop a comprehensive care plan for patients. To address this problem, case managers are now being placed between providers and patients to develop an appropriate, cost-effective care plan. Theoretically, at least, case managers can influence the kinds and amounts of services provided and the order in which they are rendered to achieve optimal efficiency (i.e., the highest quality at the lowest cost).

Although case management can potentially alter the type and quantity of medical services delivered to patients, it does not attempt to usurp the role of the attending physician. The cooperation and support of this provider is crucial to the successful implementation of the case management plan. Physician cooperation is essential at three points in the case management process. First, physicians (and frequently nurses and other providers) serve as the primary source of information in determining the patient's appropriateness for management. Second, the attending physician's attitude toward case management often influences whether or not the patient and family will accept the service. Third, because case managers are not medical practitioners, most services and supplies rendered to patients must be ordered by a physician. Thus physician approval is critical to the implementation of an alternative treatment mode.

So far, case management programs have experienced little resistance by physicians. In fact, Brandeis researchers found that while other cost management programs such as mandatory second opinion and utilization review are viewed as "all stick and no carrot," physicians see case management in a positive light. Case management programs often have more complete sources of information on treatment alternatives than hospital discharge planning or social service departments do. More importantly, physicians see case management as a means to insure patients for services that otherwise would not be reimbursable.

IMPACT ON QUALITY OF CARE

The quality of the case management process has a direct impact on how effectively the patient's physical health, mental health, and social well-being will be improved (Donabedian, Wheeler, & Wyszewianski, 1982). Quality of care is typically measured in terms of three care dimensions: structure, process, and outcome. Case management can affect each of these dimensions.

Case Management and Care Structure

Structural measures of quality of care relate to the personnel and facilities used to provide services and the organization of service delivery. In this regard, the case manager can greatly influence the quality of care by finding the most appropriate treatment facility for the patient.

A common problem in the current health care system is that patients who have experienced traumatic illness or injury often are not transferred to the most appropriate treatment setting in a timely manner. Patients can languish in a general acute care hospital long after the condition has been stabilized, thus delaying rehabilitation and the provision of specialized services needed to maximize recovery. In the Brandeis evaluation of a major insurer's case management program, it was found that the case management program was instrumental in arranging for the referral and transfer of a patient to a more intensive (and, on a per diem basis, more expensive) inpatient setting in several instances. This activity was noted to occur particularly often for head and spinal cord injury patients. In less populated areas, some providers may not be aware of the availability of specialized, intensive treatment centers for these individuals. In addition to suggesting the referral, the case management program often paid for the transportation of the patient and the patient's family to the treatment facility.

The case management program evaluated by Brandeis also helped patients obtain services and see providers that they would not have had access to otherwise. For example, in many instances the program instigated the referral of young children with developmental problems to a developmental disabilities specialist. In addition, specialized services like speech and occupational therapy for accident victims were often arranged and paid for through the case management program. Finally, the program frequently paid for equipment for patients that providers otherwise may not have ordered due to uncertainty about the patient's ability to pay. This equipment (e.g., an apnea monitor for a high-risk infant or a specialized feeding apparatus for an AIDS patient) often allowed the patient to be discharged more quickly to home. Table 13-1 presents the percentage of cases in which different types of benefit exceptions were made (such as payment for uncovered services arranged through the case management program) for 30 cases in each of the 4 diagnostic categories studied thus far in the Brandeis evaluation.

TABLE 13-1. PERCENT OF CASES MANAGED BY A MAJOR INSURER WITH BENEFIT EXCEPTIONS BY DIAGNOSIS

Type and Number of Benefit Exceptions	High-Risk Infant (*N*=30)	Cancer/ AIDS (*N*=30)	Head Traumas (*N*=30)	Spinal Cord Injuries (*N*=30)	All Cases (*N*=120)
Home nursing/aide care	53%	67%	30%	43%	48%
Uncovered services (e.g., counseling, speech and occupational therapy, tutoring, rehabilitation)	30%	32%	47%	47%	37%
Medical supplies, equipment, home modifications, and vans	53%	55%	23%	64%	49%
Specialist consultations	13%	13%	33%	53%	27%
Transport and accommodations	23%	29%	43%	13%	27%

Case Management and the Process of Care

The process of care is described by Donabedian as "what is done" to patients (Donabedian, 1968). This concept had been elaborated upon by DeGeynt to mean how well the patient is moved through the system (DeGeynt, 1970). "Process" thus denotes the sequence and coordination of care activities. Process can be measured in a "macro" sense (e.g., how the patient moved through the system from the onset of the problems to their resolution) or a "micro" sense (e.g., how well the patient moved through one care setting from arrival to departure) (Brook & Williams, 1975).

Clearly, case management is concerned with improving the process of care in the "macro" sense. All case management programs emphasize involvement with the patient at the earliest possible opportunity. The case manager then remains involved until the highest level of functional health status is achieved. This continuous involvement is especially important for many high-cost or "catastrophic" diseases whose hallmark is the long-term or chronic nature of the problem. In the Brandeis evaluation study, several high-risk infant cases were studied in which the case management program became involved with the patient at birth and remained involved for years. Case managers contacted the patients' families at regular intervals and reactivated management to address problems as they arose.

Given the fragmentation of the current health care system, the case management program may act as the only organization whose purpose is to be involved with the patient over the full course of a health problem. Table 13-2 lists the types of services case managers perform for patients who have different diagnoses. As the table shows, an average of 30% of case managers' time was devoted to simply monitoring the appropriateness of patient

TABLE 13-2. AVERAGE PERCENTAGE OF CASE MANAGER HOURS SPENT IN VARIOUS ACTIVITIES BY DIAGNOSIS*

Activity	High-Risk Infant	Cancer/ AIDS	Head Injury	Spinal Cord Injury
Researching patient condition and treatment resources	12%	8%	14%	9%
Monitoring appropriateness of patient care	32%	32%	30%	32%
Arranging and coordinating case management interventions	6%	8%	9%	7%
Benefits management	11%	13%	10%	14%
Documentation	37%	37%	36%	37%
Other	2%	2%	1%	1%
Total**	100%	100%	100%	100%

*For a case management program offered by one major insurer.

**Columns may not add up to 100% due to rounding of subtotals.

care (Henderson et al., forthcoming). Quite possibly case management improves the process of care through exerting a "sentinel effect"; that is, providers and institutions involved with the patient may alter their behavior in a positive way merely because they are being watched.

Case Management and Care Outcomes

Outcomes of care reflect the net changes that occur in health status as a result of care provided. The final outcome of care depends on

The correctness of the diagnosis
The appropriateness of the treatment ordered
The effectiveness of the treatment
The patient's adherence to the treatment regimen

Case management influences care outcomes primarily through affecting the appropriateness of treatment ordered and the patient's adherence to the treatment regimen.

Case management programs are quick to state that they leave decisions about the medical content of care to physicians. However, the fact that case managers can and do make suggestions to physicians about treatment alternatives makes them active participants in the kinds of care patients receive. One of the most important ways that case management positively influences treatment and care outcomes is through the establishment of an appropriate home care program for patients who might otherwise have had to remain in a hospital. Home care enables patients to avoid exposure to a host of nosocomial infections, iatrogenesis, and other risks encountered in the hospital setting that can result in further injury and illness. Thus, home care may result in improved outcomes for eligible patients.

Case management programs also claim to increase patient adherence to treatment regimens through regular contact with the patient and family. Hard data on this point are lacking, but given the amount of time case managers spend communicating with patients and families, it is reasonable to assume that case managers can ascertain whether or not patients are receiving care ordered and can encourage and monitor patient compliance with a treatment regimen.

Case management can also affect treatment outcomes in at least one other indirect way. It is well-recognized that the provision of preventive care is associated with better long-run outcomes. Case management programs emphasize that because of both their direct involvement with the patient and family and their holistic approach to care, case managers are sensitized to the need for providing preventive services. Examples include early intervention programs for high-risk infants, skin care regimens for the paraplegic or quadriplegic patient, and psychological counseling for the caretaker-spouse of a traumatic head injury patient. By giving high-cost patients access to these services, risk of later complications is reduced and the likelihood of a positive outcome is thus increased.

QUALITY OF CASE MANAGEMENT SERVICES

Like other services, it is likely that case management programs vary in effectiveness. Procedural and organizational differences among programs will affect how well the twin goals of cost containment and improved quality of care are met. Because of the newness of the service, quality and cost standards have not yet been developed. However, more attention has been focused on measuring cost-effectiveness than on quality, perhaps because cost savings are more easily measured.

The results of the Brandeis study suggest that it is important to focus at least equal attention on developing measures of quality improvement. In the study, cost savings were documented in roughly one-fourth of the 120 cases studied. In contrast, it was possible to document activities associated with higher quality medical care or improved quality of life in more than two-thirds of cases. Case management-directed activities led to numerous improvements in the process of medical care. For instance, the case manager often facilitated patient transfer to a more appropriate care facility and arranged for consultation by a specialist or the provision of specialized services. The program also enhanced the patient's quality of life by paying for respite care, funding transportation or home modifications that increased patient independence, and providing patients with access to pain control programs.

These results represent only an initial, "broad brush" approach to measuring case management's impact on quality of medical care and quality of patient and family life. Standards for measuring the quality of the case management process and its effect on patient outcomes are now sorely lacking. The systematic development of such standards is clearly necessary. Of the 23 case management programs surveyed by Brandeis researchers, none was able to provide evidence of structured quality assurance mechanisms although most reported that these were being developed. The survey results did reveal features of the structures and processes of different programs that potentially could serve as indicators of the quality and effectiveness of case management services.

Structural Factors Affecting Quality

The personnel and organization of case management services can significantly influence the quality of a program. Clearly, the competence of case managers is critical to effective service delivery. Most programs use registered nurses

(RNs) as case managers. However, programs may vary in terms of the case manager's average number of years' experience in nursing and case management and the number of nurse managers specializing in the care of a particular type of patient. Continuing education opportunities available to case managers may also vary from one program to another. Some programs are staffed by other types of professionals as well, such as rehabilitation counselors and social workers. These providers may serve as important resources for managing some cases or for consultation by nurses in other cases.

The frequency with which case managers consult specialist physicians appears to vary among programs offered by insurers and health management firms surveyed. Some programs surveyed had several physicians on staff, either full-time or part-time, whereas other programs had no physician on staff, and case managers' contact with outside physicians was infrequent. Currently, it appears that there are not standards governing the relationship between case managers and physicians. To assure the clinical validity of treatment plans developed by case managers, some type of review mechanism directed by physicians and/or nurses is needed.

Workload measures provide another source of information about differences in program structure. Wide variation exists in the ratio of case managers to patients. In HMO plans, for example, the ratio of case managers to those eligible for services can vary from 1 to 15,000 to 1 to 40,000 (Beswick, 1987). In addition to managing high-cost cases, these HMO-based case managers conduct many preadmission and utilization review functions. Estimates vary as to how many active cases (i.e., high-cost cases requiring attention several times weekly) can be handled adequately by one case manager. Although some programs claimed only three active cases could be managed simultaneously, others had no problem with managing up to ten (Henderson, Collard, & Mattson, 1987).

Procedural Factors Affecting Quality

Many structural and procedural measures of quality are interactive. For example, the number of active cases a manager can effectively handle is dependent on a process variable: whether or not site visits are a regular part of a program's process. In programs that require site visits as part of their standard operating procedures, case managers are responsible for fewer active cases.

To evaluate the impact of site visits on cost savings, Brandeis researchers compared cases with and without site visits in similar diagnostic categories for one case management program. Findings indicated that site visits were not associated with reduced costs. It has been suggested that very complex cases may be managed more cost-effectively if a site visit is performed. Moreover, the correlation between the presence of a site visit and increased quality, in terms of a patient's improved physical outcome and quality of life, may be significant. This issue remains to be explored. It may very well be that certain patient characteristics determine whether or not a site visit would be beneficial. Empirical research is needed to establish these relationships.

The process of care is typically monitored in one of two ways. In one approach, a case manager would periodically review the program's case documentation using a checklist that includes the elements of appropriate care (Dershewitz, Gross, & Williamson, 1979). A more sophisticated method would be criteria-mapping, which employs a set of criteria for appropriate care in a variety of clinical situations (Kaplan, 1978). In this approach, the presence or absence of certain diagnostic and other markers determines the criteria used for evaluating appropriateness. One or both of these approaches to monitoring the process of care can be developed easily for case management. A criteria-mapping method may be particularly appropriate since the need for certain case management activities depends on the presence or absence of key patient or case characteristics. For example, research may establish that site visits should only be performed under a set of specific conditions (e.g., when the patient has experienced a traumatic head injury, when there is a history of repeated admissions, and if there are poor family supports).

CASE STUDY

To date, no formal evaluation has been done to document essential care components for a quality case management program. However, the Brandeis study indicates that several key components are pivotal to assuring the effectiveness of such a program. Some of these components are

Early patient identification and intervention

A patient's timely discharge from the acute care institution

A cooperative and supportive relationship between the case management program and the client, client's family, and care providers

The existence of a mechanism to monitor patient progress over time

Coordination of care providers and services as well as coordination of benefits restructuring, if applicable

The following hypothetical case study embodies many components of quality case management. This example illustrates how a superior case management program would function.

John, a premature infant weighing 3.6 pounds at birth, was born after 33 weeks' gestation. At birth, John exhibited signs of respiratory distress syndrome. A radiologic exam also revealed changes that were consistent with hyaline membrane disease. The infant was born in the maternity unit of a rural community hospital in New Mexico but was immediately transferred to the neonatal intensive care unit of the University of New Mexico teaching hospital in Albuquerque via air ambulance. There John was placed [illegible] mechanical ventilator and given supplemental oxygen to stabilize his co[illegible]tion. During this time, John experienced periodic episodes of apnea and bradycardia, especially during feedings. After 5 weeks in the neonatal intensive care unit, John was discharged home at 5 pounds, 8 ounces with an apnea/bradycardia monitor which was to be used on a 24-hour basis.

Medical case management became involved in this case within several days of John's birth. In this example, the utilization reviewer notified the insurer that a high-risk infant with an expected hospitalization stay of six weeks had been born. The insurer then notified the medical case management program and a case manager was assigned to the case.

The case manager was an RN with a bachelor's degree in nursing and clinical experience in pediatric intensive care nursing. Throughout John's hospitalization, she made regular calls to the attending neonatologist to receive updates on John's progress and began planning for his discharge home. During this time, the case manager also initiated contact with John's family. The family was found to be a close, supportive unit composed of a mother, father, and two other siblings aged six and three. Discharge plans were coordinated by the case manager. Prior to John's discharge home, the case manager made a site visit to the family home to assess the physical plan of the home and identify any special needs of the family.

The case management program provided John and his family with several subsidized services not usually covered by their insurance plan. The program approved reimbursement for the air ambulance and paid for the parent's stay near the hospital during John's hospitalization. The case manager also approved funding for a breast pump for John's mother, thus enabling her to supply mother's milk, which is beneficial to the baby's immune system and is more easily digested than formula, for John's feedings. Reimbursement was also approved for the apnea/bradycardia monitor that John required continually postdischarge.

After John's discharge, the case manager assisted the parents in coordinating the baby's regular follow-up visits to the pediatrician and in arranging a high-risk clinic evaluation within two months of discharge. (Parents of high-risk infants frequently encounter difficulties in trying to coordinate care from multiple providers. In this area, medical case management performs a valuable service by eliminating some of the fragmentation of care parents often find when they have to deal with numerous providers.)

The case manager felt that John's parents would require assistance at home once John was discharged from the hospital. For the first two weeks, 24-hour nursing care was provided by registered nurses. Nursing care was then tapered to nights (10:00 PM to 8:00 AM) for the next four weeks, thus allowing the mother to rest at night so that she would be fit to care for John and her other two children during the day. During this time, the case manager monitored the case on a weekly basis. Monitoring was then reduced to monthly phone calls and the case was terminated six months after John's birth. At this time the child was progressing well, showed no evidence of chronic respiratory or neurologic problems, and no developmental problems were noted. The parents were encouraged to call the case manager if any problems or concerns arose.

OUTCOME MEASUREMENT FOR CASE MANAGEMENT

Outcomes of care that can be linked to case management interventions fall into two basic categories: those that are related to improvements in health status and those that are related to improvements in patient and family quality of life. Ways of measuring case management's effect on these indices are currently needed.

Case management strives to maximize a patient's health status through the timely mobilization of appropriate health services. Health status can be classified according to a variety of measures, including activities of daily living scales, presence of symptoms, presence of co-morbid conditions, frequency of complications, and presence of behavioral/psychological disabilities. Patients are referred to case management at various health status levels and with varying prognoses. Spinal cord injury patients, for example, can be paralyzed either below the waist or below the neck. A set of objective indicators of health status (e.g., mobility levels, self-care capability) could be applied to cases at referral and again at closure to measure the extent of change. Many other factors (e.g., patient motivation, family support, quality of medical care providers) make measuring the independent impact of case management difficult as well. Unfortunately, measuring the impact of key aspects of case management is the only way to effectively evaluate programs' claims of improved patient outcomes. Methods are currently needed for controlling factors unrelated to case management that affect outcomes.

The quality of patient and family life is a multidimensional concept that is difficult to measure. Brandeis and Boston University researchers have developed a survey to assess the quality of life for parents of case-managed, high-risk infants. The survey uses an interview scheduled assessing physiologic and mental health, general well-being, coping and stress, and social supports. The survey also looks at families' attitudes toward case management and the information families receive about the case management process. Analysis of the survey data will attempt to link family attitudes and case management activities (e.g., provision of emotional support, coordination of medical providers, interventions arranged) with changes in parental stress and coping levels over time. The survey will be administered to parents at two intervals: shortly after the infant's discharge from the hospital and again six months later. Although time-consuming and expensive, the use of such a survey can provide important information on how case management is viewed by patients and families and how it can lessen the strain on families at a very vulnerable time in their lives.

CONCLUSION

Hospitals seeking to expand their discharge planning services to include case management for discharged patients who are high-cost and/or technologically dependent are currently in an enviable position. First, they have access to the knowledge and experience already gained by insurers, health management firms, and employers offering case management programs. Second, because hospital-based case managers are already inside the health care system, they can obtain the support of hospital-based physicians and staff more quickly and easily than case managers working outside the health care system. Hospital-based case managers are also likely to have greater knowledge of local treatment resources than an insurance company case manager who is sometimes stationed thousands of miles away from the patient. Finally, hospitals already have systems in place for monitoring the quality of patient care that may perhaps be adapted for monitoring case management.

Case management programs need to begin to develop and implement systematic ways of measuring and monitoring the quality of their services. Industry standards should be developed in a number of areas, including workload ratios, manager qualifications, involvement of physicians and other specialists, and peer review requirements. Differences in processes of care (i.e., referral mechanisms and the ordering of site visits) between case management programs should be examined to determine how varying procedures may affect the quality of care. Finally, priority should be given to the development and application of outcome measures for patient functional status and patient/family qualify of life.

REFERENCES

Beswick, M. 1987. Complex cases: Identification and management (unpublished presentation at Group Health Association of American seminar) Boston.

Breslow, L. A. 1972. A quantitative approach to the World Health Organization definition of health: Physical, mental, and social well-being. *International Journal of Epidemiology,* 1(1):347.

Brook, R. H., & Williams, K. N. 1975. Quality of health care for the disadvantaged. *Journal of Community Health.* 1(2):132–155.

DeGeynt, W. 1970. Five approaches for assessing the quality of care. *Hospital Administration.* 15(2):21–42.

Dershewitz, R. A., Gross, R. A., & Williamson, J. W. 1979. Validating audit criteria:

An analytic approach illustrated by peptic ulcer disease. *Quality Review Bulletin.* 5(10):18–25.

Donabedian, A. 1968. Promoting quality through evaluating the process of medical care. *Medical Care.* 6(1):181–202.

Donabedian, A., Wheeler, J. R., & Wyszewianski, L. 1982. Quality, cost and health: An integrative model. *Medical Care.* 20(10):975–992.

Henderson, M., & Wallack, S. 1987. Evaluating case management for catastrophic illness. *Business and Health.* 4(3):7–11.

Henderson, M. G., Collard, A., & Mattson, J. (head injury specialist and consultant) Personal communication. Feb. 1987. Philadelphia.

Henderson, M., Souder, B., & Bergman, A. 1987. Measuring efficiencies of managed care. *Business and Health.* 4(12):43–46.

Henderson, M., et al. forthcoming. Private sector medical case management for high-cost illness. In R. Scheffler (Ed.), *Advances in Health Economics and Health Services Research, vol. 9.* Greenwich, CT: Jai Press.

Herzlinger, R., & Schwartz, J. 1985. How companies tackle health care costs: Part I. *Harvard Business Review.* 63(4):69–81.

Kaplan, S. H., & Greenfield, S. 1978. Criteria mapping: Using logic in evaluation of processes of care. *Quality Review Bulletin.* 4(1):3–7.

Rosenbloom, D., & Gertman, P. 1984. An intervention strategy for controlling costly care. *Business and Health.* 1(8):17–21.

PART IV

Case Management in Long Term Care

More Contextual Factors for Social Workers to Contemplate

Many of the themes and characteristics of the Health Care section apply to Long Term Care as well. Specifically, the cost containment basis for development of case management in long term care parallels health care in its centrality. Typical cost containment targets—rationing and/or rationalizing care—exist in both the public and private sectors. The Health Care Financing Administration (HCFA) has been the principal public policy influence in case management for recipients of long term care, creating and imposing demonstration case management programs explicitly targeted at limiting nursing home and acute care inpatient days by trying to coordinate community-based care systems.

In the long term care arena, the highest priority case management tasks involve developing efficient community-based alternatives to nursing home stays and to reduce days spent in acute care hospitals. Clients' eligibility often is based on meeting screening criteria that would justify their placement in skilled nursing facilities. Screening for eligibility is commonly cited as the first long term care case management task.

Missing from most long term care discussions is any analysis of paradigms, their direct connection to funding streams, and to the medicalization of needs. Azzarto (1986) discusses exactly this matter, demonstrating the link between continuous medicalization of the problems of the elderly and the fact that their health care is paid for by Medicare or Medicaid. The social function performed by this costly cultural practice is the elimination of larger scale social criticism of the society and its empty promises for older Americans. Austin extends this argument when she discusses the need for advocacy in the face of its absence in the Services Interaction Target for Opportunities (SITO) projects she studied. Acknowledging the need for system impact as a case management outcome, Austin states, "By itself, however, case management will achieve only limited reform if it continues to concentrate solely on case-level coordination" (1983, p. 26).

Long term care, similar to health care, involves home health services (sometimes involving sophisticated medical technology) often vital to sustaining life. This level of need emphasizes the struggle between preemptive provider-driven case management and client-driven practice. The choice of location of case management programs in long term care is hotly debated: Those who favor cost containment by rationalizing care would prefer to see case management administered (distributed) by providers; those who favor cost containment via rationing care prefer free standing case management.

The long term care case management context also contains the factor of case managers controlling the allocation of resources to providers through control over financing services. An entire national demonstration program tested outcomes comparing allocative control by case managers against basic case management practice. The Channeling Projects sought to determine outcome differences at the client and cost levels by randomly assigning clients to the two target models. As could be expected, the financial or allocative model—where case managers could control resources (i.e., directly order services from providers and pay them)—had reduced direct client contact, produced a greater facility in accessing services, and increased community-based service usage. However, the financial model showed little difference in reducing nursing home or acute care hospital stays. The basic case management model devoted more time to direct client contact, but without demonstrating reductions in cost or expensive service use. Neither model employed a client-driven concept nor did either attempt to include caregivers (family) in an empowering way. Both models remained within strictly medicalized definitions of need.

In many ways, the Channeling results parallel an earlier long term care case management demonstration effort reported by Carol Austin (1983). Austin is precise in establishing the system reform necessity that gave rise to the SITO programs of the early 1970s. She saw the allocative power potential in case management programs deriving from their presumed capacity to rearrange interorganizational resource dependencies. She devotes far more attention to organizational strategy than can be found in the vast majority of case management articles.

Kane also reflects on this issue and extends it to another common problem faced by case managers, including those committed to a client-driven orientation. How are clients who become functionally impaired to be perceived? How are goals and needs to be defined—and by whom? Is functional impairment easily determined, and how can that assessment be made? Who decides on the choice of participants in a functional impairment decision, or on what set of criteria are selected for decision? These questions recur in long term care case management and rarely are simple yes or no matters.

Seltzer, Ivry, and Litchfield bring to the foreground another fact of daily life for case managers in long term care—the role of family members. The daily direct tasks of case management are far more often acknowledged than the indirect functions families and family caretakers are expected to perform. These indirect tasks include such activities as negotiating bureaucracies for clients, advocating for their needs, and learning about medical care system functioning or financing. Question is raised about targeting families for training in these case management functions.

An additional issue in long term care involves the complex question of clients' autonomy and how that can be determined when so much of the responsibility for their care is put on family members. The complexity is pervasive, and it warrants another reading of Collopy's article on autonomy, particularly since one research finding of Seltzer, Ivry, and Litchfield was that an increased case management role for family members frequently indicated a reduced role for the elderly clients studied. Here, again, social workers along with case managers, confront the potential contradiction between the commitment to clients' self-determination and what is easiest to negotiate in a complicated situation.

As Azzarto points out, the elderly have social needs that often get medicalized out of providers' convenience and they are prevented from occupying legitimate social roles in our society. Case managers in long term care programs routinely confront the position of having to take sides between their clients and caregivers around issues related to self-determination. Since so much of daily life and its quality depend on informal networks, caregivers must be seen as having legitimate needs as well as clients and to be in need of informal social support networks. Hopefully, by thinking through the quality of life issues that surround the family context, case managers can optimize both the involvement and active participation of clients and caregivers in mutually productive ways. Partializing autonomy (see Collopy), clarifying goals and linking them to needs in open dialogue with both clients and caregivers can construct an environment where each receives validation and participates in mutually positive outcomes. Case managers practicing from a client-driven model have a responsibility for working toward this outcome and toward strengthening the informal network as participants in constructing outcomes.

This section will begin with the Azzarto article to frame the issues in a larger social and political context. The Austin piece will follow to demonstrate the interorganization dimensions to case management in long term care. Kane develops several themes and poses them as ethical confrontations for the case manager to consider when working in long term care. Finally, Seltzer, Ivry, and Litchfield report on research involving family members as case managers. I urge the reader to reexamine Collopy after reading the articles in this section for the reasons given earlier. Thematically, we maintain our focus on whether a client-driven model of long term care case management is posssible; on how it would be administered; and on whether or to what extent allocative power can produce transformation in service delivery system organization and practice paradigms. The seductiveness in thinking that controlling allocations for needed resources equates with system-changing power requires careful examination by social workers since it can *appear* to facilitate service delivery and produce reform in the delivery system.

CHAPTER 14

Medicalization of the Problems of the Elderly

Jacqueline Azzarto

At morning rounds in a community hospital, the following case was presented by a physician to teach residents about the management of diabetes:

> Mrs. B is a 72-year-old widow admitted to the hospital for uncontrolled diabetes. This is her second admission in six months. Today is her twelfth day of hospitalization. After a regimen of monitored diet and insulin regulation, her diabetes is under control. Medicare will reimburse Visiting Nurse Association services for a few weeks so that Mrs. B's condition can be watched.

However, the following notes summarize the patient's actual situation:

> Widowed five years ago, Mrs. B has become depressed recently and has neglected her diet. She lives alone on a fixed income. A cataract problem has limited her mobility, curtailed her once active involvement in church and community affairs, and made it difficult for her to administer insulin to herself. Several months ago, her only child, a son, moved to another state with his family. This was a blow to Mrs. B, who spent several afternoons a week with her grandchildren. It appears that Mrs. B's social support system is extremely limited and that her motivation to care for herself has declined. She was recently admitted to the hopsital for uncontrolled diabetes, and staff are reluctant to discharge her under the present circumstances.

Faced with the prospect of sending Mrs. B home only to have her return to the emergency room when her home nursing care was terminated, her young physician extended her stay. Concerned about his patient and frustrated with the system, he decides to take his chances with the hospital's utilization review committee and to press the social service department to come up with a better discharge plan. In doing so, he will waste hundreds of health care dollars a day. This case has helped him learn how to "medicalize" the problems of his elderly patient—how to reframe her social needs in medical terms so that they will be addressed by present health care policy rather than be shunted aside. If programs could provide Mrs. B with continuing care from home health aides, travel assistance, counseling services, and day care with an adopt-a-grandparent program, this young physician could concentrate on managing her diabetes and cataracts, secure in the knowledge that her psychosocial needs were being satisfied. In addition, the hospital would not be responsible for the costs of Mrs. B's inappropriate care. And, of course, Mrs. B would be happier and probably healthier. Instead, recent Medicare regulations will soon limit Mrs. B's hospital admissions for diabetes, and her plight and that of other patients will intensify.

The case of Mrs. B is symptomatic of a phenomenon in the United States—the "medicalization" of the problems of the elderly—that is related to inadequate policies, deep-seated attitudes and patterns of thought, and fiscal constraints. This article will define medicalization by placing it in the social context in which it takes place, provide some evidence of how it occurs, and offer some possible explanations of why it happens.

SOCIAL CONTEXT AND INFLUENCES

Comfort, a distinguished geriatrician, describes aging as a

> sociogenic process, a process by which society strips older citizens of their socially sanctioned kinship and work roles. What replaces these is a negative role of being old, of being 'unintelligent, unemployable, crazy and asexual.' (Comfort, 1976)

Comfort accuses America's youth-oriented culture of treating the old like an underprivileged minority and acknowledges that while "physical losses are serious and will ultimately kill us . . . most older people do tackle disability with as much or more courage than at any other age" (Comfort, 1976). The elderly, he contends, are suffering more from boredom and grief than from illness.

That the problems of older people are largely social in nature is also the major conclusion of Riley, a sociologist (Riley & Waring, 1978). Riley's concepts of age stratification, age inequalities, and age segregation point to social isolation, the loss of status and roles, and the negative stereotypes that accompany these factors as major causes of the problems of the elderly.

The negative stereotypes attached to old age many also result in diverging perceptions on the part of the general public and the elderly concerning the nature of older people's problems. In a Harris poll sponsored by the National Council on Aging, poor health was identified as a problem of the elderly by 51 percent of the respondents in the 18-to-64 age bracket, and inadequate medical care was identified by 44 percent (Abrams, 1976). In contrast, only 21 percent of the respondents age 65 or over mentioned poor health as a problem, and inadequate medical care was noted by only 10 percent. It is interesting that 23 percent of the respondents in the 65-and-over age group listed fear of crime, a social problem, as their major concern. In discussing the results of the poll, Abrams reached a notable conclusion concerning those older respondents who said that poor health was their reason for not working. He suggested that this was a learned excuse used to cover up other reasons, such as the feeling of not being wanted, a less acceptable and more embarrassing response.

Politicians as well as the general public have been greatly influenced by negative stereotypes of the elderly, and until recent years they have not recognized the ability and willingness of senior citizens to take part in the political process. In 1976 Abrams appealed to state legislators to understand that "a new breed of elderly is developing" that must be considered a viable political force (Abrams, 1976). In fact, Hudson and Binstock maintain that interest in politics increases with age, and Kutza reports that the percentage of older people who vote is higher than the percentage of voters in any other age group (Hudson & Binstock, 1976; Kutza, 1981). Although the elderly may have physical limitations, these conditions do not diminish their suitability for public involvement. On the contrary, the life experiences that senior citizens have undergone give them a more comprehensive perspective on public issues.

Given the pervasiveness in society of stereotypic attitudes toward the elderly, it is not surprising that these attitudes are reflected in various aspects and sectors of American life. Physicians are investigating causal relationships among social problems, negative roles, and poor health. In regard to this topic, Shanas concluded the folowing:

> There is ample clinical evidence that physical and emotional problems can be precipitated or exacerbated by denial of employment opportunities. Few physicians deny that a direct relationship exists between enforced idleness and poor health. The practitioner with a patient load comprised largely of older persons is convinced that physical and emotional ailments of many . . . are a result of inactivity imposed by denial of work. (Shanas, 1972)

Thus it appears that individuals such as sociologists, politicians, and physicians have been questioning the stereotype of older people as weak, infirm, and unable to contribute to society. A logical question, then, is why medical requirements are the needs of the elderly most consistently acknowledged by the makers of public policy. One need only look at Medicare, which will pay for skilled nursing but not for custodial care, to realize that concerns about illness overshadow those related to quality of life in the eyes of policymakers. It is reasonable to ask why policymakers are reluctant to follow the challenge posed by Butler to formulate a national policy on aging that would include in its goals older people's achievement of the right to work and the right to social roles as well as the protection of their freedom of mobility and the creation of comprehensive health and social care (Butler, 1978). However, asking this question implies an ignorance of incremental policy change, which is the method of change that prevails in the United States because of this country's political process. With incrementation, changes are small and effected cautiously because politicians do not want to upset the electorate. However, because the more efficient use of health care dollars is becoming a national imperative, a more rational approach to policy must be conceived and implemented.

NEGLECT OF SOCIAL NEEDS

How does medicalization of the needs of the elderly take place? The tendency to define and respond to social problems in medical terms can be seen in a variety of areas. For example, federal expenditures for health care reflect a narrow view of the problems of the elderly, and it is clear that specific social needs are not given appropriate attention. In a detailed examination of federal spending on programs for the elderly, Kutza found that Medicare, the most medically oriented of these programs, received the largest share of federal funds (Kutza, 1981). The least medically oriented programs, those related to housing, received the smallest share. In fact, Kutza estimated that Medicare received 12 times the funding received by housing programs.

One might argue that since the elderly receive social security benefits, they could spend some of their allotments on social services. But as Moroney has pointed out, such services are available only to those who meet certain income eligibility criteria (Moroney, 1980). Many middle-class families providing care for elderly relatives are excluded from receiving these services because they are not poor enough. These families may go without day care, homemaker services, counseling, transportation services, and other assistance, or they may struggle with limited budgets to purchase these services in the marketplace.

Not only are the social needs of the elderly often neglected in policy planning, but existing policies sometimes also pursue social goals that conflict. For example, social services that are available for the elderly who are poor are funded through Title XX of the Social Security Act, which distributes block grants to the states. A goal of Title XX is the reduction or prevention of institutionalization through community-based care, a goal that implies a concern for the social needs of individuals. However, the policy governing Supplemental Security Income, the result of other federal legislation that is also in place, seems to penalize benefit recipients for staying at home: benefits are increased by 50 percent if an individual lives in a foster home but are reduced by 33.3 percent if he or she lives at home and receives care from family and friends. Furthermore, despite the fact that Title XX addresses social needs, an astonishingly low 0.001 percent of Title XX funds are spent on programs specifically designed to provide services to the aged. In 1977 these services reached only 100,000 out of 25 million citizens over the age of 65 (Moroney, 1980).

If federal spending on social services for the elderly is low compared to spending allocated to medical services, some states, according to Abrams, are guilty of "failure . . . to put their pocketbooks where their mouths are by neglecting state matching" (Abrams, 1976). The variability in this area from state to state has been dramatic. In 1975, for example, California spent $88 million on in-home services, compared to New York, which spent $22 million. Some states have only a few social service programs. In 1980 only 36 states had adult day care programs, and only 32 provided home-delivered or congregate meals (Moroney, 1980). Given present budget cutbacks, even these programs may become extinct.

The same variability exists in public housing programs. In 1973, 1,500 elderly people were waiting for placement in publicly subsidized housing in Washington, D.C., but in New York City those waiting numbered 32,000 (Kutza, 1981). In addition, certain expenditures reflect a social welfare policy for the elderly that separates the better off from the poor. For example, elderly people in the middle and upper class receive Old-Age and Survivors Insurance. The elderly who are poor receive Supplemental Security Income and housing subsidies. Furthermore, even when the need for social services is acknowledged, fragmentation of policy leads to gaps in service: depending on their state or community, the poor may or may not have access to public programs. And, ultimately, whether older people are poor or better off, their medical needs receive much more attention than their social needs.

Another area in which the neglect of the social needs of senior citizens is seen is in that of retirement. The criterion for receipt of social security payments is typically retirement at age 65. A change in this arbitrary age is currently being examined by social security officials, and the 1983 amendments to the Social Security Act already call for a change in the primary retirement age to 67 by the year 2027. However, the motivation for extending the retirement age was not to satisfy the elderly's need to work; the extension was a response to the impending threat of bankruptcy of the social security system.

The Harris poll commissioned in 1976 by the National Council on Aging revealed that senior citizens are not alone in objecting to mandatory retirement. The poll found that "86 percent of the American public, young and old, have serious reservations about current [retirement] practices" (Church, 1976). The majority of the public believe that most older people can continue to perform as well on the job as they did when they were younger. But despite public opinion, the practice of mandatory retirement continues, which may well lead to idleness, somatization, and poor health among those forced to stop working. Thus, the secondary impact of forced retirement is felt when the older person arrives at the doctor's office. And it is ironic that although the provision of social services prior to this point might have obviated the person's need for more expensive medical services, government payment for medical care is more easy for him or her to obtain.

EXPLANATORY FACTORS

Policy Perspectives

A number of factors contribute to the pervasive emphasis on the elderly's medical problems to the detriment of their social needs. For example, the fact that Medicare is linked to the social insurance concept of social policy has been significant in the development of this society's tendency to respond to social needs in medical terrms. Medicare is viewed as medical insurance for the elderly and provides universal coverage after age 65 with no stigma or means tests attached. Derthick's analysis of policymaking for social security explains that since its inception in the United States in 1935, social insurance has been a politically and ideologically appealing concept (Derthick, 1979). Thus, Medicare was legitimated without much difficulty in 1966 and until just recently reaped the benefits of institutional protection, that is, protection by program executives, legislators, and representatives of labor, big business, and the professions. In contrast, Medicaid and social service programs require means tests, and their public image is one of administrative inefficiency and cost ineffectiveness. The resulting negative stereotype reflects the notion that programs for the poor are poor programs.

More fundamental than the negative stereotypes attached to means-tested programs are the stereotypes attached to social problems. Poverty, homelessness, and a wide variety of social ills all resound with negative connotations. The tendency to perceive the condition of the elderly in medical terms may stem from an attempt to enhance the acceptability of the social problems that old people experience (Jones, 1977). This attempt is not unique. Alcoholism, drug abuse, mental illness, and child abuse have all at some point been explained in biological rather than social terms. Given biological explanations, society can respond with medical technology, expertise that is readily available.

Medical science has always been more impressive than social science in regard to technology. In the United States, medical specialization was held in high esteem during the early 1960s, the precise time that social security policymakers were formulating new definitions of the problems of the elderly. Not only was the medical model chosen for implementation, but the medical specialist model was chosen as well. This resulted in many of the abuses—unnecessary testing, procedures, and hospitalizations—that policymakers are today attempting to reform by initiating the diagnostic related group (DRG) system. The issues surrounding the exaltation of technology in this country raise the question of why health care professionals have reinforced society's tendency to put forward medical responses to the problems of the elderly.

Dominance of Medicine

Since the time of the ancient Greeks, physicians have been viewed as scholars and scientists (despite their use of such rudimentary "scientific" methods as holding urine specimens up to the light to study them). In colonial times physicians had little to offer their patients who had smallpox, diphtheria, measles, and other diseases, but they were nevertheless highly regarded by society. According to Grob,

> As more Americans survived the dangers of infancy and childhood in ever-growing numbers, they began to identify the decline in infectious diseases with measures introduced by modern medicine. At the same time, the character of the medical profession was transformed by science and technology. (Grob, 1983)

Medicine had the answers to modern problems, and the physician was the scientific leader. Nurses, the other major group of health care professionals familiar to the public, were viewed as physicians' handmaidens, and nursing was condescendingly identified as women's work (Aiken, 1983). Social work, another profession for women, was similarly accorded low status.

In addition to witnessing the growing presence of nurses and social workers on the health care scene, the twentieth century saw the birth and development of many allied health professions, whose members include physical and occupational therapists, dietitians, physician assistants, and speech pathologists. Today, physicians constitute one of 16 categories of health care providers that have been identified, but they are the group residing at the top of a large and complex health care hierarchy (Ginzberg, 1983). What keeps them in this position in the United States is not only their scientific knowledge and skills but also their political power base and entrepreneurial role and style. In countries such as England and Israel, where physicians make less money than in this country, there is less of a discrepancy between the role and status of physicians and those of other health care professionals.

There are many differences between the health care system in America and those in other nations. In Israel, for example, teams consisting of a family physician, a nurse, and a social worker are responsible for a designated nurse territory. Members of a given team may work in different settings, but they meet weekly to discuss the problems of the families living within their territory. These problems are social as well as medical. This system contrasts sharply with the one used here, in which such coordination is rare. In addition, the health insurance system in this country differs from those used elsewhere. By often reimbursing only the physician, the American insurance system may encourage the overdiagnosis of medical problems (Monneckendam, 1984).

Reliance on the medical system is reinforced in the United States in a variety of ways, such as when it becomes legitimate for physicians to determine patients' nonmedical needs like needs for job training and disability status. It is further reinforced by such practices as waiting for a physician to pronounce someone officially dead when the person died several hours earlier and the physician has been detained. This sanctioning of the medical profession's exclusive right to handle all issues related to life and death has become burdensome to many modern physicians. In the author's experience, many young physicians like the one in the case study described earlier would willingly share their responsibilities with other health professionals. If public policy reinforced the sharing of responsibility, patients such as Mrs. B would be reimbursed for securing social services, and her physicians would be reimbursed for providing her with medical care.

Related to the issue of shared responsibility is that of the credentialing of health care providers and how it indirectly contributes to medicalization. As many states continue to deny licensure to social workers, third-party payments from insurance companies are withheld for social work services. This can discourage potential clients from using these services and perpetuate the entrenched position of other health care professionals. Also, restricting the practice of social workers may affect the way in which patients' problems and needs are defined. Provided that social workers remain committed to the philosophy of their profession and its focus on psychosocial needs (rather than a narrower concern with mental health), the profession must be committed to credentialism.

RECOMMENDATIONS

Medicalization, then, takes place on two levels in our society in regard to the needs of elderly citizens. The medical needs of the elderly are sanctioned and are addressed by public policy in a way detrimental to their social needs. At the same time, present policy forces professionals to reframe social problems in medical terms if service is to be provided to their elderly patients.

With Reaganomics as our present reality, the time is right for a comprehensive cost-benefit analysis of existing policy. Relevant questions require answers. Would not the frail elderly and their families benefit more from the provision of support services and respite care than from an emphasis on institutionalization? Would not senior citizens who are ambulatory be better off maintaining their independence in their own homes with the aid of travel and cleaning services, day care programs, and Meals on Wheels? And would this independence not help keep them out of their doctors' offices? Finally, should they not be allowed to work and contribute to society as long as they feel able? Research data are needed to answer these questions so that social workers can defend the benefits of social programs that foster independence and prove that program costs are appropriate for the achievement of long-term goals.

Happier endings are needed for the story of Mrs. B and for patients like her. Society must acknowledge both her need to contribute and her lack of social support; federal and state policy must provide her with programs that address all her needs; and professionals must work as a team to keep her out of the hospital. Only then will society have met its challenge and fulfilled its responsibility.

REFERENCES

Abrams, A. J. 1976. *Implications for State Policy and the Aging: A Guide for State Legislators,* Aging in America, no. 8. Washington, DC: National Council on the Aging, p. 5.

Aiken, L. H. 1983. Nurses. In D. Mechanic (Ed.), *Handbook of Health, Health Care, and the Health Professions.* New York: Free Press.

Butler, R. N. 1978. Toward a national policy on aging. In R. Gross, B. Gross, & S. Seidman (Eds.), *The New Old.* Garden City, NY: Anchor Books.

Church, F. 1976. *Implications for Federal Policy,* Aging in America, no. 4, Washington, DC: National Council on the Aging, p. 9.

Comfort, A. 1976. *A Good Age.* New York: Crown, p. 10.

Derthick, M. 1979. *Policymaking for Social Security.* Washington, DC: The Brookings Institution,

Ginzberg, E. 1983. Allied health resources. In D. Mechanic (Ed.), *Handbook of Health, Health Care, and the Health Professions.* New York: Free Press.

Grob, G. N. 1983. Disease and environment in american history. In D. Mechanic (Ed.). *Handbook of Health, Health Care, and the Health Professions.* New York: Free Press, p. 20.

Hudson, R. B., & Binstock, R. H., 1976. Political systems and the aging. In R. H. Binstock, and E. Shanas (Eds.), *Handbooks on Aging and the Social Sciences.* New York: Van Nostrand Reinhold.

Jones, C. O. 1977. *An Introduction to the Study of Public Policy* (2nd ed.). Belmont, CA: Wadsworth.

Kutza, E. A., 1981. *The Benefits of Old Age: Social Welfare Policy for the Elderly.* Chicago: University of Chicago Press, p. 79.

Monneckendam, M. (professor of family medicine at Tel Aviv University), 1984. Interview. Summit, NJ.

Moroney, R. M. 1980. *Families, Social Services, and Social Policy: The Issue of Shared Responsibility.* Washington, DC: U.S. Department of Health and Human Services, p. 106.

Riley, M. W., & Waring, J. 1978. Most of the problems of aging are not biological, but social. In R. Gross, B. Gross, & S. Seidman, (Eds.), *The New Old: Struggling for Decent Aging.* Garden City, NY: Anchor Books.

Shanas, E. 1972. Social myths regarding isolation of the elderly. *Journal of the American Medical Association.* 219:1147.

CHAPTER 15

Case Management in Long Term Care

Options and Opportunities

Carol D. Austin

Experimentation with various reforms in the financing and delivery of longterm care is an important agenda item for the 1980s. A number of financial reforms, ranging from cash and benefit approaches to block grants for longterm care and the creation of Social/Health Maintenance Organizations (S/HMOs) have been offered and examined by several analysts (Callahan & Wallack, 1981; Meltzer, Farrow, & Richman, 1981).[1] Some reform options appear to be more economically and politically feasible than others, but almost all will require the continued need to coordinate delivery of long termcare services to individual clients (Gottesman, 1981). Perhaps the most generally accepted tool for such coordination is case management, and this article proposes that case management can also be a tool to reform the delivery system as well.

Case management is widely viewed as a mechanism for linking and coordinating segments of a service delivery system (within a single agency or involving several providers) to ensure the most comprehensive program for meeting an individual client's needs for care. Case management frequently involves one person or a team that has responsibility for managing comprehensive assessment, planning, procurement or delivery, monitoring, and evaluation of services to meet the identified needs of the client. The particular approach to case

[1] S/HMOs are four demonstration projects funded by the Department of Health and Human Services to explore prepaid health and social services for the elderly.

management that is implemented varies from case to case in several important respects, including who has responsibility for which cases under what circumstances, whether or not the case manager may also be the service provider, conditions under which case management responsibilities may be transferred, and how services are requisitioned or arranged. The principal functions of case management in long term care are the following: (1) screening and determining eligibility; (2) assessing the need for services and related needs; (3) care planning (developing a service plan); (4) requisitioning services; (5) implementing the service plan, coordinating service delivery, and following up; and (6) reassessing, monitoring, and evaluating services periodically.

Although social work professionals are familiar with and accept the goals of case management to a large extent, the role of case manager is implemented with considerable variation and has different meanings in various agencies. Nonetheless, the role of case manager is so widespread that it is unusual to find a health or social service agency that does not claim to provide case management services for its clients. An important feature of the role and one that has received little attention is the authority of the case manager to allocate services. The extent to which case managers have authority for allocation can affect their capacity to act as change agents in local systems for service delivery.

Perhaps case management has enjoyed widespread acceptance because it has not been viewed as a systematic reform but as a function that can be incorporated into ongoing delivery systems without changing structural relationships among service providers. In the past, case management emphasized assessing, care planning, and providing services to individual clients, but today, a view of case management limited to its capacity for directly serving clients is too narrow. Case management can become a powerful strategy for altering the market behavior of providers and for shaping the character of systems for the delivery of long term care. Guidelines for such a strategy can be found in the resource dependence theory of interorganizational relationships (which will be discussed below). This theory becomes useful when care planning, a major case management function, is viewed as a process of resource allocation in which important decisions are made in regard to what extent and from which providers the client will receive services.

This article briefly discusses the resource dependence theory of interorganizational relationships as it pertains to case management and follows with a discussion of case management research. It also addresses the dimensions program designers should consider when structuring case management in long term care in ways that could enhance case managers' power to intervene in local delivery systems. The author concludes with an explanation of the implications of case management for social workers in health care.

INTERORGANIZATIONAL DEPENDENCE

It has become axiomatic in interorganizational theory that organizations seek to protect and strengthen their autonomy and resist efforts to increase their dependence on other organizations (Thompson, 1967; Yuchtman & Seashore, 1967; Levine & White, 1961). Efforts to increase coordination among agencies providing services cause them to become interdependent. Because coordination constrains the capacity of service providers to operate independently, it entails financial and time costs to those agencies, requires interaction and consultation with other agencies, and increases the level of uncertainty by introducing uncontrollable elements into agencies' internal operations. Agencies, which spend considerable time and energy negotiating their dependencies in local delivery systems, aim to minimize the disruption introduced by environmental uncertainty. At the same time, paradoxically, if an agency wants to gain some control over the action of other organizations, it must give up some of its own autonomy.

Pfeffer and Salancik assert, "If behavior [of organizations] is externally controlled, then the design of the external system of constraints and controls is the place to begin to determine organizational actions and structures" (Pfeffer & Salancik, 1978). Any system of constraints and controls at the level of service delivery requires supportive structures at the institutional and managerial levels if it is to operate with optimal effectiveness (Aiken et al., 1975; Callahan, 1981). For many, however, one of the virtues of case management as a policy reform in long term care is precisely that it can be placed within the ongoing delivery system and does not require restructuring of interorganizational relationships. This view, however, diverts attention from the potential of case managers to alter agencies' behavior. Case management can modify the way provider organizations interact by influencing their patterns of interdependence (that is, if policymakers grant case managers adequate authority and centralized control of resources).

Pfeffer and Salancik specify three factors that are critical in determining the level at which one organization depends on another: the extent to which specific resources are required by an organization for its continued operation and survival; the extent to which an external actor has discretion over allocation, use, and regulatory authority concerning critical resources; and the extent to which the organization has few alternatives for acquiring the required resources. These factors suggest that if case management is to alter the market behavior of providers by increasing their interdependence in the delivery system, then it should be deliberately structured as a system of constraints and controls along the following lines: (1) the case manager would control resources seen as important by service providers, (2) the case manager would have authority over resource allocation and regulate use of resources, and (3) the case manager's control of resources would reduce the discretion of service providers.

Although researchers have recognized the need to increase interdependence among providers to reduce fragmentation in service delivery, few have suggested case management as a tool for so doing (probably because they were mainly concerned about coordination of services to individual clients). The emphasis on clients is evident in the data collected about case management in projects to integrate federal services, in studies conducted by the Andrus Center at the University of Southern California, and in demonstration projects for long term care.

INTEGRATION OF SERVICES

The emergence of case management as an important mechanism for coordinated service delivery can be traced to the Allied Services Act, which was proposed in 1971, by Elliot Richardson, Secretary of the Department of Health, Education, and Welfare (HEW), in recognition of the need to improve coordination among HEW's own programs at the state and local levels. To this end, HEW initiated a series of demonstration projects, the Services Integration Targets for Opportunity (SITO) sites, designed to test a variety of mechanisms for integrating services primarily at the local level.[2] Integration techniques included newly developed information and referral systems, client-tracking systems, comprehensive service centers, and case management procedures. In 1974, HEW initiated the Partnership Grants program, which represented an expansion of the SITO concept, to include capacity building for integrating services at the state and local levels. Projects begun with these grants focused on comprehensive planning and management components, elements seen as necessary to support improvements in coordination of services at the level of service delivery. Forty-one sites were involved in the Partnership Grants program by June 1975 (Morrill, 1976).

This federal initiative of SITO combined with the Partnership Grants program represented an ambitious effort on two fronts: administrative reform at the state level (including the development of Comprehensive Human Resource Agencies, or CHRAs) and integration of services (focusing attention on the clients—individuals of families—that frequently requested assistance from more than one categorical program). The intent of these efforts was to break down barriers among providers and to create a delivery system that was more responsive to clients' total needs.

An example of the SITO experience is provided by Florida's reorganiza-

[2] For a comprehensive discussion and analysis of the integration of services experience, see *Evaluation* (entire issue), 3, Nos. 1 and 2 (1976); Penelope Caragonne, "Bibliography on Service Integration Literature" (Austin: University of Texas, Center for Social Work Research, School of Social Work, December 1977) (mimeographed); and *Evaluation of Services Integration Demonstration Projects,* Human Services Bibliography Series No. 1 (Rockville, Md.: Project Share, June 1976).

tion of the Department of Health and Rehabilitative Services in accordance with three principles: services were integrated through one-stop service centers with the application of a case management approach, administration and delivery of services were decentralized to the regional level, and professional policymaking and quality control were to occur at the state level (Lynn, 1976). The Florida SITO project sought to integrate diverse programs—youth services, services for the retarded, services for the aging and other adults, mental health services, vocational rehabilitation, income maintenance, social services, and health services—with their service delivery structures. When a client entered a local service center, he or she was placed in the hands of a single case manager, a generalist with knowledge of available resources. In consultation with a professional team for diagnosis and evaluation, the case manager conducted a comprehensive assessment and developed a service plan, as well as supervised follow-up and monitored progress in the case.

The SITO projects produced several significant integrative features:

Case management

Client's pathway: the route a client followed in an agency through intake, triage, information and referral, problem assessment, service planning, case assignment, monitoring, follow-up, reassessment, and termination

Data units: which provided service-delivery and management staff with information about profiles of clients, outcomes for clients, costs, resource inventories of services, and the total performance of the system

Service provider contracts: a set of contracts that bound providers to deliver to clients the services specified by the case manager

The most common element in the projects for integrating services was the case management. The authors's computer search of the Project Share data base revealed the following information about the SITO projects: eighteen projects included case management as a component, eighty-seven included case management in their implementation, and fourteen produced recommendations for improvements in case management. Case managers in SITO projects assisted clients in effective and efficient negotiation of the delivery system and served as the single point of accountability for performance of the system. Case managers—human services generalists responsibile for organizing resources for clients in the SITO demonstration—varied in their function, status, responsibility for clients, role in the client's pathway, and responsibility for reporting (Mittenthall, 1976).

The SITO projects highlighted the complex relationships between state and local administrative structures and the capacity to provide coordinated services to clients. Both administrative structures and delivery of services were shaped by funding; however, only one of the SITO projects attempted to change the flow of funding significantly, and that project achieved only temporary success in improving integration of the system.[3] Experiences at the SITO sites suggest that unless the structure of funding is modified, the progress toward integrated delivery systems will be thwarted. A primary cause of fragmented services is fragmented funding.

ANDRUS GERONTOLOGY CENTER

A team of researchers at the Andrus Gerontology Center of the University of Southern California (USC) has examined case coordination in programs for the vulnerable elderly across the nation. This investigation has produced an extensive bibliography, a census of case-coordination programs generated by a national survey, a comprehensive list and analysis of practice guidelines drawn from the operational experience of case coordinators, and an assessment of the ways in which case coordination has been evaluated (*Complete Case,* 1978; *1979–80 National Directory,* 1980; Steinberg & Carter, 1982; Steinberg, 1979).

This ambitious effort has analyzed the case manager as coordinator, advocate, and counselor; has examined the relationship between the client's pathway, assessment, and case management; and has investigated the impact of case coordination on senior centers and an Area Agency on Aging (Downing, 1979; Steinberg, 1978; 1979). The research has highlighted the complexity of the case-coordination function and the case management role.

At a symposium sponsored by the Andrus Center, front-line practitioners in case coordination discussed the following: roles of the coordinator, agency setting, practice, the importance of being able to differentiate among clients with varying levels of need, necessary background and training of coordinators, and values held by individuals who perform case coordination (*Case Coordination,* 1979). Symposium participants came from twelve case-coordination agencies whose programs had operated for a minimum of two years and whose target population was the elderly.[4] Participants were employed by a variety of programs for the vulnerable elderly: a government agency focusing on the visually handicapped, sectarian family service agencies, multiservice centers, a

[3] The Hartford SITO Project pooled funds from the State Department of Welfare, State Division of Aging, City of Hartford, United Way, and private foundations and created a new organization, The Community Life Association.

[4] Participating agencies were Multi-Service Center, Wheeling, WVa: Project Independence for the Elderly, Paducah, KY; Metropolitan Family Services, Inc., Portland, OR; Monroe County Long Term Care Program-ACCESS, Rochester, NY; Senior Information and Outreach Service, Houston, TX; Triage, Inc., Plainville, CT; Jewish Family and Children's Services, Miami, FL; Cambridge-Somerville Home Care Corporation, Somerville, MA; Visiting Nurse Association of Milwaukee, Milwaukee, WI; Family Counseling Agency, Tucson, AZ; Department of the Visually Handicapped, Richmond, VA; and Jamaica Service Program for Older Adults, Inc., Jamaica, NY.

visiting nurse association, and two experimental demonstration projects that provided community-based long term care. The agencies represented at this symposium provided long term care programs in the overlapping area of health and social services. Each participant had a minimum of two years of job experience and was employed as a direct service coordinator. The proceedings of the symposium reported how often participants performed each case management task (*Case Coordination,* 1979).

Table 15-1 categorized the tasks into three groups: those related to the client, those related to relationships among agencies or to the delivery system, and those related to knowledge or reporting. These categories are not meant to be mutually exclusive, since some tasks have consequences for both individual clients and the delivery system. For example, the task of authorization of a service affects the individual client as recipient, the agency that is to be the service provider, and the local delivery system (to the extent that the system regulates availability). Analysis reveals that reported case management tasks tend to relate primarily to clients and to relate considerably less frequently across agencies or to the delivery system. Only two of the reported tasks (authorizing service provision and following up clients in nursing homes) involve authority of case managers (and these tasks were reported as being done by less than half the symposium participants).

The dominant theme in case management of client-centered activities is discussed in a book from the USC research team (Steinberg & Carter, 1982). The basic categories for an analysis of program functioning at the client level are entry, assessment, goal setting and service planning, implementation, and review and evaluation of the status of the client and the program. At a more general level, the USC researchers have identified five fundamental dimensions of case-coordination design (Steinberg & Carter, 1982):

Primary mission: client-centered brokering, service coordination, resource distribution or change of the local system, or improvement of policy and practice

Organizational base: "freestanding" special unit within an operating agency, or consortium or federation

Authority base: extent of control over funding to service providers

Professional reference group: medical and health, mental health, social welfare, aging network, or other

Target population: most vulnerable, frail elderly, catchment area, those in need, or universal eligibility

These design elements suggest dimensions along which future case-coordination efforts can be developed. Although the USC project found wide variation in the practice of case management, a consistent theme was an emphasis on interactions of case managers with individual clients.

TABLE 15-1. CASE MANAGEMENT TASKS REPORTED BY FRONT-LINE PRACTITIONERS

Case Management Tasks	All Participants Reported	Most Participants Reported	Less than Half the Participants Reported
Related to the client	Referral Assessment Development of a service plan 1. Arranging for services 2. Coordinating service providers 3.. Developing resources for individual clients Follow-up and reassessment Alteration of the service plan Advocacy Support and encouragement about use of services	Written service plan Maintaining ongoing contact with clients Monitoring clients' medications Consultation on cases with other agencies Monitoring provision of services to individual clients Educating clients about services Reviewing and setting priorities for cases in workers' caseloads	Initiating case conferences Providing direct services for clients Termination when goals are achieved Authorizing service provision before it begins Follow-up of clients in nursing homes
Related to relationships among agencies or to the delivery system		Identifying and reporting gaps in services to the community Working supportively with service providers Community education, training, and public relations Consultation on cases with other agencies	Authorizing services provision before it begins Follow-up of clients in nursing homes Developing resources for groups of clients Initiating case conferences
Related to knowledge and reporting	Knowledge of community resources Knowledge of regulations and policies of service providers and funders		Reporting by cost per unit of service

Source: Adapted from *Case Coordination with the Elderly: The Experiences of Front Line Practitioners,* 1979. Proceedings and summary findings from a symposium held January 20–22, 1979, Los Angeles: Andrus Gerontology Center, University of Southern California, February 1979, pp. 76–77.

LONG TERM CARE

Over the past decade, the federal government has supported experimental demonstration projects designed to test and evaluate a variety of approaches to meeting the growing needs of our elderly population for health and social services. Some of these projects incorporated innovative funding arrangements, including waivers permitting states to use more flexible funding earmarked for Medicare and Medical Assistance State Plans (respectively, Titles XVIII and XIX of the Social Security Act). A project operating with a waiver of the Medical Assistance program could use these funds to provide a broader range of services for long term care. Another significant feature of these demonstrations efforts has been cost analyses of nursing home care compared to cost analyses of services designed to maintain the elderly in their homes as long as possible. Given the increasing number of older citizens in this country, the need to develop cost-effective long term care will continue to be a pressing public policy issue. Some of the demonstration projects attempted to develop a continuum of care for the elderly in their local communities, identifying gaps along the continuum and using flexible funding to fill those gaps. Specification of target populations, determination of methodology of assessment, and development of structures to improve coordination of services to clients were also common elements in these demonstration efforts.

Demonstration Projects

Findings from a recent review of nine long term care demonstrations illuminate the role of case management in the delivery of community-based long term care (Greenberg, Austin, & Doth, 1981).[5] The group of demonstrations examined were a mixed bag: some had limited goals (such as the National 222 projects that primarily sought to increase the availability of day care and homemaker services in local delivery systems) while others (such as Triage) operated with a broad set of programmatic waivers, and still others (such as ACCESS) included components for managing delivery systems (such as preadmission screening for placement in nursing homes). What the demonstration projects did share, however, was a primary focus on a narrow but crucial set of issues: outcomes for individual clients and costs of services. Review of documents and interviews with staff indicated that most of the projects focused on intervention at the client level.[6] Demonstration projects conducted

[5] The projects reviewed were Alternative Health Services, Atlanta, GA; Alternatives to Institutionalization, Worcester, MA; Community Based Care Systems, State of Washington, Olympia; Community Care Organization, Madison, WI; Effects and Costs of Day Care and Homemaker Services (six projects located in Los Angeles, CA; San Francisco, CA; Lexington, KY; White Plains, NY; Syracuse, NY; and Providence, RI); Highland Heights, Fall River, MA; Monroe County Long Term Care Program—ACCESS, Rochester, NY; On Lok Health Center, San Francisco, CA; and Triage, Inc., Plainville, CT.

[6] For a more thorough discussion of this distinction, see Greenberg, Austin, and Doth (1981).

in the future need to document their experiences on the level of the service delivery system as well as on the level of the client. (Case management links the two.) This information would allow researchers to monitor the effectiveness of various strategies for system-level change, which has not been the focus of previous demonstration projects and which could significantly influence outcomes and costs for the clients.

Staff of the nine projects consistently pointed to the case management process as the most important part of their demonstration model. Comparisons of projects soon revealed that the concept of case management meant different things from one project to the next. To discover any common patterns among the various notions, a generic model of client-level intervention or case management was developed. The model is composed of five discrete phases of work with clients: intake and inquiry, assessment, determination of eligibility, care planning, and provision of services and follow-up.

Each project identified potentially appropriate clients through a referral and screening system. The character of the network and sources of referral, criteria for initial referral, and responsibility for prescreening varied among the projects in the intake and inquiry phase. Comprehensive assessment, the focus of the second phase, involved timing (when the assessment took place), instrumentation, organizational location (where the assessment took place), characteristics of the assessors, and presence of reliability checks—features that varied across projects. Two forms of eligibility, program and target, were determined in phase three, at which time assessing the client's risk and need also took place. The major activity in the phase of care planning was the translation of data collected during assessment into a package of services for the client. Here projects different in characteristics of the care planners, organizational location, relationship of care planning to assessment, and the nature of rules for making decisions about care planning. The last phase of the generic case management model is service provision and follow-up. Projects varied with respect to who had responsibility for implementation, the nature of the interface between those responsible for service provision and follow-up and those responsible for assessment and care planning, services provided as opposed to purchased, and responsiblity for monitoring. These phases and variables are summarized in Table 15-2.[7]

These demonstration projects made conscious efforts to alter existing patterns of service delivery. Unfortunately, most evaluations of the projects did not document their experiences at the system level. Some of the projects (such as Wisconsin Community Care Organization) attempted to fill gaps in the existing continuum of care in their local communities, whereas others (such as ACCESS) controlled access to high-cost services through preadmission screening. Projects operating with waivers (Wisconsin, Washington, Triage,

[7] For an in-depth discussion of the ways in which the reviewed projects varied on these dimensions of the generic case management model, see Greenberg, Austin, and Doth (1981).

TABLE 15-2. GENERIC CASE MANAGEMENT MODEL TAKEN FROM LONG TERM CARE DEMONSTRATION PROJECTS

Phase of Work with Clients	Sources of Variation
Intake and inquiry	Networks of referrals
	Sources of referrals
	Criteria for initial referral
	Responsibility for prescreening
Assessment	Timing
	Instruments
	Organizational location
	Who performs the assessment? individual or team with what professional training
Determination of eligibility	Program eligibility
	Target-group eligibility
	Methods for assessing the client's risk and need
Care planning	Who performs care planning? individual or team professional training
	Organizational location
	Relationship to assessment
	Rules for making decisions about care planning
Provision of services and follow-up	Who implements the plan? do they interface with those responsible for care planning? do they interface with those responsible for assessment?
	What services are provided?
	What services are purchased?
	Responsibility for monitoring

Source: Adapted from Greenberg, J., Austin, C. D., & Doth, D. 1981. *Comparative Study of Long Term Care Demonstrations: Lessons for Future Inquiry.* Minneapolis: University of Minnesota, Center for Health Services Research.

ACCESS, Georgia, On Lok, and 222 Demonstrations) had the potential to alter the flow of funding for long term care, and thereby change the character of their local delivery systems.[8] A review of the experiences of the long term care demonstrations concluded that most projects had no significant effect on

[8] The demonstrations reviewed included projects operating with "1115" waivers in the Medical Assistance program or "222" waivers in the Medicare program. (Enabling legislation of the Social Security Act permits 1115 and 222 waivers that allow experimentation and documentation projects to occur.)

their delivery systems because the projects did not possess the requisite authority. Future demonstration projects should be designed to influence local service delivery systems, and in evaluating their effects on the systems, it will be important to consider the amount of authority that is built into the projects. Greenberg, Austin, and Doth have identified two dimensions of such authority to be scope and span, which are discussed later in the article on p. 25 (Greenberg, Austin, & Doth, 1981).

Although a project's scope and span of authority are important dimensions in the service delivery system for long term care, authority alone is not enough to shape the market behavior of providers, which must be reinforced with incentives and sanctions. The demonstration projects reviewed in this study did not have potent financial incentives or sanctions and instead had to rely on informal influence, persuasion, and voluntary cooperation from the diverse providers of long term care in their local areas.[9]

CASE MANAGEMENT

The distinction made by Greenberg, Austin, and Dorth between interventions at the client and at the system levels in long term care demonstrations is somewhat artificial. Its purpose is to highlight the complex task facing demonstration projects that are attempting to accomplish change in patterns of service delivery at several levels simultaneously. In reality, conditions within a local service delivery system have significant consequences for clients, such that the system level and the client level are never autonomous. Case management models can alter the character of the local delivery system by filling gaps in the continuum of care, by increasing the volume of scarce services, or by controlling access to high-cost services.

Case management has greater potential to influence the character of service-delivery at the system level than has been demonstrated to date. Beatrice asserts,

> The purpose of case management inherently implies provider change. Reducing the skewing toward institutional service guarantees that both the noninstitutional and institutional-market segments will be affected. Case management functions as a long term care policy option only if these changes are effectuated over time. Therefore, successful case management, by definition, alters provider organization. (Beatrice, 1981, p. 156)

This means that case management could be a useful tool for moving away from institutional dominance in long term care.

---

[9] For a description of the variety of approaches that can be taken to design long term-care demonstrations with increased authority and financial incentives, see Greenberg, Austin, and Doth (1981).

Screening, assessment, and care planning are tasks that are routinely identified as core case management activities. Effective and efficient targeting of client populations is the objective of screening.[10] Assessment is a comprehensive data-collection effort, designed to identify and accurately report clients' functional capacity, social supports, living arrangements, level of disability, and economic dependence. Care planning—essentially, translating assessment information into a service plan for the client—entails making a set of decisions that produces a package of services. Fundamentally, developing a care plan is a resource allocation process involving a range of decisions about how many of what kinds of services a client will receive from which service providers.[11] A case manager, with responsibility for developing care plans involving multiple providers in a local delivery system, is operating as a resource allocator, and case management can be designed to enhance the manager's authority for this task. The resource dependence view of interorganizational relationships discussed earlier provides a useful perspective for understanding how case management can be structured to affect providers' market behavior through resource allocation.

RESOURCE ALLOCATION

Two categories of variables appear to affect the ability of a case manager to shape the market behavior of provider agencies through resource allocation. One category is the nature of the local delivery system in which the case manager operates, and the other is the degree of authority and control given to the case manager. These are summarized in Table 15-3.

It is important to remember that case managers function within an ongoing delivery system and that characteristics of local networks of services vary from one community to another. Because of this variation, no single model of case management will work in every delivery system. To develop the appropriate model for a particular system, planners must assess the system's comprehensiveness (How complete is the continuum of care? What gaps exist?), its bias (How sharply is the system skewed toward institutionally based long term care?), its complexity (How dense is the population of providers? How much duplication and overlapping of service delivery exist in the system?), and its quality (How high is the quality of care and of service provision?). The case management model ultimately implemented in any local network of services

[10] For a discussion of the distinction between effective and efficient targeting, see Fredrick W. Seidl, Kevin Mahoney, and Carol D. Austin, 1978. Providing and evaluating home care: Issues of targeting. Paper presented at the Thirty-first Annual Scientific Meeting of the Gerontological Society, Dallas, TX, November.

[11] For a discussion of the service allocation process within the organizational context of provider agencies, see Carol D. Austin, 1981. Client assessment in context, *Social Work Research and Abstracts,* 17 (Spring), pp. 4–12.

TABLE 15-3. VARIABLES AFFECTING CASE MANAGERS' CAPACITY TO SHAPE THE MARKET BEHAVIOR OF PROVIDERS

Variables	Sources of Variation
Delivery Systems	
Capacity of the system	Completeness Bias Complexity Quality
Service providers' control over critical resources	Referrals Assessment data
Case Management	
Discretion over allocation and use of critical resources	Span of authority Scope of authority Financial incentives
Centralization of control of resources	Fragmented funding Financial reform

will be a product of that network's characteristics and the functions case management is intended to perform.[12]

A second significant characteristic of the delivery system is the providers' power to resist case management controls. That power revolves around control of the critical resources: clients, information, and funding. The case manager's control over providers' market behavior may be limited by the extent to which case managers are dependent on providers for appropriate referrals and assessment data. If identification of clients and assessment are decentralized to a variety of locations in the community and performed by staff of provider agencies, case managers will depend on those agencies for clients and information.[13] A more centralized case management system with a single point of entry would minimize the power of service providers to resist case management controls. Because providers can be expected to try to protect whatever power they possess in dealing with case managers, centralization is a key issue.[14]

In addition to the issues of control of referrals to clients and of information, the case manager's discretion over the allocation and use of funding is key and will fundamentally affect his or her capacity to change providers' behavior. The case manager's degree of discretion over the allocation of funds is made up of three elements: span of authority, scope of authority, and financial incentives (Greenberg, Austin, & Doth, 1981). To define this term, span of authority refers to the width of the range of services over which the

[12] For a thorough discussion of the contingencies of locale, see Beatrice (1981).

[13] Greenberg, Austin, and Doth (1981) discuss variations in organizational location of screening, assessment, care planning, and service provision and monitoring.

[14] For an examination of an option for service delivery of long term care that maximizes centralization (the single agency approach), see Callahan (1981a).

case manager has control. A wide span would entail the authority to allocate funds for acute care, home care, and nursing home care, for example. Case managers operating with the widest span would control allocation of all funds available to members of a specific population from a variety of different sources (for example, Titles XVIII, XIX, and XX of the Social Security Act and Title III of the Older Americans Act).

Scope of authority in the allocation of funds refers to the breadth of impact the case manager has in different portions of the delivery system (for instance, the manager's influence on, access to, and use of funds for nursing home services and acute care). Case managers operating with a broad scope would control funds, for example, for prior authorization, preadmission screening, discharge planning from hospitals, and follow-up of clients admitted to nursing homes. These mechanisms enhance the case manager's ability to target services to identified subpopulations of clients effectively and efficiently by controlling access to and use of high-cost services. Case managers with a narrow scope would only control funds to monitor the development of service plans and contracts with providers.

Case management can be designed to use financial incentives and sanctions to produce desired market behavior of providers and to change characteristics of the market. Such incentives might be used to develop services missing in the local continuum of care. Sanctions that would serve as cost-control measures would include target budgets, limits on budgets for individual clients, or ceilings on budgets for specified catchment areas. Capitation of service costs (a system of prepaid fixed costs for services) is another cost-containment mechanism.

The extent to which case managers have discretion over the allocation of resources is closely related to the degree to which control of the resources is centralized. In the current system of fragmented funding, case managers are likely to control only a portion of the resources for any given client. Medicare and Medicaid waivers—like those operating in some of the long term care demonstrations discussed earlier—were necessary to create a pool of funds that case managers could control. Fragmented funding in a fee-for-service system allows providers to charge the costs of services received by eligible clients directly to those programs for which the client is eligible. This makes it difficult to contain costs. Case managers could control use of and access to services if they had the authority to say who gets served through mechanisms such as prior authorization and preadmission screening.

An expansion of the case management role to emphasize resource allocation and "gatekeeping" is not without potential dilemmas. This aspect of case management may cause unmanageable strain by asking the case managers to both advocate for and possibly deny services to their clients. Callahan suggests that a Professional Standards Review Organization (PSRO) might be a more appropriate gatekeeper of allocations for long term care (Callahan, 1981b). The tenuous current status of PSROs, however, may make this system of agencies an unlikely choice. Furthermore, case managers, many of whom are human services generalists at the bachelor's level, may not command enough respect in their local communities to perform authoritative gatekeeping tasks. Will health care and social services professionals accept case managers' decision about the authorization of services and scope of service delivery? Planning for care, the basic set of resource allocation decisions, has often been the responsibility of an interdisciplinary team composed of representatives of professional groups providing long term care. Case managers will still need the authority necessary to implement plans for care. The extent to which different people or agencies are responsible for planning and implementing care will remain an important variable in designing the case management function.

Several analysts have cautioned against having high expectations for effective case-level coordination in the absence of coordination of programs and resources (Aiken et al., 1975; Agranoff, 1979; Callahan, 1981a). Although many agree that a fundamental restructuring of policies and programs is necessary to eliminate the fragmentation and duplication with which case management deals, it is unclear whether federal and state policymakers will improve the coordination of programs and resources. By itself, however, case management will achieve only limited reform if it continues to concentrate solely on case-level coordination.

"CHANNELING" DEMONSTRATION PROJECTS

The most recent federal initiatives in research on service delivery for long term care are known as the National Long Term Care Channeling Demonstration Projects. They are being implemented at demonstration sites at the county level across the country. The channeling demonstrations are based on the idea that it is necessary to direct clients to a set of services that meet their assessed needs more appropriately. These projects are experimenting with a variety of approaches to organizing and coordinating services and structuring funding through case management.

The National Long Term Care Channeling Demonstration Projects fall into two groups—basic and complex. Basic channeling models provide case-level coordination (case management) and will have some control over social services funding (such as funds for community services block grants and Title III of the Older Americans Act). Channeling projects can engage in minimal expansion of services but will receive no additional funding. Under basic channeling, case management emphasizes the activities at the client level (outreach, screening, assessment, planning for care, arranging for services, follow-up, monitoring, and reassessment) (Gottesman, 1981).[15]

[15] Basic channeling was implemented in Middlesex County, New Jersey; eight rural counties in eastern Kentucky; Baltimore, Maryland; Houston, Texas; and an urban/rural site in Maine.

Channeling models that are complex are being developed and may provide an opportunity to experiment with a broader notion of case management.[16] Complex channeling projects present an opportunity to test an approach to case management that includes authority for resource allocation in which case managers have some leverage with service providers. Inclusion in the complex channeling projects of mechanisms (such as prior authorization and preadmission screening) that control access to high-cost services, budgets that place spending limits on services for individual clients or catchment areas, or protocols that attempt to standardize decision making for care planning would provide valuable experience for reforms of long term care.

IMPLICATIONS FOR SOCIAL WORKERS

There is consensus among social workers that one of the difficulties in the service delivery for long term care has been the "medicalization" of social needs. This trend has occurred primarily because funds for health care (largely under Medical Assistance funding) have been more readily available than support for social services. Nevertheless, it is important for the public to remember that many of the services that help to maintain the elderly in the community are supportive social services. It will become increasingly apparent as society continues to explore ways to provide alternatives to nursing home care that the expertise of social workers is essential in the development of services that address elderly people's social needs. Psychosocial assessment and evaluation of the strengths of existing informal support systems—crucial components of individualized care planning—are core social work skills. There are identifiable points in the case management process in assessment and in care planning in which this expertise is required.

This article has presented the thesis that care planning (the translation of assessment information into a package of services) is a process of resource allocation (a set of decisions that distribute funds to various providers in local delivery systems). The author has suggested that practitioners who make decisions about care planning can change providers' market behavior, stimulate the development of new programs, and alter the distribution of funding. Care planning provides an opportunity for social workers to operate as change agents in their local communities by developing case management for the elderly. Social work professionals bring needed expertise in the form of their assessment skills and bring important knowledge about how to change the system through program development, exercising influence, and creative plan-

---

[16] Complex channeling was implemented in Miami, FL; Philadelphia, PA; Greater Lynn, MA; Rensselaer County, NY; and Cuyahoga County (Cleveland), OH. Current plans call for the complex channeling projects to include a Medicare Waiver (222), a means test, cost sharing with participants, and case management.

ning. If the provision of services is to move from a narrowly medical approach to long term care toward a perspective that more accurately addresses elderly people's needs for social services, social workers will have to play a central role in the future development of community-based long term care.

As resource allocators, community-based case managers may find themselves in conflict with other professionals in thier local areas. Hospital-based social workers, particularly those with responsibility for discharge planning, may resist efforts to centralize assessment and care planning. This may be a particular problem when the expertise of community case managers who are generalists in human services is questioned by experienced practitioners with weightier professional credentials who are working in community agencies. What productive courses of action are open to social workers in these circumstances?

First, it is useful to view case management as a phased process (intake and inquiry, assessment, determination of eligibility, care planning, and provision of services and follow-up). In this way it is possible to identify which parts of the process require the expertise of social workers and which do not. For example, it might be productive for social workers to attempt to influence the way assessment and care planning are developed and implemented and allow those case managers who are community-based to have more direct control over other management tasks. Second, social workers can assist in planning the development of resources for community-based long term care by identifying gaps in the existing continuum of care in their communities and by designing creative programs to fill those gaps. Third, social work practitioners need to monitor the design and implementation of case management activities to make sure that clients' interests are being addressed. It is possible that case management procedures can operate in a manner that denies services to needy clients or that creates additional barriers for clients in gaining access to the delivery system. Concerns for cost containment need to be balanced by an awareness of the need to protect vulnerable individuals and ensure equity in decisions about care planning. Providing the full continuum of care means offering social service programs that maximize independence for the aged. Now and in the future, social workers in health care need to move into positions in which they influence the development of policy for long term care, program design, and decision making—areas in which they can make valuable contributions.

CONCLUSION

Case management in programs for the elderly has focused on the interactions between the case manager and the client. This has obscured the fact that care planning is crucial to resource allocation in a local delivery system. A view of interorganizational relationships that emphasizes their interdependence on resources is a useful perspective for analyzing the capacity of case managers to change market conditions by altering the behavior of service providers. If the capacity of case managers to act as change agents is to be expanded, control of resources must be centralized and managers must be given more discretion.

Case management has been described as a middle-ground option for policy reform of long term care. Its implementation does not require fundamental changes in funding patterns for interorganizational relationships. Perhaps this is why it is so widely accepted, particularly when its major emphasis has been on coordination at the case level. The middle ground in which case management can be developed as a reform option is broader, however, than present experience suggests. Models that expand case management to include authority for resource allocation and implementation of financial incentives to influence market conditions deserve greater attention.

REFERENCES

Agranoff, R. 1979. *Dimensions of Service Integration,* no. 13. Rockville, MD: Project Share, April.

Aiken, M., et al. 1975. *Coordinating Human Services: New Strategies for Building Service Delivery Systems.* San Francisco: Jossey-Bass.

Beatrice, D. F. 1981. Case management: A policy for long term care, In J. J. Callahan & S. S. Wallack (Eds.), *Reforming the Long-Term-Care System: Financial and Organizational Options.* Lexington, MA: D.C. Health & Co., Lexington Books.

Callahan, J. J. 1981a. Single agency options for long term care. In J. J. Callahan & S. S. Wallack (Eds.), *Reforming the Long-Term-Care System: Financial and Organizational Options,* Lexington, MA: D. C. Heath & Co., Lexington Books.

Callahan, J. J., Jr. 1981b. Delivery of services to persons with long term care needs. In J. Meltzer, F. Farrow, & H. Richman (Eds.), *Policy Options in Long Term Care.* Chicago: University of Chicago Press.

Callahan, J. J., Jr., & Wallack, S. S. (Eds.). 1981. *Reforming the Long-Term-Care System: Financial and Organizational Options.* Lexington, MA: D. C. Heath & Co., Lexington Books.

Case Coordination with the Elderly: The Experience of Front Line Practitioners. 1979. Proceedings and summary of findings from a symposium held January 20–22, 1979. Los Angeles: University of Southern California, Andrus Gerontology Center, February.

Complete Case Coordination Bibliography. 1978. Los Angeles: University of Southern California, Andrus Gerontology Center.

Downing, R. 1979. *Three Working Papers: An Exploration of Case Manager Roles: Coordinator, Advocate and Counselor; Issues of Client Assessment in Coordination Programs; Client Pathway.* Los Angeles: University of Southern California, Andrus Gerontology Center, March.

Gottesman, L. D. 1981. Client level functions of the long term care demonstration: The base intervention. Philadelphia: Temple University Institute on Aging, April. (Photocopied.)

Greenberg, J. Austin, C. D., & Doth, D. 1981. *A Comparative Study of Long Term*

Care Demonstrations: Lessons for Future Inquiry. Minneapolis: University of Minnesota, Center for Health Services Research.

Levine, S. & White, P. E. 1961. Exchange as a conceptual framework for the study of interorganizational relationships. *Administrative Science Quarterly.* 5.

Lynn, Jr., L. E. 1976. Organizing human services in Florida. *Evaluation.* 3(1, 2):58–78.

Meltzer, J., Farrow, F., & Richman, H. 1981. *Policy Options in Long Term Care.* Chicago: University of Chicago Press.

Mittenthall, S. D. 1976. A system approach to human services integration. *Evaluation.* 3(1, 2):142–148.

Morrill, W. A. 1976. Services integration and the Department of Health, Education and Welfare. *Evaluation.* 3(1, 2):52–57.

1979–80 National Directory of Case Coordination Programs for the Elderly. 1980. Los Angeles: University of Southern California, Andrus Gerontology Center.

Pfeffer, J., & Salancik, G. R. 1978. *The External Control of Organizations: A Resource Dependence Perspective.* New York: Harper & Row, p. 281.

Steinberg, R. M. 1978. Case service coordination: Senior center issues. Paper presented at the Annual Conference of the National Council on Aging, Los Angeles, CA.

Steinberg, R. M. 1979. *Area Agencies on Aging: Case Study of a Controversial Purchase of Service Contract.* Los Angeles: University of Southern California, Andrus Gerontology Center.

Steinberg, R. M. (Ed.). 1979. *Case Coordination and Service Integration Projects: Client Impact, Program Survival and Research Priorities.* Three papers delivered at the National Conference on Social Welfare, Los Angeles, May 1978. Los Angeles: Andrus Gerontology Center, University of Southern California.

Steinberg, R. M. & Carter, G. W. 1982. *Case Management and the Elderly: A Handbook for Planning and Administering Programs.* Lexington, MA: D.C. Heath & Co., Lexington Books.

Thompson, J. D. 1967. *Organizations in Action.* New York: McGraw Hill.

Yuchtman, E., & Seashore, S., 1967. A system resource approach to organizational effectiveness. *American Sociological Review.* 32:891–903.

CHAPTER 16

Case Management

Ethical Pitfalls on the Road to High-Quality Managed Care

Rosalie A. Kane

Case management in long term care (LTC) has proliferated without full agreement about its appropriate definition, purpose, auspices, or authority. Nevertheless, a consensus is emerging in favor case management, not only in LTC for the elderly, but also in programs serving other populations (e.g., the chronically mentally ill or the developmentally disabled) and in comprehensive programs that deliver both acute care and LTC to the elderly on a capitated basis.

The current enthusiasm for case management may be justified by outcomes for those served. Under the proper circumstances, case management can be a powerful tool to improve the quality of care and the fairness and appropriateness of its allocation. But safeguards and adequate forethought are necessary to ensure that managed care meets often subtle ethical challenges. This article suggests a framework for examining the ethical issues raised by case management.

In the vague language of the 1980 Budget Reconciliation Act (which permitted states to apply for Medicaid waivers to offer a broad array of community-based LTC services, with case management at the top of the list), case management is coordination of a specific group of services on behalf of a specific group of people. Case management can also be defined by listing its component processes. By widespread agreement, these processes include screening or case finding; comprehensive, multidimensional assessment; care planning; implementation of the plan; monitoring; and reassessment (at regular intervals to restart the process and as requested by both client and care providers). Case management often also includes authority to purchase services for the client, authorize third-party reimbursement, and/or establish eligibility for public entitlements based on the client's functional impairments (Austin, 1985).

ADVOCACY VERSUS RESOURCE CONTROL

Case management represents a convergence of two distinctive approaches to improving care. One approach stresses client advocacy; the other emphasizes resource allocation. The first position holds that users of health care—particularly the vulnerable elderly and disabled in the midst of a health crisis—need skilled and specialized help to find the resources that match their needs. Thus, a case manager does a detailed assessment of those needs, clarifies the range of options, explains the mysteries of fragmented public entitlements, helps the client and family make a decision, and acts as an advocate in helping the client find affordable services of adequate quality. The roots of these approaches are deep in the traditional perspectives of social work, public health nursing, and other helping professions—so much so that some skeptics claim that not much is new about case management. Arguably, case management has been and is performed by hospital social workers at discharge, by nurse coordinators of home health agencies, and by a host of others.

A second perspective on case management stems from a variety of efforts to allocate services appropriately in a community, use resources wisely for those most in need, document inadequacies of total resources for planning purposes, and introduce systemwide incentives to improve the quality of all care providers in the community. Case managers with this perspective generally are found in positions where they can exert real control over resources, for example, in community-based LTC programs funded by Medicaid waivers (Kemper et al., 1986), in capitated, prepaid health care systems such as health maintenance organizations with enriched LTC components (Leutz et al., 1985), and in private LTC insurance (Meiners, 1982). Such case managers are sometimes considered "gatekeepers" to care programs.

At first blush, a gatekeeper is at variance with an advocate. A gatekeeper controls entry to programs and intensity of service within them, whereas an advocate strives to gain the most for each client. An extreme position in favor of the pure advocacy role conceives the case manager as a broker, whose ethical obligations are solely directed toward the functionally impaired client. Indeed, a brisk cottage industry of private, fee-for-service case management has sprung up, particularly in retirement areas, to provide just this type of attention and advocacy to those who can afford it (Secord, 1987).

The first ethically tinged question to be resolved, then, is whether it is possible for a case manager to simultaneously serve as an advocate for a client or patient and as an agent of "the system." If one takes the position that this dual stance is impossible, one either develops procedures to ensure that each client has an independent case manager as adviser, or one abandons, as a fiction, the idea that case managers with control over resources can truly be client advocates.

Fortunately, the role of advocate and the role of gatekeeper can be reconciled ethically as long as the case management program is designed to serve an entire population at risk with a finite set of resources. In that case, the community of actual and potential LTC users in a geographic area or a defined population group is the clientele. The case manager becomes an advocate for identifying and meeting the needs of the entire group fairly and well, as well as for meeting the needs of any given individual. Moreover, even case managers with no gatekeeping authority face the problem of mixed loyalties whenever their advocacy extends to the well-being of the client's family. [Conflict of interest most likely occurs in situations where a fee-for-service case manager is hired and paid by a family member to manage the case of an elderly relative (Bermel, 1986).]

The difficulties of balancing advocacy and gatekeeping challenge the case manager, often contributing to stress and uncertainty in the job. Arguably, however, no irreconcilable ethical problem prevents this model of service. Moreover, as will become apparent from the remainder of this article, severe conflicts of interest can emerge when case managers are also service providers rather than relatively disinterested allocators of service.

AUTONOMY VERSUS BENEFICENCE

Biomedical ethics, particularly in the United States, has been preoccupied with reconciling the principle of autonomy—that is, the right of persons to be protected from unwanted force or interference—and the principles of beneficence or nonmaleficence—that is, the moral obligation to do good and not do harm (Childress, 1982; Englehardt, 1986; Gorovitz, 1982). The principle of autonomy obliges case managers to refrain from interfering with decisions that competent persons make about their own lives unless those decisions harm others. The principles of beneficence and nonmaleficence oblige case managers to act in the best interest of the clients.

Regardless of whether the case manager has a mixed gatekeeping/advocacy role or a pure advocacy role, the reconciliation of autonomy and beneficence creates ethical dilemmas. These are similar in kind to those faced in clinical care by physicians, nurses, social workers, and others who struggle to balance their professional judgment about what is good for the patient with respect for the patient's autonomy. The case management function introduces some new and subtle elements to this familiar problem.

Autonomy

Case management is fraught with dangers to the client's autonomy, some inherently perplexing and others resolvable by conscious informed-consent procedures and other autonomy-enhancing processes.

Many autonomy issues arising in case management are not limited to that function but occur in all work with the elderly in LTC. Among the intractable but rather generic problems is the issue of deciding when a person is competent to make various types of decisions. Most LTC users who are said to be impaired in decision making have not undergone a judicial process to establish legal competence. Indeed, such a process may not even serve the best interest of the functionally impaired person; legal competence is an either-or-attribute, whereas decisional capacity is relative to the type of decision that needs to be made and the fluctuating abilities of the patient (Collopy, 1986). In LTC, there is an ever-present danger that patients are discounted as competent decision makers merely because they judge the situation differently from the professionals. A case manager may view a patient's risk taking or refusal of professional advice as evidence of incompetence, whereas to the patient, it represents a conscious, rational choice.

Another difficult issue is balancing the autonomy of family members who care for the frail elderly with the autonomy of the functionally impaired persons themselves. A client may adamantly prefer living in the community, but exercise of this autonomous choice may impose heavy constraints on a spouse or adult offspring (Frankfather, Smith, & Caro, 1981). Case managers with control over resources typically cannot authorize expenditures in the community that are higher than the cost of nursing home care for the same person. The more impaired the client's functioning, the more likely that a plan of community care will engage clients in expressing preferences and making their own trade-offs. Arguably, however, the policy could also increase costs by promoting a belief that each client *should* use the maximum allowable dollars in a given time period.

Beneficence

Deciding when and to what extent a case manager should set aside the principle of autonomy is difficult. Once a principle of beneficence is acknowledged, even greater difficulties arise. If case managers are to do good, they must be able to choose the good course of action accurately. But what is good for a functionally impaired person? Is it even possible to reach a hierarchy of "the good" that ranks, say, physical well-being and safety? Is it better to seek present benefits of increased freedom of movement and independence at the risk of increased future disability and dependence—for example, as the result of a fall? Can a ranking of the good be developed to apply to all clients of a program, or must the preferences of each individual client be consulted? The

LTC field is replete with unresolved dilemmas because little public dialogue has taken place regarding how outcomes should be valued (Kane & Kane, 1983).

Then, too, the beneficent case manager would need to develop a hierarchy of good that ranks the well-being of the client (whatever priorities are given to the facets of well-being) with the well-being of spouses, adult children, and other relatives. What if the values traded off are the contentment of the client versus the economic interests of the family member? The beneficent case manager might also wish to consider the taxpayer's interests. Perhaps the case manager would act differently on behalf of a well-to-do client compared to one whose care plan is implemented at public expense.

JUSTICE AND CASE MANAGEMENT

Thus far, the discussion has largely revolved around the ethical principles of autonomy and beneficence. A third important principle concerns justice. For case management, this includes fair decisions about who needs care, fair allocation of benefits and services (including the use of the case manager's time), and equitable ways to resolve disputes.

Just Use of Resources

In large-scale case management programs, resources are typically limited. The case manager is expected to contain program costs by controlling clients' access to services, particularly high-cost services. If decision rules are routinely applied to the client assessment data to determine the care plans, then the decisions will be fair in the sense that an exact translation is made from disability to service. But care planning by rote is likely to drive up costs while driving out flexible, innovative, client-centered plans. When left to their own imagination, clients will find ways to involve neighbors or nearby restaurants in providing care, sustenance, or transportation. Similarly, clients may find a "live-in" arrangement that (because of room and board considerations) would cost no more than a much less intensive service purchased from an agency.

In the interest of fairness, case managers puzzle over whether it is appropriate to acquiesce to clients' wishes for a particular form of care not only if the net result is greater costs but also if the likelihood of quality control is less. They also worry that the more demanding clients receive a disproportionate amount of service.

Some case managers have been accustomed to calculating costs carefully and interpreting cost constraints directly to clients. Some case management programs generate profiles of patient costs so that case managers can compare typical resource consumption among persons with comparable disability levels. In the view of one program administrator, such profiles prevent "a particularly demanding or a particularly likeable client from acquiring excessive services to the detriment of the program as a whole" (Coale, 1985). Along those lines, one might even argue that effective and fair advocacy as well as gatekeeping requires use of modern information technology to determine who is getting what from the common pot.

Once high-cost clients are identified, case managers find themselves on ethical thin ice. Typically, the case manager may discuss these costs with the client. The client may be told that although costs can temporarily rise above the norms, the situation cannot continue indefinitely. If the costs at home exceed the costs of a nursing home, the client may be urged to consider relocating. The major difficulty occurs when the client refuses the nursing home. At this juncture, some case managers would withdraw home-based services entirely because of an unwillingness to be responsible for a service plan that is less intense than they consider necessary. Other case managers would leave to the client the decision about whether to persist at home with less than optimal service and whether to take the associated risks. (Arguably, after all, a move to a nursing home is not risk free to the client, even though the case manager is less likely to consider those risks in advance or learn about the outcomes afterward.)

Clearly, case managers should not impose their own views of acceptable risk on clients and families. But what are a case manager's rights when he or she cannot in good conscience accede to the plan the client prefers? Does the case manager have a duty to refer the case to another case manager? If several case managers and their supervisors agree that the client's choices are dangerous to self or society, is this a test of truth?

Case Finding versus Serving Current Caseload

Case finding—that is, identifying from a larger population those who need services—is one of the functions of case management. A question arises about how to distribute resources between promoting the program and screening potential clients in contrast to arranging services. Money spent in case finding can be well spent if it permits preventive actions that minimize later problems. Case finding also is consistent with an obligation to identify the extent of need. Arguably, even if all needs cannot be met, the information forms the basis for reallocation of resources at a higher administrative level.

The problem is determining how far a program should go in case finding. Is it ethical, for example, to stop accepting new clients for a period in order to catch up on monitoring and reassessment of current clients? When this was done in Vancouver, British Columbia, for a citywide LTC program, case managers identified substantial numbers of clients served at too high a level and, thus, theoretically freed resources to be used to serve new enrollees better (Kane & Kane, 1985). Logical as it sounds, however, curtailing intake is a drastic step for a community program.

Potential Conflicts of Interest

Many agencies sense that case management is a growing market. Indeed, a diverse cast of organizations is doing case management. Agencies often argue against a "single-entry," case-managed system—that is, a system requiring that all those seeking subsidized community care apply to or be referred to a single agency, such as the local health department or the local area agency on aging, for assessment and ongoing case management. Often, community agencies prefer viewing case management as a reimbursable service that can be offered equally resonably by a number of agencies and that can be purchased by public programs.

In a middle position, some argue for separating gatekeeping from the clinical functions (e.g., assessment and care planning) and the advocacy functions. In such a scheme, there could still be a single point of accountability, but the case managers, acting as gatekeepers, would rely on data supplied by contracting agencies to determine initial eligibility and to approve changes in service plans. If multiple agencies perform case management in a given community, however, this ironically introduces duplication and fragmentation into a service that is expected to be a unifying and rationalizing force.

Public policy probably should not prevent any agency from offering a service it perceives as necessary and that it can finance from fees or charitable contributions. On the other hand, it may be irresponsible for those that finance programs to delegate the case management and, with it, the allocation of services. Most important, a conflict of interest is possible when agencies that provide services also do the assessments of need for service and make care plans. This encourages case managers to identify a need for the services their own organization provides and to direct toward their agency the most desirable or profitable clients.

COMPETENCE AND CASE MANAGEMENT

Standards for Case Management

Ethical practice must, at the least, meet standards of competence. A case management program is unethical if it permits case managers to be derelict in their duties or to function without adequate training or skill. Here we encounter the difficulty that no particular standard has been established for case management. Anyone can set himself or herself up as a private case manager, and agencies have widely varying hiring practices and expectations for performance. Moreover, a credentialing approach to standard setting (e.g., insistence that all case managers be qualified social workers or nurses) would hardly guarantee competence but would definitely raise costs.

Competence in case management is better defined by the ability to perform the tasks required and, eventually, by the outcomes achieved, rather than by arbitrary training requirements. For the sake of discussion, the following abilities and attitudes might be expected of case managers:

Knowledge about services in the community, including both the range of available services and the quality of different providers.

Technical skill in conducting a comprehensive assessment of a client's functioning and social well-being, including the ability to discern when more specialized assessments are needed (e.g., from a geriatric physician, a psychiatrist, a lawyer, or a home inspector).

Commitment to improving the inherent capabilities of clients when possible, which in turn means undertaking the more time-consuming and difficult task of trying to rehabilitate and improve functioning when possible rather than offering services to compensate for a remediable impairment.

Ability to anticipate the likely costs of care and to keep an accurate, ongoing record of actual costs. Especially when a maximum amount may be expended annually, the case manager has a duty to the client not to squander resources; competence includes an ability for sound economic planning.

Prompt attention to referrals, requests for information, monitoring, and reassessment. The program may have a computerized system to aid in tracking the caseload, but the individual case manager must be well-enough organized to use it.

This list represents a beginning only. Other capabilities could be proposed, and eventually all structural and process criteria retained should be associated with desirable outcomes for the clients. It will also be desirable over time to develop a standard range of case management so that each case manager need not invent the response to common situations and so that the adequacy of the case manager can be audited. Schneider, in particular, has advocated such procedural guidelines to answer questions about the desirable case management response to circumstances such as a client on six or more medications who is not under regular medical care or a moderately confused client who lives alone (Schneider, in press). Although one must guard against becoming rigid or rule bound, some guidelines to "good practice" would surely be helpful to case managers.

Monitoring the Quality of Care Plans

Along with case finding, assessment, and care planning, monitoring care is one of the functions of case management. Although potentially an important force for improving the overall quality of care, monitoring is one of the least well-specified aspects of case management. Even the frequency of desirable monitoring is unclear, let alone the type of verification the case managers should seek to assure themselves of the adequacy of service. At the minimum, the case manager should know that the services ordered are delivered reliably, but beyond that they surely have some obligation to monitor the quality of the services they plan. Case management programs vary in the degree to which the case manager attempts to maintain a personal relationship with the client. But one can also ask whether case managers can be effective in monitoring care unless they enjoy a relationship of trust with the client.

The agencies contracted by case managers usually bear the legal responsibility for things that go wrong. But what is the moral responsibility of the case manager? How seriously should the client's complaints be taken? What are reasonable precautions for the case managers to take? Should the case manager be expected to monitor with particular vigilance certain types of providers (e.g., nonagency providers) or under certain circumstances [e.g., when the client is in the hospital and thus likely to be subject to hastily formed plans by a new cast of discharge planners (Peters, 1986)]?

A case management program can be a powerful force for improving care in the community, particularly if it enjoys considerable purchasing power and uses that power to gradually exact higher standards from vendors of care. One possibility, however, is that case managers will become so liability conscious that they shy away from flexible care arrangements and insist on purchasing care from agencies so that the liability can be diffused. Yet community care can often be arranged less expensively and more satisfactorily from the consumer's perspective by using other than the established agency vendors. Therefore, it is useful to ask whether the case manager's monitoring responsibility is discharged by contracts with bonded agencies hiring licensed personnel or whether the monitoring function requires direct surveillance of the care.

CONCLUDING NOTE

This article has presented numerous issues and questions and few answers. The discussion has amply illustrated that many technical aspects relating to case managers and management agencies are unsettled. Some might argue that it is premature to focus on ethics in a field that is ill defined and ever changing. Far from being premature, however, early discussion of ethical issues may suggest an appropriate direction for public policies and may even help us determine which models of case management to endorse and which to avoid.

REFERENCES

Austin, C. D., et al. (Eds.). 1985. *Case Management: A Critical Review.* Seattle: University of Washington Long Term Care Gerontology Center.

Bermel, J. 1986. Taking care of mother: When social services become a business. *Hastings Center Report.* 16(2):2–3.

Childress, J. 1982. *Who Should Decide? Paternalism in Health Care*. New York: Oxford University Press.

Coale, C. D. 1985. Care for the elderly: Fiscal accountability in a case management system. In C. D. Austin et al. (Eds.), *Case Management: A Critical Review*. Seattle: University of Washington Long Term Care Gerontology Center.

Collopy, B. 1986. The conceptually problematic concept of autonomy in long term care. (Unpublished manuscript prepared for The Retirement Research Foundation, Chicago.)

Englehardt, T. 1986. *The Foundations of Bioethics*. New York: Oxford University Press.

Frankfather, F., Smith, D., & Caro, F. 1981. *Family Care of the Elderly: Public Initiatives and Private Obligations*. Lexington, MA: DC Heath.

Gorovitz, S. 1982. *Doctors' Dilemmas: Moral Conflicts and Medical Care*. New York: Oxford University Press.

Kane, R. L., & Kane, R. A. (Eds.). 1983. *Values and Long Term Care*. Lexington, MA: DC Heath.

Kane, R. L., & Kane, R. A. 1985. *A Will and a Way: What the United States Can Learn From Canada About Caring for the Elderly*. New York: Columbia University Press.

Kemper, P., et al. 1986. *The Evaluation of the Long Term Care Channeling Demonstration*. Princeton, NJ: Mathematica Policy Inc.

Leutz, W., et al. 1985. *Changing Health Care for an Aging Society: Planning for the Social Health Maintenance Organization*. Lexington, MA: DC Heath.

Meiners, M. 1982. *The State of the Art of Long Term Care Insurance*. Washington, DC: National Center for Health Services Research.

Peters, B. 1986. The ten commandments of case management during hospitalization. In A. O. Pelham & W. F. Clark (Eds.), *Managing Home Care for the Elderly*. New York: Springer.

Schneider, B. in press. Care planning. *Generations*, special issue on case management.

Secord, L. 1987. *Private Case Management for Older Persons and Their Families*. Excelsior, MN: Interstudy.

CHAPTER 17

Family Members as Case Managers

Partnership between the Formal and Informal Support Networks

Marsha Mailick Seltzer
Joann Ivry
Leon C. Litchfield

Sussman (1976) conceptualized two roles families play in the care of the elderly, namely direct and indirect care provider. Contained in the literature are numerous descriptions and analyses of the important contribution made by the family in direct care provider roles (see for example Brody, 1985; Bordy et al., 1978; Lowy, 1983; Shanas & Maddox, 1976). Although the family as indirect care provider has been mentioned in the literature (Silverstone & Burack-Weiss, 1983), this case management function has received considerably less attention despite the fact that it is usually the family who is called upon by the elerdly person to deal with the formal service system and is thus placed in an "interstitial position between the elderly individual and the organization" (Sussman, 1976). The family serves as facilitator, protector, advocate, buffer against the bureaucracy, and source of information about

Support for this research was provided by the Permanent Charities Fund of Boston, the Blanchard Foundation (managed by the Boston Safe Deposit and Trust Company) and the Fox Memorial Fund. The authors wish to gratefully acknowledge the contributions made by Judith Gonyea, Richard Levin, Louis Lowy, and Mildred D. Mailick, who commented of an earlier version of this manuscript and by Rose Ann Ariel, Renee Hecht, Elaine Mittell, Harriet Pearlman, and Kathryn Simmons who collected the data and implemented the demonstration project. An earlier version of this paper was presented at the 38th Annual Scientific Meeting of the Gerontological Society of America, New Orleans, LA, November, 1985.

housing, pensions, medical care and other service options. Although the formal service sector can fulfill all these functions, the history and continuity of a family member's interest in an elderly relative enhances the family's potential to serve as a case manager. Indeed, Lowy (1985) noted that case management (which he calls care management) is the most important care providing function that a family can fulfill on behalf of an elderly relative.

Case management has emerged as a useful strategy with which to respond to a fragmented and complicated service delivery system (Austin, 1981; Brody, 1979; Monk, 1981; Steinberg & Carter, 1983; Wylie & Austin, 1978). Case management is a service coordination mechanism designed to provide multiple services to clients with complex needs. It is an attempt to reach out to clients, promote service awareness, provide a needs assessment, develop a service plan, and finally, ensure that clients receive prescribed services. Among the activities included in the case management function are screening, assessment, care planning, service arrangement, service provision, service monitoring, linkage, and reassessment. The essence of the case management approach is to establish responsibility for the coordination of services within a single locus of control. Service control is retained by the case manager, who acts as consultant and facilitator, integrating and individualizing services and establishing an ongoing personal relationship with the client.

In their review article on case management, Cantor et al. (1981) noted that families are often called upon to plan services on behalf of relatives and to perform other case management functions. Many families, however, are insufficiently aware of community entitlements and resources, and hence require information and training to make them effective consumers and case managers of community services (Silverstein et al., 1985). Schlesinger et al. (1980), Tuzil (1978), and Walz (1975) have noted the need for social service agencies to provide direct training to families in case management. Although the literature is replete with exhortations for professionals to cooperate, collaborate, and coordinate their services with the informal support system, there is little specific guidance on how sharing is to be accomplished. Smyer (1980) observed that currently there is a paucity of information about the best methods of collaboration between the formal and informal service systems.

As a response to the need to form a partnership between the formal and the informal support systems of elderly persons, the Jewish Family and Children's Service of Greater Boston and the Boston University School of Social Work collaborated in a research and demonstration project designed to train family members of elderly persons as case managers. The purpose of this paper is to present findings relevant to the following questions: Can family members be trained to increase their responsibility for the case management of services for their elderly relatives? Can the training of family members in case management be accomplished without increasing costs for the social service agency that conducts the training? Are the service needs of elderly persons adequately met when their case management is provided by family members in partnership with a social worker? What are the characteristics of family members who are most likely to assume case management responsibility for their elderly relatives?

METHOD

Sample

Starting on January 1, 1982, and continuing for 2 full years, all elderly persons who were referred to the Jewish Family and Children's Service, with several exceptions, were invited to participate in the study. The exceptions consisted of individuals requiring information and referral only, emergencies requiring a response within 24 hours, and persons unable to understand the informed consent form.

In total, 264 elderly individuals qualified as appropriate candidates for the study. They were told that if they elected to participate in the study, a family member or close friend of their choice would be interviewed by a social worker and, in some cases, would work with the social worker on case management. Those reluctant to have a family member participate in case management were encouraged not to volunteer for the study. In all, 202 (77%) agreed to participate and were randomly assigned to either the experimental or control groups. Subsequently, 45 cases were dropped from the study due to unavailability of family members (n = 17) or early termination of agency services (n = 28). The final sample consisted of 81 experimental group and 76 control group elderly clients and their designated family members.

As shown in Table 17–1, the two groups did not differ on any of the measures taken at the point of pretest (intake). The elderly clients were predominantly female, Jewish (96.1%), averaged over 80 years of age, and were moderately impaired in health and mental status. Although relatively independent in their personal activities of daily living, they had more difficulty with instrumental activities of daily living. At pre-test (prior to the onset of agency service), these elderly clients received an average of two formal services.

The family members were related to the elderly clients as child (57%), sibling (10%), spouse (6%), other relative (21%), or friend (6%). Their average age was 62. Almost all family members were married and employed in either full- or part-time jobs. In addition, they had very frequent in-person or telephone contact with their elderly relatives, averaging in-person contact once a week and telephone contact several times per week. Case management was not a new function for these family members because they had performed an average of six case management tasks on behalf of their elderly relatives prior to participating in the study.

TABLE 17-1. CHARACTERISTICS OF THE SAMPLE AT PRETEST[a]

	Experimental Group ($n = 81$) Mean	Control Group ($n = 76$) Mean
I. Elderly person		
sex (% female)	90%	79%
age	83.6	82.4
marital status (% married)	22%	28%
income (monthly)	501.2	576.1
health status[b]	3.7	3.8
mental status[c]	3.7	3.8
ADL skills[d]	46.1	45.7
IADL skills[e]	31.5	30.3
educational level completed[f]	1.8	2.0
number of services received at pretest	2.0	2.3
II. Family member		
sex (% female)	70%	64%
age	62.0	61.6
marital status	73%	78%
income (monthly)	2732.9	1978.2
employment status (% currently employed)	66%	61%
frequency of contact with elderly person[g]		
by phone	5.7	5.8
by visit	4.8	5.1
number of case management services performed prior to agency contact	5.7	5.9

[a]The experimental and control groups were compared using two-tailed *t*-tests. There were no significant pretest differences ($p < .05$).
[b]Measured on a 5-point scale with 5 signifying good health.
[c]Measured on a 5-point scale with 5 signifying intact mental function.
[d]Measured on the Barthel Index (Mahoney & Barthel, 1965); scores range from 16 to 64 with 64 signifying totally independent.
[e]Scores range from 14 to 56 with 56 signifying totally independent.
[f]0 = none, 1 = grammar school, 2 = high school, 3 = college, 4 = graduate school.
[g]1 = once/year or less, 2 = several times/yr, 3 = monthly, 4 = several times/month, 5 = weekly, 6 = several times/week, 7 = daily.

Procedures

In both the experimental and control groups, elderly clients and their families received the usual services provided by the agency, including counseling, crisis intervention, and concrete services. All services were provided by master's level social workers. In addition, those families who were assigned to the experimental group received the family-centered training, which was delivered individually through contact between the social workers and the family member. The training program, which has been described in detail elsewhere (Seltzer et al., 1984; Simmons et al., 1985), consisted of four components. First, it was expected that the participating family member, who was identified by the elderly client, would assume responsibility for the performance of at least one new case management task, dictated by the needs of the elderly client, during the course of agency service.

Second, the social worker and family member collaborated on the development of a case management service plan for the elderly client, including allocation of case management tasks between family member and social worker. This plan was to be signed by both the social worker and the family member as an indication of their willingness to share responsibility. There was space on this form to keep track of who performed each task (social worker, family member, elderly client, other) and the status of each task (successfully completed or not).

Third, family members were provided with information on community resources and entitlements in the form of five training booklets specifically developed for the project: *Guide to In-Home Services, Guide to Housing, Day Care, Respite Care and Nursing Homes, Guide to Transportation and Social Opportunities, Guide to Financial Entitlements and Legal Protective Services;* and *Guide to Advocacy.*

Fourth, there was regular contact between social worker and family member via telephone or in-person meetings on a bi-weekly basis or more often. The objectives of systematic contact between the caseworker and the family member were to provide individualized consultation on how to perform assigned case management tasks, to monitor case mangement performance, to provide supportive counseling, and to ensure ongoing assessment of client needs.

Family members in the experimental group were not asked to deliver additional concrete services to their elderly relatives, but rather to increase their involvement in the coordination of such services via case management. Because the family centered intervention was delivered in the form of a training program, experimental group family members were viewed as partners with the social worker. One of the underlying goals of this intervention was to strengthen the partnership relationship between the formal and informal support systems.

Members of the control group were not exposed to any of the four components of the training program. Specifically, there was no minimum expectation of family performance of case management services in the control group. Furthermore, the control group families did not participate in the case management service planning meeting with the social worker and they did not formally review the case management needs of their elderly relative or sign the form which for experimental group family members served as a partnership contact with the social worker. Furthermore, control group families did not receive any of the training booklets. Finally, although the social workers in the experimental group had contact with families at least once every 2 weeks throughout the study, in the control group there was no such minimum frequency of contact and, in fact, they averaged one contact every 5 weeks. Thus, there were substantial differences between the experimental intervention and the services received by the control group.

It should be emphasized that no services were withheld from the control group. Rather, the specific needs of each elderly individual dictated the pattern of service delivered to him or her. As noted earlier, all elderly participants received counseling, professional case management, and concrete services. No attempt was made, however, to formally train family members in the control group to serve as case managers for their elderly relatives.

The purpose of the control group in this study was to provide an indication of how the family members in the experimental group would have functioned if they had not received the training. It is common for families of elderly persons to perform some case management functions without the benefit of any special agency involvement. The control group revealed whether the experimental intervention altered the level of a family member's case management involvement from where it would have been had training not been provided.

Two social workers were assigned to the control group and two to the experimental group, with no mixed caseloads. All data were collected by the social workers themselves. Interrater reliability, as measured by percentage of agreement, was 93%.

Measures

Examination of posttest differences between the experimental and the control groups was focused on three domains of outcome variables: performance of case management tasks by social workers, family members, and elderly persons; duration of service provision; and the extent of unmet service needs of the elderly participants. In addition, three additional sets of posttest comparisons were made between experimental and control groups: the size and level of contact with the informal support network; the elderly participant's level of health and functional abilities; and the elderly participant's residential status as either in noninstitutional or institutional settings. Data were collected about these latter three domains for descriptive purposes and to detect unanticipated positive or negative effects of the experimental intervention. The research of Blenkner et al. (1971) has highlighted the need for monitoring unanticipated consequences of social gerontological interventions.

The three domains of outcome variables were measured as follows:

Case Management: The extent of case management (CM) performance by social workers, family members, and elderly persons was assessed by ten measures: (1) performance of at least one new CM task by family member; (2) performance of at least one new CM task by elderly person; (3) number of new CM tasks performed by family member; (4) number of new CM tasks performed by social worker; (5) number of new CM tasks performed by elderly person; (6) number of new CM tasks completed by family member; (7) number of new CM tasks completed by social worker; (8) number of new CM tasks completed by elderly person; (9) total number of new CM tasks performed; and (10) total number of new CM tasks completed. The first two measures reflected the minimum level of case management performance. Measures 3, 4, 5, and 9 reflected the number of case management tasks which family members, elders, and social workers agreed to perform. Measures 6, 7, 8, and 10 indicated the success of case management performance by each of these individuals as defined by satisfactory task completion prior to agency termination of service to the client. New case management tasks were defined as those which were not being performed at the time of service initiation by the agency. Those included tasks never performed on behalf of the elderly person and those performed in the past but not at the point of case intake.

Duration of Service: the duration of service was measured by the number of days between case intake and termination of service.

Unmet Service Needs: the extent of unmet service needs of the elderly person was measured by (1) the number of services received by the elderly person at the time of case termination, and (2) the number of unmet service needs as defined by the number of needed services minus number of received services. Judgments about the need for each service category were made by the social worker assigned to the case.

RESULTS

As shown in Table 17–2, the experimental group showed the hypothesized changes for all three dependent variable domains. Family members in the experimental group were significantly more likely to perform at least one case management task than control group family members (88% vs. 62%, respectively). They also performed and completed significantly more case management tasks than those in the control group.

As additional evidence that the training intervention facilitated the sharing of case management responsibility between family member and social worker, the social workers in the experimental group were found to perform significantly fewer case management tasks than those in the control group. Unexpectedly, the elderly clients in the control group were found to be more likely to perform at least one new case management task than those in the experimental group (53% vs. 22%, respectively) and to perform and to complete significantly more case management tasks than those in the experimental group.

There were no differences between the experimental and control groups in the total number of case management tasks performed or completed. Of interest was that the total number of case management tasks actually performed during the intervention period (4.8 tasks for the experimental group and 4.2 for the control group) was greater than the number planned at the

TABLE 17-2. POSTTEST COMPARISONS BETWEEN EXPERIMENTAL AND CONTROL GROUPS (MEAN SCORES AND *t* TESTS)

Case Management (CM)	Experimental (n = 81)	Control (n = 76)
Performance of at least one new CM task—f.m.	0.88	0.62[c]
Performance of at least one new CM task—e.p.	0.22	0.53[c]
No. of new CM tasks performed—f.m.	3.17	1.58[c]
No. of new CM tasks performed—e.p.	0.46	0.88[a]
No. of new CM tasks performed—s.w.	1.99	2.68[a]
No. of new CM tasks completed—f.m.	1.83	1.03[b]
No. of new CM tasks completed—e.p.	0.19	0.55[b]
No. of new CM tasks completed—s.w.	1.25	1.70
Total no. of new CM tasks performed	4.79	4.20
Total no. of new CM tasks completed	3.01	2.67
Days between intake and termination	226.77	305.49[b]
Unmet needs		
No. of services received by the elderly person	2.33	2.95[a]
No. of unmet service needs of the elderly person	0.57	0.93

[a]$p < .05$.
[b]$p < .05$.
[c]$p < .001$.

beginning of service (3.1 tasks in the experimental group and 2.4 tasks for the control group). This increase was largely due to the emergence of newly identified case management needs during the time between the pretest and the posttest, not an uncommon phenomenon for individuals in this stage of life.

The duration of service was significantly shorter for the experimental than for the control group by nearly 80 days per case, on the average. Further, although control group cases received significantly more services than experimental group cases, there was no difference in their number of unmet service needs.

The experimental and control group were also compared with respect to their health, functional abilities, mortality rate, and residential arrangements at posttest to detect any unanticipated effects of the training program. No differences were expected or found in these domains.

Three hierarchical multiple regression analyses were conducted in which the dependent variables were the number of new case management tasks performed by the designated family member, the social worker, and the elderly client, respectively. The same set of independent variables was used in each regression analysis, including five background characteristics of the elderly client (age, sex, health status, mental status, and ADL skills), four background characteristics of the designated family member (age, sex, frequency of visits with the elderly person, and number of case management tasks performed prior to agency contact), and experimental versus control group status. The first nine of these variables were assessed at pretest and were selected because they represented the type of information usually available to health and social service agencies at the point of client referral. These variables possibly could be useful in identifying predictors of case management performance by family member, elderly person, and social worker. By entering the experimental versus control group status variable last into the equation, it was possible to estimate the unique variance associated with participation or nonparticipation in the case management training program.

Together the 10 independent variables explained 39% of the variance (R^2) in the number of case management tasks performed by family members. The two largest predictors were the mental status of the elder and whether the family member was in the experimental or control group (explaining 18% and 9% of the variance, respectively). A low score on the mental status rating and the family member being in the experimental group were associated with more case management performance by the family member. The number of case management tasks performed by family members prior to agency contact explained less than 1% of the variance in the number of case management tasks performed during agency contact. Thus, past experience was considerably less powerful a predictor of case management performance than participation in the training program.

The 10 independent variables accounted for 27% of the variance in the number of case management tasks performed by social workers. Social workers were likely to perform more case management when the family member was older, when the elder had poorer ADL skills, and when there was less contact between the elderly person and the family member. Family participation in the training program was not a significant predictor of social workers' level of case management performance, once all other variables were controlled.

Fully half the explained variance in the number of case management tasks performed by elderly clients on their own behalf was accounted for by the age of the elderly person (10% of the variance), with younger clients found to perform more case management tasks. Not unexpectedly, a higher mental status rating was also predictive of more case management performance by the elderly clients (explaining 4% of the variance).

DISCUSSION

Although the literature contains a number of references to the potential for families of elderly persons to assume case management responsibility on behalf of their elderly relatives, there is little specific information available on the extent to which families actually fulfill this important function. The distribution of case management performance among family members, social worker, and elderly person during a period of formal service provision was described in this study. The control group, in which there was no agency training or elevated expectation for family performance of case management, provided an estimate of the typical level of case management performance by each of these potential partners. Surprisingly, as many as 62% of the control group family members performed at least one new case management task while their elderly relative was receiving service from the agency social worker. The average number of new case management tasks performed by control group family members was 1.6. These tasks were in addition to the 5.6 case management functions that they had performed on behalf of their elderly relatives prior to the beginning of agency service. Thus, the performance of case management seems a normative function for family members of elderly persons, especially when the elders reach their 80's.

The comparison between the level of case management performance in control and experimental group family members gives an indication of the impact of the training intervention. Fully 88% of the experimental group family members performed at least one new case management task during the study period (an increase of 40% over the control group). Furthermore, the average experimental group family member performed twice as many case management tasks as his or her counterpart in the control group. Thus, the training intervention substantially boosted the level of family performance of case management.

As noted earlier, the goal of the family-centered training was to increase the involvement of family members without increasing their responsibility for direct service provision. There was no significant difference between the experimental and control groups in the number of hands-on services they provided at either pretest or posttest. Thus, the case management training program did not have the effect of increasing family responsibility for direct service provision for their elderly relatives. Instead, indirect service provision (i.e., case management) was increased for family members.

A complementary finding was that social workers in the experimental group performed significantly fewer case management tasks than control group social workers, without resulting in a higher level of unmet service needs for the elderly client. Another positive effect of the agency–family partnership was the substantial difference in the duration of agency service between the experimental and control groups, with the experimental clients completing service nearly 80 days earlier than control group clients. Although the agency must assume the responsibility (and the costs) associated with conducting the training program, the shorter duration of services may make the effort worthwhile from a management as well as a service point of view.

The shorter duration of service was not found to impact negatively on clients, as the two groups did not differ in residential status, health, or functional abilities at posttest. It was interesting that the control group elderly clients received significantly more services during the course of agency service than those in the experimental group. In light of the comparability of the two groups in number of unmet service needs, residential status, health status, and functional status, one explanation for the greater number of services received by the control group might be that nonessential services were provided to them during the extra 80 days that they were carried as cases of the agency.

The elderly client in this study, though not a targeted partner in the family-centered intervention, was found to be an active partner in case management. In the control group, fully 53% of the elderly clients performed at least one new case management task during the period of agency service even though there was no special expectation that they should do so. Only 22% of the elders in the experimental group, however, performed at least one new case management task, perhaps because the experimental group social workers' focus on the family member unintentionally resulted in a diminution of the role of the elderly person.

Two points are noteworthy regarding the role of the elderly person in case management. First, whereas some recognition of the role of the family member as case manager in conjunction with the formal service system is contained in the literature, the elderly person as case management partner has received less attention. The need for case management ordinarily arises when a person is no longer able to coordinate services on his or her own behalf. Yet, it may not be necessary for an elderly person to completely relinquish this role to either the formal or informal support system. The fact that over half the elders in the control group performed new case management tasks in the absence of special training or support suggested that elders should be seen as potential case management partners who can share responsibility with social workers and family members. Their willingness and ability to do so could perhaps be increased if elders, like family members, were involved in a training program.

Second, the risks and benefits of expecting elderly people, particularly the oldest old, to do their own case management should be explored. Although on the face of it, increasing an elderly person's autonomous performance of case management appears desirable, there undoubtedly will be instances in which elders are too frail. Investigators should thus examine not only the feasibility but also the desirability of extending the family-centered training to the elder.

The results of the multiple regression analyses suggested that different types of elderly persons and their families may have different levels of success in carrying out case management. For example, when elderly individuals are confused, have poor functional skills, and when there is frequent contact between elder and family member, it seems most appropriate for the social service agency to reach out to family members and provide case management training and support to them. In contrast, when the elderly client is younger and not confused and when there is less frequent contact between the elder and the family member, the best approach may be to provide case management training and support directly to the elderly person. Finally, when the elderly person has impaired functional skills, has less frequent contact with a family member, and when that family member is elderly, it may be necessary for the social worker to take primary responsibility for case management.

One caution is warranted in the interpretation of the findings of this study, namely that the elderly persons and their family members were a targeted group. Nearly all elderly clients were Jewish and most family members were middle class. Further, the sampling methodology excluded certain types of elderly persons, including those who felt that they did not need case management, who had emergency needs that could not wait for the pre-test to be administered, who had mental impairments so extreme that they were unable to understand the informed consent form, or who had no family available even by telephone. The impact of these selection criteria was that the family-centered training was targeted away from both the least and the most impaired elders. The family-centered training program may indeed be very effective with families of extremely impaired elders in community settings if the intervention can begin quickly enough to respond to emergencies and if there is no informed consent form to sign, both of which were requirements imposed by the research process that would not be ordinarily applicable to service delivery situations.

There are a number of interesting and important issues that were not addressed in this study but which warrant future examination. In particular, it is undoubtedly the case that family dynamics have an impact on the selection by the elderly person of one family member to be trained and on his or her success in carrying out assigned tasks. Any intervention involving one family member may well result in some change in overall family interaction patterns. An understanding of how the family-centered intervention affects family dynamics would potentially strengthen the clinical use of this partnership model. In a related vein, not examined was whether particular types of family members, such as spouses, adult children, or siblings, are better able to assume case management responsibilities than are others.

The findings suggested four additional research questions, each of which is currently being investigated. First, are the effects of the family centered training durable? Do trained family members continue to assume responsibility for case management once the formal service sector is no longer involved? A follow-up study of half of the sample has been conducted to address these issues (Seltzer et al., 1986). Second, how generalizable are the findings of this study to the general population of elders and their family members? Because almost all participants were Jewish and family members were generally middle-class, it is not known whether the same pattern of findings would emerge with different racial, ethnic, or socioeconomic status groups. A replication study with a more heterogeneous sample is being conducted. Third, can the case management training be delivered in formats other than individual case-by-case training conducted by social workers? The efficacy of a group training format, as well as individual training, will be examined in the replication study. Finally, can the elderly person be trained to serve as a member of the case management team along with the family member? This question will also be examined in the replication study.

REFERENCES

Austin, C. D. 1981. Case management: Let us count the ways. Paper presented at the 34th Annual Scientific Meeting of the Gerontological Society of America, Toronto, November.

Blenkner, M., Bloom, M., & Nielson, M. 1971. A research and demonstration project of protective services. *Social Casework.* 52:489–499.

Brody, E. 1979. Message from the president. *The Gerontologist.* 19:516.

Brody, E. M. 1985. Parent care as a normative family stress. *The Gerontologist.* 25: 19–29.

Brody, S. J., Poulshock, S. W., & Masciocchi, C. F. 1978. The family caring unit: A major consideration in the long-term support system. *The Gerontologist.* 18:556–561.

Cantor, M., Rehr, H., & Trotz, V. 1981. Workshop II: Case management and family involvement. *The Mount Sinai Journal of Medicine.* 48:566–568.

Lowy, L. 1983. The older generation: What is due, what is owed. *Social Casework.* 64:371–376.

Lowy, L. 1985. The implications of demographic trends as they affect the elderly. Paper presented at the 25th Annual Scientific Meeting of the Boston Society for Gerontologic Psychiatry, Boston, MA, November.

Mahoney, F. I., & Barthel, D. W. 1965. Functional evaluation: The Barthel Index. *Maryland State Medical Journal.* 14:61–65.

Monk, A. 1981. Social work with the aged: Principles of practice. *Social Work.* 26:61–68.

Schlesinger, M. R., Tobin, S. S., & Kiely, S. R. 1980. The responsible child and parental well-being. *Journal of Gerontological Social Work.* 3:3–16.

Seltzer, M. M., Litchfield, L. C., & Lowy, L. L. 1986. Family members as case managers: A longitudinal study. Paper presented at the 39th Scientific Meeting of the Gerontological Society of America, Chicago, IL, November.

Seltzer, M. S., Simmons, K., Ivry, J., & Litchfield, L. 1984. Agency–Family partnerships: Case management of services for the elderly. *Journal of Gerontological Social Work.* 7:57–71.

Shanas, E., & Maddox, G. L. 1976. Aging, health and the organization of health resources. In R. Binstock & E. Shanas (Eds.), *Handbook of Aging and the Social Sciences.* New York: Van Nostrand Reinhold.

Silverstein, N. M., Michelson, S., & LoCastro, S. 1985. Adult children and aging parents: How knowledgeable are the elderly's key informal supports? Paper presented at the 38th Scientific Meeting of the Gerontological Society of America, New Orleans, LA, November.

Silverstone, B., & Burack-Weiss, A. 1983. *Social Work Practice with the Frail Elderly and their Families.* Springfield, IL: Charles C Thomas.

Simmons, K. H., Ivry, J., & Seltzer, M. M. 1985. Agency-family collaboration. *The Gerontologist.* 25:343–346.

Smyer, M. A. 1980. The differential usage of services by impaired elderly. *Journal of Gerontology.* 35: 249–255.

Steinberg, R. M., & Carter, G. W. 1983. *Case Management and the Elderly: A Handbook for Planning and Administering Program.* Lexington, MA: Lexington Books.

Sussman, M. B. 1976. The family life of older people. In R. H. Binstock & E. Shanas (Eds.), *Handbook of Aging and the Social Sciences.* New York: Van Nostrand Reinhold.

Tuzil, T. 1978. The agency role in helping middle-aged children and their parents. *Social Casework.* 59:302–305.

Walz, T. H. 1975. The family, the family agency, and the post-industrial society. *Social Casework.* 56:13–20.

Wylie, M., & Austin, C. 1978. Policy foundations for case management: Consequences for the frail elderly. *Journal of Gerontological Social Work.* 1:7–17.

PART V

Evaluating Case Management

Contexts and Service Factors for Social Work Involvement

Both articles in this section pose a series of questions in program evaluation research that apply directly to case management. Both insist on the necessity of beginning evaluative research in any program area by being precise about exactly what services are being offered; about how the values guiding programs are being operationalized; and about how outcomes are defined and directly related to interventions or how they confuse program outcomes with other systemic or context-based factors.

Conceptual and operational clarity, and the internal consistency between them and outcomes measures, form the central research questions. After reviewing examples of community support systems programs and evaluation literature about them, Bachrach concluded, "Fuzziness in program design and program direction begets fuzziness in investigation" (1982, p. 47). Differentiating evaluations of client outcomes from system deficits and dysfunctions complicates the issue. Social work practice acknowledging the dual practice commitments discussed earlier must be able to make this differentiation.

In the introductory essay and in Part I, we discussed the relative lack of clarity about how and where advocacy fits into case management in different models. Defining the necessity for advocacy at the individual client and systems or issue level and operationalizing advocacy as a legitimate case management function permit thorough analysis of a case management program. Without accountability for the systems reorganization dimension to case management, or with only the capacity to evaluate direct client–case manager interaction on service-use issues, program evaluation become a provider-driven or funding-stream-driven tool.

Output measures that only count units of delivered services confuse service availability or accessibility with appropriateness to clients' needs. This common practice, also typically flowing from provider-centered evaluations, confounds the problems faced by case management clients through collapsing effectiveness measures into efficiency measures; through confusing agency outputs (units of services) with client outcomes; through reducing quality of life factors to quantity of service indicators. These typical provider-driven practices, when embodied in program evaluation research, obstruct clarity of vision and cricial assessment of service design, impede system reorganization strategy, or obscure critical reflection on practice paradigms. Simple service utilization or cost measures obstruct the dual focus of psychosocial practice in case management or other social work interventions by ignoring systemic or contextual inputs that shape clients' lives and agency practice. These simple measures also fail to contribute to system impact analysis or to progressive policy development.

The two articles that follow try to address the types of issues and questions that must be reflected in psychosocial interventions. The urgent need to generate both program design clarity and evaluative methodologies for assessing system interventions and creating system impact are examined. Both require examination of quality of life factors that are more than attitudinal measures of clients' satisfaction with service delivery. Wilson has the courage to say that structural aspects shaping the quality of clients' lives must be seen as indicators of system or program effectivness. I try to challenge conventional concepts of effectiveness tied to recidivism rates or simple cost accounting of service output in relation to functional improvement.

Both authors also raise the question of how researchers can factor in nonsystem variables such as the intensity and scope of clients' informal supports; the weight of involvement in social networks as a factor in determining clients' outcomes on measures of service effectiveness; and the role of system deficits in shaping the quality of life variation in clients' experience over time. Case managers must ask the kinds of questions and pose the conceptual issues raised in the two articles, if they are to develop a client-driven concept of practice.

Ignoring responsibility for carefully conducting research or program evaluation most often results in provider-driven formats that focus on output measures of quantity of services provided and their cost per client as the entire universe of meaning. Evaluations of the long term care case management projects (Capitman et al., 1986; Mathmatica Policy Research, Inc., 1986) already demonstrate the potential for generating quantitative studies that entirely by-pass the involvement of clients and even their families in establishing their own goals or identifying their own needs. Parallel studies exist in mental health where even the research showing positive outcomes reduces the quality of a person's life to the length of time he or she has stayed out of a hospital or reduces the value of case management to the recidivism rate of its clients.

Often, case managers or social workers in other intervention approaches are fearful of research or are intimidated by its usual quantitative forms. This will have to be confronted by those of you who want to pursue client-driven case management.

Programs with these values in the public sector, or in the voluntary sector (usually under contract to some public authority), are going to be evaluated, and almost always in simplified quantitative form. Staff and administrators attempting to create a client-driven practice model will need to generate some alternative; to construct some way to integrate qualitative data that presents what they are doing with quantitative measures to demonstrate their impact. The two articles presented here attempt to assist in that process.

CHAPTER 18

Community Support and Community Integration

New Directions for Client Outcome Research

Susan F. Wilson

This article was prepared under contract with the National Institute of Mental Health's Community Support Program. Its purpose is to stimulate discussion about current and future directions for the mental health field to measure the impact of its work with consumers, and more broadly, its impact on how consumers' lives change over time. The content of the article is the result of an extensive review of the outcome literature related to adults with severe psychiatric disabilities and a series of discussions with a number of expert researchers across the United States.[1] Although a number of methodological issues are raised within this article, no attempt is made to discuss them in fine detail. Instead, the literature and the sometimes-conflicting views of experts are used to propose a new set of directions for outcome research, one that refers to an emerging shift in the field from seeing people with psychiatric disabilities principally as service recipients, to seeing them as having the potential for full community membership.

[1] This article was prepared with the assistance of a number of other researchers. Paul J. Carling, Ph.D., Director of the Center for Change through Housing and Community Support, was particularly helpful in the overall conceptual design of the paper and in thoughtfully editing several drafts. The content on research/evaluation implications was enhanced through a two-hour conference call discussion involving the following national experts: William Anthony, Ph.D. (Boston University Center for Psychiatric Rehabilitation), Gary Bond, Ph.D. (Purdue University), Sue Estroff, Ph.D. (University of North Carolina), Courtney Harding, Ph.D. (Yale University), Phillip Leaf, Ph.D. (Yale University), Mary Ann Test, Ph.D. (University of Wisconsin), and Jacqueline Parrish (CSP Program Director, NIMH). The author wishes to thank these individuals for the insightful comments, and for the generous contribution of their time. Any limitations of the article, of course, are the sole responsibility of the author.

TRADITIONAL APPROACHES TO OUTCOME RESEARCH

Historically, client outcome research has been based on the then-current assumptions about the needs of people with mental illness. For example, until the last few decades it was assumed that most people with mental illness would never recover and that they therefore needed long term institutional care. During the mid fifties to mid sixties, the introduction of psychotropic medications, along with increasing economic and ethical incentives to reduce institutional size, resulted in people with mental illness beginning to live in community settings (Bachrach, 1983; Bell, 1980). Without adequate resources, support services or follow-up, however, many people did not fare well, a situation which fueled an ongoing debate about the appropriateness of community living (Bachrach, 1982b; Talbott, 1981; Turner & TenHoor, 1978). As community treatment programs developed, empirical research studies began to address this debate by comparing the effects of hospital versus community-based treatment on client outcome. These empirical studies compared outcomes of institutional care versus community-based care after long periods of hospitalization (e.g., Linn, Caffey, & Klett, 1977; Marx, Test, & Stein, 1973; Weinman & Kleiner, 1978); outcomes of institutional care versus community-based services as alternatives to institutional care (e.g., Mosher & Menn, 1978; Pasamanick, Scarpitti, & Dinitz, 1967; Stein, Test, & Marx, 1975); and the efficacy of different community-based approaches (e.g., Caffey, Galbrecht, & Klett, 1971; Fairweather et al., 1969; Hogarty et al., 1974; Lamb & Goertzel, 1972). Overviews of this research by Braun et al. (1981), Kiesler (1982), and Test and Stein (1978) concluded that although the studies' methodological designs and measures varied tremendously, the findings were remarkably similar: Community treatment was effective in reducing hospitalization, and the effects on symptomatology and psychosocial functioning were at least equal for people living in community and people living in hospital settings. As such, community-based care came to be seen as a viable treatment alternative, and in fact, as the preferred approach.

During the 1970s, the explicit goal of community treatment was to keep people out of hospital settings (i.e., community maintenance) and recidivism was used as the primary measure of system effectiveness. As more people lived in the community for longer periods of time, however, expectations about the abilities of people with mental illness began to change (Bachrach, 1986; Turner & TenHoor, 1978). The mental health community began to shift from a model of viewing mental illness as either acute or chronic (i.e., people will either get well or will need custodial care forever) to a model in which every person was seen as having potential for overcoming the negative effects of the disability if given appropriate supports (Anthony, Cohen, & Vitalo 1978; Anthony & Farkas, 1982; Estroff, 1987; Kanter, 1985; NASMHPD, 1987).

EMERGENCE OF THE COMMUNITY SUPPORT APPROACH

In 1977 the introduction of the National Institute for Mental Health (NIMH) Community Support Program (CSP) reflected this shift in thinking about the capabilities of people with mental illness and the role of community-based services. Designed to help states develop more comprehensive community-based service systems, the CSP model stresses "the potential of these people and builds on their strengths and abilities by providing opportunities for rehabilitation and growth" (Brown & Parrish, 1987, pp. 17–18). The CSP model has been adopted by virtually all state mental health authorities as their preferred services approach (NASMHPD, 1984). Based on these changing assumptions about consumers, community-based services began to focus both on keeping people out of hospital settings and on enhancing their abilities; the goal was no longer community maintenance, but one of client growth.

The comprehensive community support system (CSS) model was conceptualized as having the mandate and capacity to provide all of the supports that were once provided by hospitals, such as shelter, food, and clothing, as well as clinical treatment, social support, and leisure activities (Bachrach, 1982a; Dickey et al., 1981; Rosenfield, 1987). Thus, the original intention of CSS was that they be designed to attend to all aspects of clients' lives (Turner & TenHoor, 1978).

NEW LEARNINGS

Since the introduction of the CSP initiative in 1977, our knowledge about the capabilities and needs of people with severe and persistent psychiatric disabilities has grown tremendously. This increased knowledge has resulted from the practical experiences gained through actually trying to support people in the community who previously were or would have seen institutionalized, from the increasing willingness of clients and their family members to speak out about their abilities and needs, and from the various learnings gained through research on the impact of services. Some of these learnings that have direct relevance to how we think about outcome research can be summarized as follows:

> Mental illness is not necessarily a life-long, degenerative process that progresses in a predictable, linear pattern (Brooks, 1988; Gardos, Cole, & LaBrie, 1982; Harding et al., 1987a,b; Morrison & Bellack, 1987; Rogers, 1987). For example, Harding et al. (1987b), in a 20-year follow-up of severely disabled hospital patients, found that "widely heterogeneous patterns of social, occupational and psychological functioning evolved over time" (p. 732), and they concurred with Vaillant (1978) that "diagnosis and prognosis should be treated as different dimensions" (p. 733).

People with severe mental illness can maintain jobs, housing, and positive relationships with friends and families regardless of the presence of psychiatric symptoms and with various levels of mental health support (Anthony, Cohen, & Vitalo, 1978; Bond et al., 1988; Harding, 1986).

Mental health services must be designed to be flexible and responsive to different individual's needs within any given environmental context (Carling et al., 1987; Minkoff, 1987; O'Brien, 1981; Turner & Shifren, 1979).

People with mental illness can and should have a choice about the type and intensity of services they receive (Minkoff, 1987; Mitchell, Pyle, & Hatsukami, 1983; Prager, 1980; Solomon, Gordon, & Davis, 1986; Strauss, 1986).

Most people with mental illness do not view themselves as chronic mental patients, and they value independence and productivity more highly than any other treatment outcome or aspect of life (Bigelow et al., 1982; Chamberlin, 1987; Estroff & Patrick, 1987; Minkoff, 1987; Solomon, Gordon, & Davis, 1986).

Although our understanding of the implications of these learning continues to grow, taken together they appear to suggest that, on a long-term basis, the mental health service system should no longer be expected to meet all needs of clients, or in effect to function as a closed system of care for people who become totally dependent on it to survive. People with mental illness are increasingly viewed as people who live within and are influenced principally by the ecology of their community. As noted by Minkoff (1987), "unlike the "old chronic patients, whose identities as patients were imposed on them in the state hospital, patients in the post institutional 1980's have the freedom to struggle, on their own, to develop their identities in the community—identities not just as patients but as people, people with chronic mental illness" (p. 946). Thus, mental health researchers, administrators, and service providers are increasingly discarding the concept that the service system should assume total responsibility for all aspects of clients' lives. Instead, the service system is seen as responsible for assisting the individual and his or her surrounding community to be connected in whatever ways the person might choose.

IMPLICATIONS OF NEW LEARNINGS FOR RESEARCH AND EVALUATION

The Shift from Service-Users to Community Participants

The implications of this philosophical shift toward using client outcomes to measure service quality and effectiveness are profound. Over the past decade, outcome measures have broadened to include indicators of quality of life (such as employment status, income, living situation, social activities and networks, leisure time activities, satisfaction with life), as well as the more clinically oriented indices (such as recidivism, mental health services use, medication use, and degree of symptomatology) (Bellack & Mueser, 1986; Lehman, Ward, & Linn, 1982; Mechanic, 1987; Plum, 1987; Rogers, 1987; Rosenfield, 1987; Schulberg, 1979). A review of this outcome research, however, shows that the consistent focus has been on how well people are doing *within* the CSS, rather than on measuring success in terms of how mental health services are assisting people to attain or maintain community membership. For example, in a completed NIMH follow-up study of CSP clients, the authors concluded that "the CSP project is meeting its goals of avoiding rehospitalization, keeping clients enrolled in community programs, maintaining clients in satisfactory residential settings, enhancing the quality of life (QOL) for participants, and improving client functioning," even though they also note that "clients did not seem to change dramatically . . . with respect to behavioral indicants" and they "tended to remain socially isolated" (Rogers, 1987, p. 17).

There are a number of reasons why success continues to be measured in terms of service-related indicators:

1. These indicators are much easier for both researchers and service providers to use and understand than are "soft" indicators that reflect the various aspects of quality of life.[2]
2. The elements associated with quality of life have primarily been viewed as predictor variables for the more treatment-oriented outcomes rather than as important outcomes in their own right.
3. There has been no clear consensus about the goal of CSS (Bachrach, 1982a; Carling et al., 1987; Cometa, Morrison, & Ziskoven, 1979; Tessler & Manderscheid, 1982).

Thus, the mission of the service system is often still viewed as *maintaining* people in *community services,* rather than assisting them whenever needed to achieve or maintain roles as regular community members.

Redefining the role of the mental health system based on our new learnings over the past decade, however, necessitates changing our focus from how well individuals use the service system to how well individuals are actually functioning in communities on the same dimensions that we would use to

[2] Although numerous authors have pointed out the problems with using recidivism as a primary outcome indicator (e.g., Bachrach, 1976, 1982b; Beiser, Shore, & Peters, 1985; Kruzich, 1985; Plum, 1987; Smith & Smith, 1979; Test & Stein, 1978), it is a remarkably enduring measure, perhaps because it is the easiest to quantify and understand. As noted by Anthony and Farkas (1982) and Setze and Bond (1985), recidivism is used because it is a "hard" criterion that is highly reliable, has face validity, reflects cost savings, has implications for prognosis (i.e., evidence suggest that each successive rehospitalization diminishes a favorable prognosis), and can be compared across studies.

measure the success and satisfaction of any other group. A key component of such a focus is how these individuals evaluate their own experiences and life situations. There are a number of compelling reasons to shift the focus from simply looking at mental health service use to looking at more generic outcomes. Increasingly, service systems are defining their goals in terms of people living in stable housing with supports and people having expanded options related to education and employment (NASMHPD, 1984, 1987). However, a focus on such concrete benefits to consumers is by no means a simple process. For example, assessing "vocational success" involves conflicting views about what constitutes work (e.g., competitive employment, full-time versus part-time versus other "productive" activity, earnings versus satisfaction, and so forth).

Beyond these increasingly common indicators, there also are more subtle outcomes that, while rarely measured, may be highly significant. For example, specific outcomes such as marriage and regaining child custody may reflect "success" in the general population, but we rarely include such data in services-focused research. As noted by Bond et al. (1988), these tangentially reported outcomes present "evidence of client movement . . . from merely meeting basic needs to making long-term commitments to life changes" (p. 416). These are the types of outcomes that may be truly representative of CSP philosophy and goals; if so, they are the outcomes toward which our service system must strive.[3] Thus, we appear to be moving toward a research approach that goes beyond the concept of "success" and "failure" and instead focuses on overall, long-term quality of life.

Quality of Life: Research Dilemmas

Focusing on quality of life as a primary indicator of system effectiveness poses a number of research dilemmas. First, this concept is values-based in that it assumes that enhanced quality of life is the outcome for which the service system should be striving. Values-free research, on the other hand, would focus on testing this very assumption. While this is the cause of some debate in the research community, it is important to have studies that are directed by CSP values, which measure broad outcomes and which also examine the validity of those values. A second dilemma is the difficulty in empirically defining quality of life. In what is perhaps the most commonly used approach, Flanagan (1978) has attempted to define quality of life by developing an

[3] A note of caution is important here, however. Simultaneous with this long-term shift in research to different outcome measures, we also must continue to struggle with the more short-term need to demonstrate the effectiveness of our current CSP programs by examining changing patterns of service use, such as the impact of certain services on reducing high-cost hospitalization. Without this evidence, it is clear that we will neither have the information we need to improve our programs, nor will we be able to secure public and political support for even implementing CSP services in more than a few communities in the United States.

empirically derived conceptual schema based on responses from a broad sample of the general American public. This schema outlines fifteen critical components of quality of life collapsed into five categories (physical and material well-being; relations with other people; social, community, and civic activities; personal development and fulfillment; and recreation) (see Table 18-1). It could be argued that it is not appropriate to expect people with mental illness to achieve a similar degree of "success" in each of these areas, as would be expected by the general public. A different way of framing this issue, however, is to examine "success" based on the discrepancy between individuals' expectations and goals in each of these domains and in their current situation. In this approach, then, a mental health systems' effectiveness would be measured according to each persons' own definition of successful community living. Practically, this entails a high degree of individualization that typically does not occur in most systems-level outcome research. Nevertheless, this appears to be a highly relevant way to truly measure the success of mental health services in terms of actual impact on consumers' lives. Attending to quality of life schemas like that developed by Flanagan points out an important bias inherent in most existing research: Many aspects of life that have a strong impact on most "nondisabled" people are typically ignored when assessing the status or quality of life of mental health consumers. For example, the role of religion and spirituality, menopause, parental death,

TABLE 18-1. FLANAGAN'S 15 EMPIRICALLY DERIVED COMPONENTS OF QUALITY OF LIFE

I. Physicial and material well-being
   A. Material well-being and financial security
   B. Health and personal safety
II. Relations with other people
   C. Relations with spouse (girlfriend or boyfriend)
   D. Having and raising children
   E. Relations with parents, siblings, or other relatives
   F. Relations with friends
III. Social, community, and civic activities
   G. Activities related to helping or encouraging other people
   H. Activities relating to local and national governments
IV. Personal development and fulfillment
   I. Intellectual development
   J. Personal understanding and planning
   K. Occupational role
   L. Creativity and personal expression
V. Recreation
   M. Socializing
   N. Passive and observational recreational activities
   O. Active and participatory recreational activities

Source: Adapted from Flanagan, J. C. 1978. A research approach to improving our quality of life. *American Psychologist. Feb.:* 139–140.

victimization, and having or not having a spouse or children are all issues with which most people struggle during their lives. Yet these important issues and events are rarely considered in studies focused on mental health consumers, perhaps in part due to our own stigmatized learning about the capabilities of people with mental illness. The impact on an individual's opportunities that results from living in the very restricted role of a mental patient also needs to be incorporated into research on client outcome (Estroff, 1981).

Relationships and leisure-time activity are indicators of quality of life that are increasingly included in outcome research, although there is much confusion about which aspects of these concepts are most relevant. To demonstrate this confusion, one need only examine what appears to be a simple concept, that of social relationships. In practical terms, however, it is difficult to determine the optimal number of relationships for a given individual; relationship quality often is not considered (i.e., whether relationships are positive or negative); the role(s) that each relationship plays in an individual's life may vary tremendously; the number of reported relationships might be inflated due to the person's living situation (e.g., in a congregate mental health setting); people who represent important supports, but who live far away, are rarely included; the importance of interdependency and reciprocity of relationships is often overlooked; and individuals' satisfaction or subjective feelings about aspects of their relationships need to be explored. Many of these same issues also apply when trying to assess the quality of an individual's leisure-time activities.

Related Methodological Quandries

A related research dilemma concerns the concept of "outcome" itself. It has been argued that this term is merely a research artifact that assumes some final point in a person's progression along a certain life dimension, and that it does not take into account the ups and downs of everyday life (Harding, 1986). In addition, most research incorporates short follow-up timelines which limit the capacity to assess changes in complex areas (Bachrach, 1982b; Bond et al., 1988; Carling et al., 1987; Morrison & Bellack, 1987; Mueller, 1980; Schulberg & Bromet, 1981; Tessler & Manderscheid, 1982). To assess with any degree of accuracy the impact of services on the lives of consumers, however, it will be necessary to conduct longitudinal studies that can monitor change over an extended period of time. Similarly, when short-term outcome studies are undertaken, it is important that the results be interpreted with an explicit focus on this serious methodological limitation.

It is clear from much of this discussion that a number of methodological issues limit the comparability and generalizability of existing research studies. This situation is further confounded by incorporating quality of life, which is composed of multiple indicators, as a major outcome measure. Methodological problems detailed in the literature include the use of different instruments to measure each particular variable (Test & Stein, 1978); variation in the reliability and validity of the instruments used (Anthony & Farkas, 1982; Bachrach, 1982b); most outcome variables (in addition to quality of life) are vague and hard to empirically define (Anthony & Farkas, 1982; Cometa, Morrison, & Ziskoven, 1979; Stevenson & Longabaugh, 1980); target groups across studies are not standardized in terms of clinical and demographic characteristics (Bachrach, 1976, 1982b; Schulberg & Bromet, 1981; Smith & Smith, 1979); and, causal linkages between treatment and outcome are difficult to establish because of these methodological problems, because of confounding effects of multiple interventions, and because many of the factors involved in examining quality of life are interrelated (Anthony, Cohen, & Vitalo, 1978; Bachrach, 1982b; Bradley et al., 1987; Lebow, 1982; Schulberg, 1981; Spaniol et al., 1981; Strauss & Carpenter, 1974; Tessler et al., 1982).[4]

These methodological problems are further complicated because many, if not most, researchers create new measures or adapt existing instruments to fit their particular study. This highlights the need for opportunities for national researchers to collaborate on research design and instrument development. In order to have a solid foundation of information about effective services, the development of comparable, meaningful methods for outcome measurement must be given the same priority as conducting the actual studies. This is particularly critical given the very early and evolutionary nature of much of the research in this area.

There also is a need to collect both quantitative and qualitative information about client outcome. As indicated in the previously mentioned study by Bond et al. (1988), both types of information are important in interpreting the impact of services on clients' lives and omitting either can result in erroneous conclusions. The technology for qualitative data collection and analysis has grown tremendously in the past few years (e.g., there is now computer software available for qualitative data analysis), and researchers are beginning to include open-ended questions in quantitatively focused questionnaires.

In addition, more research needs to be focused on specific groups of people, many of whom are often neglected. Outcome studies concerning elders or minorities might produce different findings from those focused on the overall population of clients. Furthermore, retroactive studies are needed to examine the true "failures" of our services (i.e., people who have committed suicide), as are studies of those people who were once defined as mentally ill who no longer need to use mental health assistance. It also cannot be assumed

---

[4] As a result of these methodological issues, using a client outcome focus has become seen as more appropriate for specific *program* evaluations (in which it is easier to incorporate well-defined outcomes and methodological controls) than it has for *service system* evaluation (where it is difficult to control the many extemporaneous factors) (Bachrach, 1982b; Hargreaves, 1982; Spaniol et al., 1981). Yet, the use of client outcome measures to evaluate system effectiveness is extremely important (Bachrach & Lamb, 1982; Ciarlo, 1982; Fiester & Neigher, 1979; Newman, 1982; Schulberg & Bromet, 1981).

that attrition is a random event: Thus, studies should routintely report information on people who leave services. This group of people may be an important focus of research on their own, given the implication that their leaving may well reflect a dissatisfaction with the type of services currently available, or with the type of outcomes they perceive themselves deriving from these services.

Finally and fundamentally, client outcome research can be greatly enhanced by incorporating consumer perspectives into all aspects of design, implementation, and interpretation. These individuals and their family members struggle with the effects of a mental illness diagnosis on a day-to-day basis, and they are the recipients of the services we are trying to assess. As such, their knowledge is extremely useful for assisting our ongoing thinking about the important questions that need to be asked, and about the best methods for achieving valid and reliable answers.

REFERENCES

Anthony, W. A., & Farkas, M. 1982. A client outcome planning model for assessing psychiatric rehabilitation interventions. *Schizophrenia Bulletin.* 8(1):13–38.

Anthony, W. A., Cohen, M. R., & Vitalo, R. 1978. The measurement of rehabilitation outcome. *Schizophrenia Bulletin.* 4(3):365–383.

Bachrach, L. L. 1976. A note on some recent studies of released mental hospital patients in the community. *American Journal of Psychiatry.* 133(1):73–75.

Bachrach, L. L. 1982a. Assessment of outcomes in community support systems: Results, problems, and limitations. *Schizophrenia Bulletin.* 9:39–61.

Bachrach, L. L. 1982b. Young adult chronic patients: An analytical review of the literature. *Hospital and Community Psychiatry.* 33:189–197.

Bachrach, L. L. 1983. *Deinstitutionalization.* San Francisco, CA: Jossey-Bass.

Bachrach, L. L. 1986. Dimensions of disability in the chronic mentally ill. *Hospital and Community Psychiatry.* 37(10):981–982.

Bachrach, L. L., & Lamb, H. R. 1982. Conceptual issues in the evaluation of the deinstitutionalization movement. In G. J. Stahler, & W. R. Tash (Eds.), *Innovative Approaches to Mental Health Evaluation.* New York: Academic Press.

Beiser, Shore, Peters. 1985. Community care for the mentally ill. *American Journal of Psychiatry.* 142(9):1047–1052.

Bell, L. V. 1980. *Treating the Mentally Ill: From Colonial Times to the Present.* New York: Praeger.

Bellack, A. S., & Mueser, K. T. 1986. A comprehensive treatment program for schizophrenia and chronic mental illness. *Community Mental Health Journal.* 22(3): 175–189.

Bigelow, D. A., et al. 1982. The concept and measurement of quality of life as a dependent variable in evaluation of mental health services. In G. J. Stahler & W. R. Tash (Eds.), *Innovative Approaches to Mental Health Evaluation.* New York: Academic Press.

Bond, G. R., et al. 1988. Assertive case management in three CMHCs: A controlled study. *Hospital and Community Psychiatry.* 39(4):411–418.

Bradley, V. J., et al. 1987. *Evaluating psychosocial rehabilitation programs: What next?* Cambridge, MA: Human Services Research Institute.

Braun, P., et al. 1981. Overview: Deinstitutionalization of psychiatric patients, a critical review of outcome studies. *American Journal of Psychiatry.* 138(6):736–749.

Brooks, G. W. 1988. Reflections on the Vermont story or foresight, insight and hindsight. *Psychiatric Journal of the University of Ottawa.* 13(1):21–24.

Brown, N. B., & Parrish, J. 1987. Community support and rehabilitation of the mentally disabled in the United States. *International Journal of Mental Health.* 15(4):16–25.

Caffey, E. M., Galbrecht, C. R., & Klett, C. J. 1971. Brief hospitalization and aftercare in the treatment of schizophrenia. *Archives of General Psychiatry.* 24:81–86.

Carling, P. J., et al. 1987. *Housing and community integration for people with psychiatric disabilities.* Washington, DC: DATA Institute.

Chamberlin, J. 1987. *On Our Own: Patient-Controlled Alternatives to the Mental Health System.* New York: McGraw-Hill.

Ciarlo, J. A. 1982. Accountability revisited: The arrival of client outcome evaluation. *Evaluation and Program Planning.* 5:31–36.

Cometa, M. S., Morrison, J. K., & Ziskoven, M. 1979. Halfway to where? A critique of research on psychiatric halfway houses. *Journal of Community Psychology.* 7:23–27.

Dickey, B., et al. 1981. A follow-up of deinstitutionalized chronic patients four years after discharge. *Hospital and Community Psychiatry.* 32(5):326–330.

Estroff, S. E. 1981. *Making It Crazy.* Berkeley, CA: University of California Press.

Estroff, S. E. 1987. Taking issue: No more young adult chronic patients. *Hospital and Community Psychiatry.* 38(1):5.

Estroff, S. E., & Patrick, D. L. 1987. *Disability, income maintenance and severe, persistent mental illness.* Chapel Hill: University of North Carolina School of Medicine. (Unpublished manuscript.)

Fairweather, G. W., et al. 1969. *Community Life for the Mentally Ill.* Chicago, IL: Aldine Publishing.

Fiester, A., & Neigher, W. 1979. Client outcome: Overview. *Evaluation in Practice.* Bethesda, MD: National Institute of Mental Health.

Flanagan, J. C. 1978. A research approach to improving our quality of life. *American Psychologist. February:*138–147.

Gardos, G., Cole, J. O., & LaBrie, R. A. 1982. A 12-year follow-up study of chronic schizophrenics. *Hospital and Community Psychiatry.* 33(12):983–984.

Harding, C. M. 1986. Speculations on the measurement of recovery from severe psychiatric disorder and the human condition. *Psychiatric Journal of the University of Ottawa.* 11(4):199–204.

Harding, C. M., et al. 1987a. The Vermont longitudinal study of persons with severe mental illness; I: Methodology, study sample, and overall status 32 years later. *American Journal of Psychiatry.* 144(6):718–726.

Harding, C. M., et al. 1987b. The Vermont longitudinal study of persons with severe mental illness, II: Long-term outcome of subjects who restropectively met DSM-III Criteria for schizophrenia. *American Journal of Psychiatry.* 144(6):727–735.

Hargreaves, W. A. 1982. Outcome evaluation or treatment research?: A response to Ciarlo (1982). *Evaluation and Program Planning.* 5:357–358.

Hogarty, G. E., et al. 1974. Drug and sociotherapy in the aftercare of schizophrenic patients. I. Two year relapse rates. *Archives of General Psychiatry.* 31:603–618.

Kanter, J. 1985. The process of change in the long-term mentally ill: A naturalistic perspective. *Psychosocial Rehabilitation Journal.* 9(1):55–68.

Kiesler, C. A. 1982. Mental hospitals and alternative care. *American Psychologist.* 37(4):349–360.

Kruzich, J. M. 1985. Community integration of the mentally ill in residential facilities. *American Journal of Community Psychology.* 13(5):553–564.

Lamb, H. R., & Goertzel, V. 1972. High expectations of long-term ex-state hospital patients. *American Journal of Psychiatry.* 129(4):471–475.

Lebow, J. 1982. Models for evaluating services at community mental health centers. *Hospital and Community Psychiatry.* 33(12):1010–1014.

Lehman, A. F., Ward, N. C., & Linn, L. S. 1982. Chronic mental patients: The quality of life issue. *American Jounral of Psychiatry.* 139(10):1271–1276.

Linn, M. W., Caffey, E. M., & Klett, C. J. 1977. Hospital vs. community (foster) care for psychiatric patients. *Archives of General Psychiatry.* 34:78–83.

Marx, A. J., Test, M. A., & Stein, L. I. 1973. Extrahospital management of severe mental illness: Feasibility and effects of social functioning. *Archives of General Psychiatry.* 29:505–511.

Mechanic, D. 1987. Evolution of mental health services and areas for change. In D. Mechanic (Ed.), *Improving Mental Health Services: What the Social Sciences Can Tell Us.* San Francisco, CA: Jossey-Bass, pp. 3–13.

Minkoff, K. 1987. Beyond deinstitutionalization: A new ideology for the post institutional era. *Hospital and Community Psychiatry.* 38(9):945–950.

Mitchell, J. E., Pyle, R. L., & Hatsukami, D. 1983. A comparative analysis of psychiatric problems listed by patients and physicians. *Hospital and Community Psychiatry.* 34(9):848–849.

Morrison, R. L., & Bellack, A. S. 1987. Social functioning of schizophrenic patients: Clinical and research issues. *Schizophrenia Bulletin.* 13(4):715–725.

Mosher, L. R., & Menn, A. Z. 1978. Community residential treatment for schizophrenia: Two year follow-up. *Hospital and Community Psychiatry.* 29:715–723.

Mueller, D. P. 1980. Social networks: A promising direction for research on the relationship of the social environment to psychiatric disorder. *Social Science and Medicine.* 14A:147–161.

National Association of State Mental Health Program Directors. 1984. *Position Statement: The Chronically Mental Ill.* Alexandria, VA: NASMHPD.

National Association of State Mental Health Program Directors. 1987. *Position Statement: Housing and Support for People with Long-Term Illness.* Alexandria, VA: NASMHPD.

Newman, F. L. 1982. Outcome assessment in evaluation and treatment research: A response to Ciarlo and Hargreaves. *Evaluation and Program Planning.* 5:359–362.

O'Brien, J. 1981. *Community Support Systems for People with Severe Mental Disabilities: A Framework for Definition.* Atlanta, GA: Responsive Systems Associates.

Pasamanick, B., Scarpitti, F. R., & Dinitz, S. 1967. *Schizophrenics and the Community.* New York: Appleton-Century-Crofts.

Plum, K. C. 1987. Moving forward with deinstitutionalization: Lessons of an ethical policy analysis. *American Journal of Orthopsychiatry.* 57(4):508–514.

Prager, E. 1980. Evaluation in mental health: Enter the consumer. *Social Work Research and Abstracts.* 5–10.

Rogers, E. S. 1987. Community support program client follow-up study. *Community Support Network News.* 4(1):17.

Rosenfield, S. 1987. Services organization and quality of life among the seriously mentally ill. In D. Mechanic (Ed.), *Improving Mental Health Services: What the Social Sciences Can Tell Us.* San Francisco, CA: Jossey-Bass, pp. 47–59.

Schulberg, H. C. 1979. Community support programs: Program evaluation and public policy. *American Journal of Psychiatry.* 136(11):1433–1437.

Schulberg, H. C. 1981. Outcome evaluations in the mental health field. *Community Mental Health Journal.* 17(2):132–142.

Schulberg, H. C., & Bromet, E. 1981. Strategies for evaluating the outcome of community services for the chronically mentally ill. *American Journal of Psychiatry.* 138(7):930–935.

Setze, P. J., & Bond, G. R. 1985. Psychiatric recidivism in a psychosocial rehabilitation setting: A survival analysis. *Hospital and Community Psychiatry.* 36(5):521–524.

Smith, C. J., & Smith, C. A. 1979. Evaluating outcome measures for deinstitutionalization programs. *Social Work Research and Abstracts.* 23–30.

Solomon, P., Gordon, B., & Davis, J. M. 1986. Reconceptualizing assumptions about community mental health. *Hospital and Community Psychiatry.* 37(7):708–712.

Spaniol, L., et al. 1981. Evaluating local CSS programs serving the chronically mentally ill: Findings, issues, and conclusions. Paper presented at the CSP Learning Conference, June. Washington, DC.

Stein, L. I., Test, M. A., & Marx, A. J. 1975. Alternative to the hospital: A controlled study. *American Journal of Psychiatry.* 132(5):517–522.

Stevenson, J. F., & Longabaugh, R. H. 1980. The role of evaluation in mental health. *Evaluation Review.* 4(4):461–480.

Strauss, J. S. 1986. Discussion: What does rehabilitation accomplish? *Schizophrenia Bulletin.* 12(4):720–723.

Strauss, J. S., & Carpenter, W. T. 1974. The prediction of outcome in schizophrenia. *Archives of General Psychiatry.* 31:37–42.

Talbott, J. A. 1981. The emerging crisis in chronic care. *Hospital and Community Psychiatry.* 32:447.

Tessler, R. C., & Manderscheid, R. W. 1982. Factors affecting adjustment to community living. *Hospital and Community Psychiatry.* 33(3):203–207.

Tessler, R. C., et al. 1982. The chronically mentally ill in community support systems. *Hospital and Community Psychiatry.* 33(3):208–211.

Test, M. A., & Stein, L. I. 1978. Community treatment of the chronic patient: Research overview. *Schizophrenia Bulletin.* 4(3):350–364.

Turner, J. E. C., & Shifren, I. 1979. Community support systems: How comprehensive? *New Directions for Mental Health Services.* 2:1–23.

Turner, J., & TenHoor, W. 1978. The NIMH community support program: A pilot approach to a needed social reform. *Schizophrenia Bulletin.* 4(3):319–348.

Vaillant, G. E. 1978. A ten-year follow-up of remitting schizophrenics. *Schizophrenia Bulletin.* 4(11):78–85.

Weinman, B., & Kleiner, R. J. 1978. The impact of community living and community member intervention on the adjustment of the chronic psychotic patient. In L. I. Stein & M. A. Test (Eds.), *Alternatives to Mental Hospital Treatment.* New York: Plenum Press.

CHAPTER 19

Surviving Abuse and Its Neglect

Toward Increasing Responsiveness of Mental Health Systems

Stephen M. Rose

Extensive violence, including incest, other childhood sexual and physical abuse, and related trauma have been reported by psychiatric researchers for a number of years (Burgess & Holmstrom, 1974; Emslie & Rosenfeld, 1983; Hussain & Chapel, 1983; Carmen, Rieker & Mills, 1984; Lindberg & Distad, 1985; Bryer et al., 1987; Jacobson & Richardson, 1987; Cole, 1988; Craine et al., 1988). Less understood, but equally well documented is the reluctance of mental health professionals and other social services workers to inquire about and to develop appropriate programs for these victims (Bryer et al., 1987; Craine et al., 1988; Cole, 1988; Rose, Peabody, & Stratigeas, 1989).

Client-driven case management, operating from an advocacy/empowerment framework, must struggle to understand the factors that shape clients' lives. These factors, reflecting a person-in-environment relationship and cognizant of the dual focus for practice on the individual *and* the system, must guide evaluative research. In the material presented earlier, the impact of abuse *and* the response of various systems must be reported. Doing so requires examination of conventional concepts of independent, dependent, and intervening variables. This will be our focus as we report on a study of hidden victimization among 89 clients of an intensive case management (ICM) program in Suffolk County, New York.

Clients were people with extensive mental health system involvement, most were considered high risk/heavy users (HR/HU) of acute inpatient and psychiatric emergency rooms. The program incorporated the advocacy/empowerment philosophy (Rose & Black, 1985) described in Part VI of this book.

RESULTS

Routine inquiry about abuse backgrounds, when done by empowerment-oriented case managers considerate of clients' rights to determine their own participation (see Figure 19-1) and sensitive to the potential explosiveness of the issues, validates abuse victims and legitimates their experience. It allows people to discuss issues and feelings previously kept secret or denied; it gives client a depth of legitimation through acknowledging the truth of their externally imposed oppression; and it constructs a dialogue between workers and clients based on clients' strengths and validity for enduring both externally inflicted damage to the person and their emotional experience. Open recognition of previous violations and traumatic domination opens the door to externalizing the repressed residue of incest or other abuses. Routine inquiry about abuse backgrounds, already recommended by a number of researchers (Bryer et al., 1987; Cole, 1988; among others) deserves serious scrutiny by social workers, mental health policymakers, and program planners as a basis for designing alternative, appropriate services.

When conducted in the ICM program, stark realities were unveiled by the ICM clients: 50% were adult children of alcoholics or other substance abusers (ACOAs) including 44% of the men and 58% of the women. We assumed a chronological sequence in which ACOA experience preceded the additional abuses indicated in the following paragraphs. Of the 44 ACOAs among the ICM clients, more than 86% became HR/HUs of mental health system services ($p \leq .01$). This group of ACOA+HR/HU ICM clients made up 43% of the total ICM caseload.

The ACOA experience appears to be a foundation for extensive additional abuse. Of the 41 (of 44) ACOA ICM clients responding to the incest questions, 37% were incest victims compared with 12% of the ICM clients who were not ACOAs ($p \leq .01$). Among the incest victims, 80% are ACOAs, including 64% of the ICM women clients from ACOA backgrounds. When all childhood sexual abuse is considered, 34% of the ICM clients were victimized. When ACOA background mediates this relationship, we learned that 70% of the ICM clients sexually abused as children are ACOAs and that 48% of the ACOA clients were sexually abused as children ($p \leq .01$). Among HR/HU clients, 77% of those coming from childhood sexual abuse backgrounds are ACOAs; 45% of the ACOAs among the HR/HU group have histories of childhood sexual abuse ($p \leq .03$).

Sexual abuse continued beyond childhood for many ICM clients. The number of clients who experienced some sexual abuse during their lives increased to 43%, with 8 of the 38 clients involved experiencing sexual abuse only after childhood. Of the entire group of sexually abused ICM clients, two-thirds are ACOAs and 57% of the ACOAs experienced some type of sexual abuse ($p \leq .01$).

The focus for ICM is building relationships with clients that identify their strengths and mobilize those strengths to work on their own goals for living. Many clients have shared with us events or aspects of their earlier lives which prevented or interfered with living in stable, desired ways. Among the barriers for many people has been the effects of coming from a background which included living in families where alcohol or drug problems existed, or where sexual and/or physical abuse took place. Other people suffered severe sexual or physical abuse while they were children or as adults from people outside their families. Many people continue to live with the impact of these abuses. Our purpose here is to learn about abuses, to understand what has happened to people, and to see the degree to which the mental health system has offered appropriate responses. For this reason, we are also asking your permission to get hospitalization information that describes admissions and discharge dates, diagnoses, and treatments supplied to you.

Your name will *never* be used or disclosed. If you look at the top of the questionnaire, you will see that only a code number appears. Any specific information you give about yourself or your family is entirely confidential and will not be seen by anyone outside the ICM program. But deciding to be a part of this evaluation is your decision. *Whatever you decide will not influence your relationship or work with your ICM.*

Participating in this research is your decision. You can decide that you either do not want to participate at all; that you don't want to participate at this time; or that you do want to participate. You can make separate decisions about the hospital information and about answering the questions the ICM has about abuse. If you want to participate, but there are questions which you do not want to answer, you can choose not to do so.

Thanks very much for considering participating. When we finish the research, a copy of everything written up will be given to you by your ICM.

Stephen M. Rose, Ph.D.
Suffolk ICM Evaluation

____
SIGNATURE

____
INTENSIVE CASE MANAGER

If you have any questions about your rights as a research subject, contact Dr. Robert Schneider, Committee on Research Involving Human Subject, 516-632-6960.

Figure 19-1. Suffolk Intensive Case Management Program; Program Evaluation–Routine Inquiry for Abuse.

Sexual abuse among the ICM clients, like the present power relationships in most families, distributes unequally between men and women. More than twice the number of women ICM clients suffered were sexually attacked as children than were the men—50% of the women compared with 22% of the men. The 2:1 ratio holds among the ACOA clients as well: 64% of the women endured sexual attacks as children compared with 32% of the men. The ACOA experience among male ICM clients appears to be a contributing factor to being sexually abused as children; for women ICM clients, ACOA background is not incidental ($p \leq .05$). When we assess all sexual abuse by gender, 58% of the women were victimized compared with 32% of the male ICM clients. Women from ACOA backgrounds were significantly more likely to have been sexually abused ($p \leq .03$) than were men. Craine et al. (1988) also found a strong correlation ($p \leq .0001$) between family history of substance abuse and sexual abuse among female state hospital patients.

Many ICM clients survived extensive physical abuse, mostly while children, by members of their families, particularly among the ACOAs. Physical abuse was counted separately from sexual abuse, even though both occurred concurrently for many ICM clients. Of the entire ICM caseload, 25% came from ACOA backgrounds that included physical abuse while children. The relationship between ACOA experience and being physically abused as a child by a family member parallels the data on sexual abuse ($p \leq .03$). Of the 44 ACOA ICM clients, 50% were physically abused as children; 65% of those physically abused as children are now ACOAs. Enduring physical abuse at some time in their lives strongly correlates with ACOA backgrounds ($p \leq .005$). Almost one-third of the ICM clients came from an ACOA background that included a history of some physical abuse.

Twenty-three ICM clients experienced both sexual and physical abuse as children ($p \leq .00001$). More than one-quarter of the ICM caseload consisted of people who were both sexually and physically assaulted as children. For incest victims, the association with physical assault as children occurred routinely ($p \leq .001$). Double abuse occurred for both male ($p \leq .00001$) and female ($p \leq .01$) clients. The *ACOA background doubles the potential for both childhood sexual and physical abuse for ICM clients ($p \leq .01$). Dual abuse, along with its neglect by service providers, seems a clear indicator for future HR/HU status ($p = .0001$).*

Thus far, our reported data reflect strong associations between ACOA backgrounds of ICM clients and a series of externally inflicted abuse factors. Now let us look at the association between ACOA life experience and self-inflicted abuses of self-mutilation and substance abuse.

Almost one-third of the ICM clients have mutilated themselves at some time. An association between being an ACOA and self-mutilation is apparent; 71% of the self-mutilating clients are now ACOAs ($p \leq .01$). The relationship is stronger ($p \leq .05$) among women than it is among men. The whole realm of self-mutilation requires far greater examination. Most often, for the

ICM clients, self-mutilation that involves cutting oneself had been diagnosed as a suicidal symptom. The clients, however, provided a contrasting account. Overwhelmed by what many researchers and clinicians have described as posttraumatic stress disorder experiences (see Figley, 1985; Patten et al., 1989), or an emotional experience of reliving an extraordinarily abusive trauma concurrently experienced as real *and* as abstract, clients cut themselves. The desperate purpose involves restoring some mastery over their experience, to constrain themselves from suicide by forcing a return to the reality required to deal with their bleeding.

None of the clients in this study had ever been asked about their self-mutilation; what was happening to them when they committed the act; or what it meant to them. Neither were they asked about being an ACOA nor were they asked about other abuse experiences. When the clients spoke about their abuse backgrounds, only 3 received some response, none appropriate to their needs for legitimation and ongoing support based on their sexual or physical abuse histories and their meaning to the clients in the present. Mental health professionals rarely inquire about abuse or often ignore its meaning when they do learn about it (see Jacobson & Richardson, 1987, among others).

More than half (55%) of the ICM clients had a history of substance abuse, including 61% of the men and 49% of the women. Among the ICM clients from ACOA backgrounds, 75% have substance abuse histories (p = .00026). None of the clients had ever participated in a mental health or substance abuse inpatient or outpatient service where the connection between an ACOA background and current substance abuse had been made and treated as such. The ACOA–substance abuse relationship holds for men (p = .00074) and women (p = .04). More than 86% of the male ACOAs had a substance abuse history compared with 64% of the women.

Table 19-1 illustrates the association between ACOA–substance abuse history and HR/HU participation in the mental health system. Among the 65 HR/HU ICM clients responding (of the total 66), 79% of the ACOAs became substance abusers while more than 70% of the substance abusing HR/HU clients came from ACOA backgrounds (p = .004). Clients with HR/HU participation patterns in the mental health system make up 42 of the 49 (86%) substance abusing people on the caseload and more than 86% of the ACOAs. *The ICM clients who are HR/HUs are much more likely to come*

TABLE 19-1. ACOA–SUBSTANCE ABUSE AMONG HR/HU CLIENTS

	History of Substance Abuse		
ACOA	***Yes***	***No***	***Total***
Yes	30	8	38
No	12	15	27
Total	42	23	65

TABLE 19-2. RELATIONSHIPS BETWEEN ACOA AND OTHER VARIABLES BY PERCENTAGE OF ICM CLIENTS INVOLVED AND *p* LEVELS

Variables	ACOA(%)	*p* Level
HR/HU status	86	.00761
Substance abuse	75	.00026
Any physical abuse	64	.00557
Any sexual abuse	57	.00981
Childhood physical abuse	50	.02858
All childhood sexual abuse	48	.00696
Self-mutilation	46	.01100
Incest	35	.01133

from ACOA backgrounds and have substance abuse histories than other ICM clients (*p* = .00415).

SUMMARY OF THE ACOA LINK TO OTHER ABUSE VARIABLES

Table 19-2 presents the relationships of the ACOA background among ICM clients to the assembled abuse factors discussed earlier. The table presents the abuse variables analyzed, the percentage of ACOA ICM clients for whom the association holds, and the *p*-scores attained in the chi-square tests administered.

In Figure 19-2, the variables are presented comparatively, examining the differences between ICM clients from ACOA backgrounds *and* those with substance abuse histories affected by the specified abuse variable with those who were not. In the comparison, a 23% mean difference in scores exists with all additional abuse variables showing higher impact on substance abuse than ACOA alone.

The ACOA experience has a complex, lasting impact on its survivors. The scope, extent, duration, and meaning of its relation to added abuses varies by individual while the totality of its impact on the ICM caseload remains undeniable.

DISCUSSION

Bryer et al. (1987), after studying childhood sexual and physical abuse among female psychiatric inpatients, conclude the following:

> The correlation of severity of adult psychiatric symptoms with childhood physical and sexual abuse is the most important finding. . . . These results

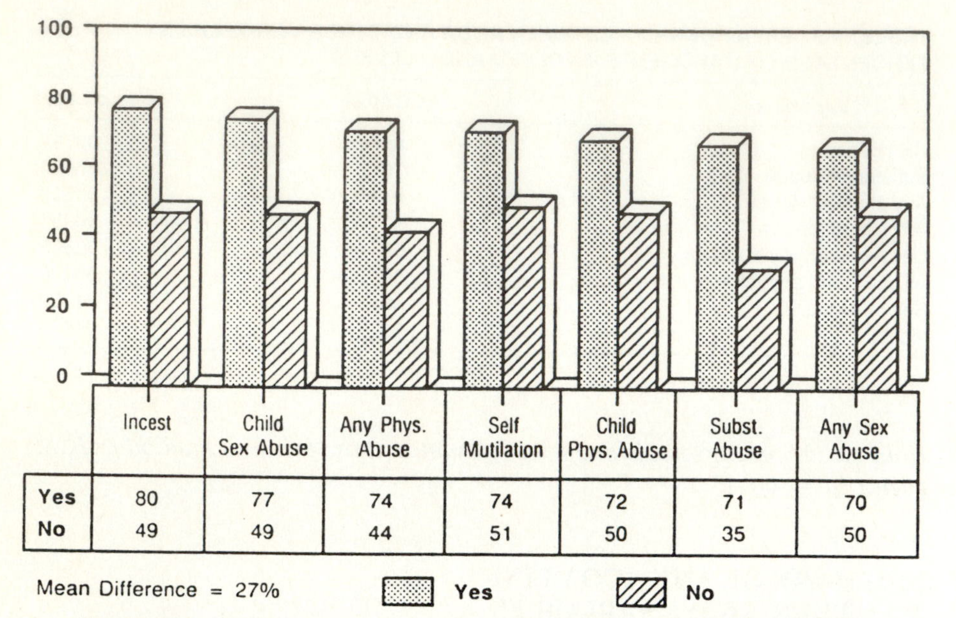

	Incest	Child Sex Abuse	Any Phys. Abuse	Self Mutilation	Child Phys. Abuse	Subst. Abuse	Any Sex Abuse
Yes	80	77	74	74	72	71	70
No	49	49	44	51	50	35	50

Figure 19-2. ICM clients from ACOA backgrounds who become HR/HU's by impact of selected abuse variables. *Note:* 80% of ACOA clients who have experienced incest became HR/HUs versus 49% of those with no experience of incest; 77% of ICM clients from ACOA backgrounds who were sexually abused as children became HR/HU's versus 49% of those who were not sexually abused as children.

> suggest that victims of childhood abuse continue to experience longstanding negative consequences of abuse. . . . The adult psychiatric problems associated with childhood abuse appear to be more severe when the patient has experienced more than one type of abuse. (1987, p. 1429)

Our data support this conclusion. The added factor of ACOA experience precipitating other abuses confirms findings by others as well.

Three outcome variables appear to be strongly associated with ACOA backgrounds and related abuse factors among the ICM clients. The three outcome variables are self-mutiliation, substance abuse, and nonproductive, downward spiraling contacts with the mental health system yielding the HR/HU status.

Three "background" variables were also documented: The constant failure of mental health and social services providers in every setting to do routine inquiry about or appropriately respond to needs arising from being an ACOA or from experiencing incest, other childhood or adult sexual abuse, or physical abuse; the success of service providers in preserving their typical practice models and classification mechanisms to the exclusion of sexually and/or physically abused clients' real needs; and the preservation of organizational boundaries, concepts of practice (Warren, Rose & Burgunder, 1974), and fragmentation between the mental health, substance abuse, and domestic violence-related agencies.

Abusive life histories characterize the existence of most ICM clients. Most often, abuse begins at home, in families where one or more people with power and authority have alcohol or other addictions. This reality establishes an ongoing experience of chronic uncertainty and the betrayal of essential trust among clients from ACOA backgrounds. Additionally, many ICM clients are reduced to powerless objects of further sexual and physical abuse, mostly at the hands of family members. Complicating the brutalization and its emotional residue are denial, secrecy, and evasion converging with clients' deeply felt shame making coherent understanding of their own experience particularly enigmatic.

Involvement of these ICM clients with the mental health system appears to heighten dysfunction. Failure to recognize abuse and respond appropriately to it, whether conscious or unintended, constitutes acts of invalidation, delegitimation, and severing of people from their contextual experience. Concluding a study of 406 patients in psychiatric hospitals, Cole (1988) found that serious consequences occurred when clinicians failed to inquire about patients' abuse backgrounds.

Neglecting to routinely inquire or failing to respond appropriately extends beyond naive errors of omission. Clients further internalize and repress the driving forces shaping their lives, a factor presumably related to the overwhelming number who become HR/HU participants in the mental health system. As Craine et al. (1988) state, "In fact, the longer the abuse goes untreated, the greater the repression and the more ingrained the symptomatology" (p. 300). Bryer et al. (1987) confirm this assessment at the conclusion or their own research:

> Professionals' not initiating a discussion of the topic can transmit a message confirming patients' belief in the need to deny the reality of their experience. Patients' attempts to deal with their distress, then, can take even more indirect paths, leading to the development of severe and confusing symptoms. . . . It follows that instituting psychological and pharmacological therapies without knowing about the original trauma would be like treating the varied and chaotic symptoms of the Vietnam veteran without knowing about Vietnam or what happened there. (p. 1430)

Abused ICM clients with histories of regular compliance with mental health system treatment plans as well as frequent rehospitalizations and emergency room visits, routinely and without conscious choice, reinforce their repression.

CONCLUSION

Routine inquiry, without appropriate follow-up supports, resolves little. Even requiring the inquiry for abuse experience poses a system problem of some magnitude. Carmen et al. (1984), after studying sexual and physical abuse among 188 psychiatric hospital patients, capture this dilemma:

> Thus, even when abuse is identified, clinicians' confusion about the role of abuse in psychiatric illness leaves them unprepared to implement special treatment approaches for what appears to be a large proportion of psychiatric patients. (p. 383)

Routine inquiry and subsequent program development can only succeed when they have a value-based conceptual capacity to envision potential human development for people whose identities can be transformed from victim to survivor, from adaptive consumer to productive participant, from objects that are known and acted on to subjects who know and act (Carmen, Rieker, & Mills, 1984; Freire, 1968; Rose & Black, 1985).

Continuing to promote or permit active denial and repression brings with it both a great human and financial toll. The continual interaction of unrecognized abuse, ACOA involvement, and isolated, unresponsive organizational operations can only yield advanced numbers of substance abusing, HR/HU of mental health services.

Client-driven research requires reconstituting the way evaluators look at independent, dependent, and intervening variables. Disease models exclude external variables as independent factors in producing behavioral outcomes. Our data attest to this: Without ACOA and other abuses identified as independent variables and system neglect seen as intervening variables, neither self-mutilation, substance abuse, nor HR/HU participation in mental health services can be envisioned as system outcomes reflected in the lives of individuals. Mental health system involvement can be seen as an intervening variable increasing the probability of reproducing itself when abuse backgrounds of participants are neglected.

Similarly, the data indicate that substance abuse among ICM clients can exist concurrently as a dependent variable (resulting from the interaction of ACOA plus other abuses plus inappropriate service system responses); as an intervening variable contributing to the hospitalization rate of neglected, abused people; or as an independent variable promoting greater frequency of recidivism. How outcomes are identified and measured has profound influence on the capacity of a program to have system impact. Contributing influences of the clients' social context, both positive and supportive of people's development *and* obstructive or preventive of it, must be factored into client-driven outcome evaluations. To do otherwise, or to simply perceive clients as more or less functional objects in a benign social world, simply reproduces the domain boundaries and practice models of conventional service providers. The very organizations and their intervention models that create the systemic dysfunctions requiring case management as a system change strategy instead become reaffirmed by it.

REFERENCES

Bryer, J. B., et al. 1987. Childhood sexual and physical abuse as a factor in adult psychiatric illness. *American Journal of Psychiatry.* 144:1426–1430.

Burgess, A. W., & Holmstrom, L. L. 1974. Rape trauma syndrome. *American Journal of Psychiatry.* 131:891–896.

Carmen, E. H., Rieker, P. P., & Mills, T. 1984. Victims of violence and psychiatric illness. *American Journal of Psychiatry.* 141:378–383.

Cole, C. 1988. Routine comprehensive inquiry for abuse: A justifiable clinical assessment procedure? *Clinical Social Work Journal.* 16:33–42.

Craine, L. S., et al., 1988. Prevalence of a history of sexual abuse among female psychiatric patients in a state hospital system. *Hospital and Community Psychiatry.* 39:300–304.

Emslie, G. J., & Rosenfeld, A. 1983. Incest reported by children and adolescents hospitalized for severe psychiatric problems. *American Journal of Psychiatry.* 140: 708–711.

Figley, C. R. (Ed.). 1985. *Trauma and Its Wake: The Study and Treatment of Post-Traumatic Stress Disorder.* New York: Brunner/Mazel.

Freire, P. 1968. *Pedagogy of the Oppressed.* New York: The Seabury Press.

Hussain, A., & Chapel, J. L. 1983. History of incest in girls admitted to a psychiatric hospital. *American Journal of Psychiatry.* 140:591–593.

Jacobson, A., & Richardson, B. 1987. Assault experiences of 100 psychiatric inpatients: Evidence of the need for routine inquiry. *American Journal of Psychiatry.* 144:908–913.

Lindberg, F., & Distad, L. 1985. Post-traumatic stress disorders in women who experienced childhood incest. *Childhood Abuse and Neglect.* 9:329–334.

Patten, S. B., et al., 1989. Posttraumatic stress disorder and the treatment of sexual abuse. *Social Work.* 34:197–203.

Rose, S. M., & Black, B. L. 1985. *Advocacy and Empowerment: Mental Health Care in the Community.* London:Routledge & Kegan Paul.

Rose, S. M., Peabody, C. G., & Stratigeas, B. 1989. Client-driven outcomes and system responses: Research report #1 (Mimeographed). School of Social Welfare, State University of New York at Stony Brook.

Warren, R. L., Rose, S. M., & Burgunder, A. F. 1974. *The Structure of Urban Reform.* Lexington, MA: D.C. Heath & Co.

PART VI

An Advocacy/ Empowerment Model of Case Management for Social Work

CHAPTER 20

Case Management:

An Advocacy/Empowerment Design

Stephen M. Rose

Advocacy/empowerment case management requires a dual commitment from case management to deliver direct services to vulnerable clients *and* to challenge dysfunctional service delivery systems. The advocacy/empowerment perspective assumes that the very existence of case management constitutes a serious indictment of system functioning. Put somewhat differently, if there were comprehensive service planning coupled with adequate and appropriate resources; if there were integration of diverse service system components; if there were highly responsive provider systems with both facility of access and appropriate modes of intervention; and if there were client-driven supportive services tied to adequate material resources such as safe, affordable housing, there would be no need for case management.

The appearance of case management in numerous service sectors attests to the universality of systems deficits, fragmentation, and irrationality. Each of the service areas discussed earlier, along with systems involved with abused children, people with acquired immunodeficiency syndrome, the elderly, and others, illustrate this point.

To ignore, deny, or deflect attention away from system shaping factors, or to neglect the many barriers to appropriate resources and services, betrays people whose life circumstances and vulnerability require case management. The most common form of betrayal exists in denigration of the advocacy function of case management or in its expression in coopted or provider-driven form. This form reduces advocacy to case specific measures to gain access to traditional service offerings; e.g., advocating to secure a Medicaid card so that the client can become a more efficient conduit for third party payments. While the client may benefit from the outcome, its central concern remains the provider system.

Empowerment also gets coopted; clients are *required* to "choose" from service menus defined and controlled by providers who determine clients' needs for them. Clients do not participate in establishing their own goals or in defining their own needs. Treatment plans or service plans either prepared by professionals or by case managers often preempt clients' active involvement. Typically, they by-pass client-directed goal formulation, substituting for it a needs assessment format controlled by providers' problem-defining paradigms, typical service modalities, and reimbursement formulas.

When clients' needs are assessed without their direct involvement in producing life directions or specific goals to pursue and implement, the planning that takes place exists within a provider-driven framework. This occurs because clients' needs and identities are being determined by the services already being delivered. In other words, clients are perceived only as functional, compliant consumers or dysfunctional categories, both defined by funding guidelines and existing service models.

The advocacy/empowerment case management sees empowerment differently. It requires clients' active involvement in producing or defining their own goals and in designing their implementation strategies. A corollary assumption values the setting for living as the most interdependent environment possible for each person. In this perspective, needs assessments comes from clients' goals. Needs establish what must be acquired, confronted, accomplished, or developed at the level of the client, the family, or the social network or systems level to produce client-defined or desired outcomes. Parallel to the advocacy dimension, the rules, roles, and routines or service providers are not the central concern.

The advocacy/empowerment design regards itself as client-driven rather than provider-driven. The distinction will be made clear in this chapter. This model articulates several explicit values which appear in following paragraphs as basic assumptions that serve as the foundation for advocacy/empowerment case management practice (see Rose & Black, 1985, for an elaboration of advocacy/empowerment theory and community mental health practice). Following the elaboration of the assumptions, the basic practice model will be developed.

ASSUMPTION 1

Case Management Clients Are Seen as Whole Human Beings Living in a Social Context

As whole human beings, clients are seen as persons who participate in an identifiable or knowable social context. The structure and values or ideology of that context can enhance, obstruct, impede, and/or sustain them. We understand the clients and ourselves similarly, as "contextual" or socially active participants. The arena for advocacy/empowerment case management functioning and responsibility is contextual, incorporating the interaction of person with context. Contextual understanding includes the concrete, material resources required to live decently along with the social as well as emotional supports necessary to grow and develop.

The client role in relation to any particular provider or the client status, as determined by providers' diagnostic systems, does not limit or confine advocacy/empowerment case management concerns. From this perspective, the dignity of the person transcends the role of client in relation to any service provider; similarly, it sees diagnosis as descriptive rather than prescriptive.

Goal setting, or defining the directions to pursue and establishing a framework for the problems to be confronted, does not confine or restrict case managers and clients to accepting the limitations of existing providers' services, eligibility requirements, or resource deficits. Functional improvement or compliance with treatment plans, the typical objectives of provider-driven case management, are replaced by purposive designation of needs as prerequisite to goal attainment and by allocation of responsibility for implementation.

ASSUMPTION 2

People Can Grow and Develop When Provided with the Necessary Material, Social and Emotional Supports, and Validation to Live Stable, Positive Lives

Adequate material resources and constructive social relationships are the foundations on which stable, positive lives are built. For this reason, advocacy/empowerment case management represents a continuous struggle to assure the availability of appropriate, supportive living environments and to assist clients to create or strengthen informal social networks where they can participate as fully valid, consciously involved human beings. Regardless of the severity of their disability or handicap, people can learn, grow, and develop when they live in materially adequate, supportive contexts. This fundamental belief in human dignity and strength constitutes the basis for the advocacy/empowerment commitment.

People who actively participate in transforming their environments, at whatever level their capacity allows, change themselves in the process. Conversely, people coerced into adapting to debilitating environments are forced into managed identities or roles that sustain their dependency. *Advocacy/empowerment case management expresses a commitment to supporting clients' change from objects, known and acted upon, to subjects who know and act* (Freire, 1968; Rose & Black, 1985). *Empowerment, the active continuous, conscious process of determining direction, of setting goals and working to produce them, or living as a subject, characterize the relationships advocacy/empowerment case managers seek to build.*

When people's handicaps do not permit full autonomy of action, the principle of optimizing the person's participation remains. In circumstances involving children or people who are clearly debilitated, where legal or individual obstacles prevent self-determination, case managers will have to make assessments about how to involve family members and other central actors from the client's support system in decision-making processes.

Advocacy/empowerment case management works to build trusting relationships, validating the struggles of clients to focus on their own goals or directions and on advocating to assure appropriate, accessible, and adequate resources. Cnaan and his associates express this commitment well: Responsibility rests with case management staff "to enlarge clients' expectations of themselves, to help them view themselves as capable of progress, and to support this process of growth" (1988, p. 63). *Operationalizing the concept of validation occurs through the case manager's efforts to assist and support the clients to focus on their goals and interests as subjects.* Often, this process will involve case managers directing dialogue toward clients' appreciating their own strengths (see Chapter 8) and coming to understand the limitations imposed on their self-concept and potential development by static diagnostic categories or provider-determined social roles. Validation also comes when case managers initiate and support the activity necessary to transform a goal-centered focus into a plan for implementation.

ASSUMPTION 3

Growth and Movement Occur in the Context of Relationships Characterized by Honesty, Clarity of Goals, and Continuity between Goals, Purposes, and Shared Plans of Action

Advocacy/empowerment case management relationships with clients are purposive and process-oriented. They are forged in the belief that people can focus on their own needs and can be assisted to develop direction plans that articulate those needs as the basis for ongoing work. Clarity of goals develops through dialogue between the case manager and his or her client, perhaps with input from significant others determined by the client to be important to the process.

Process-oriented attention supersedes achievement-based judgment. Case managers support clients to focus on operationalizing goals; to construct manageable steps that move toward the goal while continually embodying its meaning and purpose; to mutually determine implementation responsibilities by joint decision-making about who will take specific concrete steps within a jointly determined time frame.

Living stable, positive lives within supportive contexts constitutes the purpose of the direction plan. Goal definition or direction setting *always* precedes need assessment to be certain that any articulated need comes from the client's own direction and not from a service provider's menu. Inserting goal or direction planning into the array of case management task areas and assigning it top priority redirects the focus from provider-driven service consumption to client-validating activities.

Joint determination of responsibility for implementation supports the empowerment process by moving it from the realm of planning to the arena of action. Purposeful connection of goals to needs to activity replaces the more typical process of referral. Even where linkage to service providers does occur, it takes place in the context of a larger client-defined direction plan.

Clients learn to see and use their relationship with providers strategically: They work on knowing what they must use, how it fits into their own plan, and how to evaluate the effectiveness of the service from its contribution to their goal. Regular review of participation in services or programs maintains continuity of purpose and meaning and protects against routinization of involvement or cooptation into provider-driven patterns. This process becomes one dimension of monitoring, another case management task. Reviewing how the actions to be taken by the client and case management relate to client's goals and their purpose complements the monitoring function. At each meeting, a review of implementation steps occurs, with continuity linked to the goals, purposes, and needs.

Empowerment, a key organizing value, occurs by keeping the focus of intervention and interaction on goal formulation, on goal reframing where appropriate, and on purposive activity. Many people who become case management clients have a broad array of needs that crosscut multiple service providers' domains. Often, this weakens their capacity to function autonomously. Many clients can be expected to be quite vulnerable and to have very low levels of self-confidence, particularly if they have been in systems that employ stigmatizing labels. Case managers will encounter this when working on setting goals and assigning tasks to be carried out.

Identifying the optimal capacity of each client to share responsibility for implementing goals or partial tasks derived from goals constitutes the empowerment dimension of a goal. Clients who doubt their own capacity will have to decide whether the debilitating impact of their own doubt requires consideration as a goal for the direction plan. But, except in cases of absolute emergency or crisis, where clients cannot actively articulate their goals or needs, the case management process requires the active involvement, engagement, and participation of clients at every level.

Regular review of the process of case management takes place between case managers and their clients. Continuity in moving from setting goals to operationalizing them, from establishing responsibility to implementing it, from examining movement to examining its purpose, and from identifying unanticipated problems and planning for them all reflect the empowerment principle. They do this by validating the client's capacity, commitment, and accomplishment. Each aspect of the process highlights the clients' participation and validates their struggle to emerge from restrictive identities and pejorative social roles as patients or as managed objects.

ASSUMPTION 4

Diagnosis Does Not Determine the Person's Entire Future Development or Capacity to Live More Fully Than Providers' Roles Permit

Human development, the capacity for growth and change as a human being, cannot be restricted by diagnostic categories and providers' definitions of clients' roles. Advocacy/empowerment case management presumes clients' potential for development. This potential is tied to the participation of the client in producing direction and meaning centered in goals, articulated in deriving needs, and expressed through sharing responsibility for movement as discussed earlier.

Validation as a subject cannot depend on functional compliance with treatment plans or service regimens defined and operationalized by others. This belief extends even into high technology health care, where we presume that people's responsibility for self-care in accord with medical prescriptions will correspond to the degree of understanding they have about their situation and the level of involvement they have regarding their input into the process. More effective outcomes occur through informed participation or coproduction of direction plans that come from passive consumption or compliance.

Provider-driven case management models mistake functional compliance with development or stabilization. Advocacy/empowerment case managers reject this notion in favor of active coproduction of direction plans, of conscious focus, engagement, and determination of action. The most adroit consumer remains passively adaptive to provider determinations of what is best. These definitions have neither routinely served clients effectively in terms of reducing system dependency nor have they produced continuity of care, comprehensive service delivery across organizational domains, or expansions of needed material resources for most case management clients.

The principle of empowerment or self-determination becomes complicated when clients legally or physically cannot speak for themselves. Children are legally tied to parents or designated others while some elderly people may have organic impairment of their decision-making capacity which places family members or other court-appointed guardians in decision-making authority. The role of the family or significant others will have to be carefully evaluated with regard to decision-making and legal status. Effort on the part of the advocacy/empowerment case manager to stay client-centered in his or her focus may require extra legal reflection in some cases to account for people not recognized as responsible for incapacitated clients but more significant to them than family.

The degree of incapacitation must also be assessed to determine whether the identified client has some capacity to express his or her judgment. This problem of partial capacity is both physical and legal, especially when it comes to children. In these circumstances, case managers must have access to legal consultation and readily available support for themselves. On the value dimension, the discussion by Collopy (1988, Chapter 5) can be valuable to reconsider in its commitment to optimal autonomy, even in the face of immobilizing handicaps.

THE ADVOCACY/EMPOWERMENT DIRECTION PLAN

The direction plan (see Table 20-1) is the major instrument used to extend the advocacy/empowerment approach into practice. Through use of the direction plan, the goals and needs assessment developed in the case management relationship are converted into an implementation plan. This is done for each goal by establishing exactly what steps have to be undertaken to move toward accomplishing the goal. It also specifies who will do them. Existing strengths and obstacles are identified and assessed by the case manager and the client with regard to how they could influence outcomes. This is done at both the client and systems level. Changes are made routinely to reflect the relationship between client and case manager as the central meaningful component of the advocacy/empowerment case management design, one that transcends the document that it creates.

CASE STUDY

Robert is a 27-year-old man who has been in and out of a psychiatric hospital 15 times in the last 3 years. He has a severe drinking problem as well as behavior difficulties. The mental health system has identified Robert as "dually diagnosed," "treatment resistant," and a "MICA patient" (mentally ill chemical abuser). When assigned to a case manager who wanted to involve him in establishing his needs and goals, Robert's only statement was his absolute desire to stay out of the state hospital forever. This goal was taken seriously by the case manager, who entered it immediately into Robert's direction plan while talking to Robert about his goals.

Clients are given copies of each step or revision of direction plan development, countersigning it or identifying any objections. Here, the case manager reviewed

TABLE 20-1. DIRECTION PLAN

Client:

ICM:
Date:
AREA: Housing

Current Status What's Going On Now?	Personal Goals Where I'd Like To Be Is . . . ?	Perceived Obstacles What Keeps Me From Getting It?	Moving Ahead Now, I Have To Do . . .
I am now living at? with?	*I would like to live . . . ? Why?*	*I can't do this now because . . . ?*	To change this, I have to . . . ?
Prioritizing Needs What Steps Do I Take?	**Resources I Need The Supports I Need Are . . . ?**	**Managing and Monitoring How Will My Progress Be Noted?**	**Continuity and Evaluation Is This Really Where I Want To Go?**
What steps do I take?	*Each resource gets me . . . ?*	*How can I make sure it happens?*	*How am I doing? Am I on track?*

AREA: Finances

Current Status What's Going On Now?	Personal Goals Where I'd Like To Be Is . . . ?	Perceived Obstacles What Keeps Me From Getting It?	Moving Ahead Now, I Have To Do . . .
My financial situation is . . . ?	*I need how much each month?*	*I have not got it because . . . ?*	*To get what I need, I have to?*
(Identify source, amount & need)			

Prioritizing Needs What Steps Do I Take?	Resources I Need The Supports I Need Are . . . ?	Managing and Monitoring How Will My Progress Be Noted?	Continuity and Evaluation Is This Really Where I Want to Go?
What steps do I take?	*Each resource gets me . . . ?*	*How can I make sure it happens?*	*How am I doing? Am I on track?*

AREA: Social Supports and Friends

Current Status What's Going On Now?	Personal Goals Where I'd Like To Be Is . . . ?	Perceived Obstacles What Keeps Me From Getting It?	Moving Ahead Now, I Have To Do . . .
Relationships I have: + and −	*The connections I would like?*	*These things get in my way . . .*	*To change, I have to . . . ?*

Prioritizing Needs What Steps Do I Take?	Resources I Need The Supports I Need Are . . . ?	Managing and Monitoring How Will My Progress Be Noted?	Continuity and Evaluation Is This Really Where I Want To Go?
What steps do I take?	Each resource gets me . . . ?	How can I make sure it happens?	How am I doing? Am I on track?

with Robert his recent history, examining the decreasing time between hospitalizations and the lengthening time of each hospitalization. Clearly, Robert was deteriorating as long as he kept living in the welfare hotels where the hospital placed him and where his drinking problem was actively supported. This produced a confrontation where Robert's pattern of behavior and his goal to live a more stable, positive life were determined to be entirely contradictory. The case manager could support Robert's goal selection, which meant confrontation with living patterns that were counterproductive. In this case, after the case manager refused to relinquish the substance of the contradiction and continued to support Robert's strengths in choosing his goal, Robert decided to enter a detox program and participate in Alcoholics Anonymous, along with demanding a more appropriate housing option. All of these interactions were recorded in the direction plan, with the case manager continuing to show how the implementation process flowed from Robert's goal selection.

The direction plan is a dynamic document, with interactions and decisions about goals, needs, strengths, and obstacles as well as implementation and monitoring data recorded regularly with the client present. A copy of the plan, with any additions, refinements, or changes routinely goes directly to the client. (This, of course, requires simple mechanics as well—carbon copies on hand as well as minimal legibility.)

Clients' assuming the optimal level of responsibility for implementing each step in their direction plan exists as a primary value and as a target for ongoing monitoring between clients and case managers. The discussion and negotiation between case managers and clients over the designation of who will assume what level of task and function in relation to implementing the clients' goals is a basic building block of the advocacy/empowerment process. Not only does it target attention to clients' strengths, it also serves to "contextualize" problems.

The relative impact of environmental factors can be assessed; system factors shaping clients' outcomes can be delineated. Parallel to this aspect of the process, clients have to examine the factors they can control as these variables play a part in shaping their own outcomes. Clients often assume individual responsibility for system deficits or resource deficiencies by internalizing responsibility for system factors that are out of their control (e.g., for the absence of safe, affordable housing). At other times, they can deny responsibility for behavior or relationships that they can influence or shape. Either area can be documented for ongoing dialogue as part of a direction plan. Advocacy issues can be mutually defined, and clients' understanding of precisely where and how environmental obstacles or their own behavior affect them can be examined in relation to goal attainment.

The case manager and Robert had to decide who would locate detox programs and how a decision would be made to enter one of them. Time frames for

> accomplishment had to be established: The detox programs had to be identified by a set date; the visit to each program would be completed by a set date; who would call to make the arrangements, by what date, and so on.
>
> The case manager kept regular contact with Robert while he was in the detox unit of the hospital he determined was best for him. The objective was continuity and consistency with Robert's goal, so the focus of the relationship was discharge planning. Of primary import was the place where Robert would live when leaving the detox program and its proximity to AA meetings and to a psychosocial rehabilitation program that Robert had attended once before and felt was appropriate for him in that it provided both some transitional structure and skill training related to future employment.

In addition to making certain that clients' discharge planning help them realize their goals, it is equally important for case managers to be certain that clients have accurate information about service providers, benefits, or entitlement programs. At times, clients' distrust or uncertainty may require a joint visit with the case manager to a provider to gather new factual or experiential data to assess the resources and its applicability to a client's specific goals.

The case manager represents continuity, the bridge to positive, active, selective utilization of services. Had Robert not known about the program he felt was appropriate, the case manager would have arranged for him to visit it prior to discharge and to explore his perception of its applicability to his plan. The availability of the service would not determine its appropriateness as so often happens in provider-driven discharge plans.

Goal statements specify the specific needs for individually tailored environmental supports together with relationship needs and what clients have to do to secure both. Goal statements in the direction plan are temporal, successive, and dynamic—they can change as the client or the circumstances require.

> Robert moved from the community and a life of chaotic deterioration to a structured setting for stabilization as part of his goal to live in the community. At the same time, his participation in the structure of the detox unit became part of the larger process of living a more stable, independent, positive life on return. As Robert succeeded in his goal of stabilization and growth, family or friends that were alienated from him while he was actively drinking were reintroduced as the basis for creating informal supports. Supported employment became a viable alternative to continuing employment as it required greater autonomy and produced movement toward independence from mental health services.

The direction plan, used with each client, and specifically designed in accord with the pace and capacity that each client brings, emphasizes a number of previously stated values. In its focus on the needs and goals of human beings living in a social context, the person is validated as a contributor or participant. Similar to the strengths model of case management discussed in

Chapter 5, the advocacy/empowerment design emphasizes clients' capacities through focusing on what they will need to live optimally autonomous (Chapter 4) or positively interdependent lives in the most supportive environment attainable.

Community resources, including appropriate services and providers, are identified and accessed in relation to the goals established in the direction plan. System deficits, resource gaps, or provider barriers to optimal environments become targets for advocacy activities through documentation of their impact on individual clients' lives and design of appropriate strategies.

The direction plan activates the case manager's relationship to the client, through the advocacy/empowerment approach. The goal setting focus leads to another principle of direction plan development—continuity. The case manager in the advocacy/empowerment perspective does not separate the case management functions of needs assessment, planning, linking, monitoring, and advocacy into discrete tasks or a specified sequence. Clients' goals serve as the basis for integrating all tasks. Continuity exists through the case manager who creates the interface between different dimensions of the process and makes them overt. Needs come from goal-based statements of what the client would like to experience in daily life. This establishes the foundation for developing the implementation plan and the progression to mutually identified assignments of responsibility for implementation. As seen in our example, however, the process does not necessarily follow a rational, linear course. Goals may change, unanticipated problems may emerge, or previously underdeveloped strengths of the client might require reframing direction plans or rearranging of the client might require reframing direction plans or rearranging priorities within a plan. Changes such as these are expected parts of a dynamic process centered in the relationship between the case manager and the client, not reified in the plan.

The entire direction plan dimension of the case management process is reviewed routinely to assure that it is moving and purposive, while constantly subject to refinement, adjustment, or significant (but not frivolously or randomly picked) change. The reviewing component of the process constitutes the advocacy/empowerment version of monitoring. It becomes a data and experiential base for reflecting on movement toward goals.

The identification of accomplishment, whenever and wherever it exists, is "named" (Freire, 1968) and celebrated as a form of acknowledgment and growth, of validation for the client. In Robert's situation, his strength and commitment to his own growth are cited and documented in the direction plan when he enters the detox program and when he leaves. Returning to an institutional setting, rather than being experienced as a failure and as another example of Robert's lack of control, is turned into its opposite, documented and highlighted as a clear accomplishment.

Where movement either does not occur or occurs in a direction contradictory to the goals established with the client in the direction plan, advocacy/

empowerment case managers are responsible for regaining focus, clarity, and purpose. This responsibility holds whether the change is predetermined by the client and presented verbally or presented behaviorally as in a relapse for a client with alcohol problems or in a rehospitalization for a former psychiatric patient. The direction plan, as a process document or intervention strategy, can always be altered. But, when this occurs, establishing the reasons for doing so communicates the belief that change can be understood and that negative situations can be confronted. This again places the client, rather than the plan or the case manager, at the center of the process and communicates the belief that as needs and situations change, their evaluation produces the requirement for change in the direction plan.

The direction plan process does not presume a logical, linear enfolding with rational, symmetrical patterns. Chaotic processes can occur, particularly with those clients who have a history of invalidation and institutional dependency, long experience in unstable familial relationships (e.g., the adult who grew up in a home characterized by addicted family members), or addictions. Even when chaotic behaviors and setbacks occur, the case manager can assert some certainty by being there for the client, by neither abandoning the person nor the belief that she or he can be an active contributor to his or her own life course. The direction plan, when used flexibly yet assertively, can contribute to that stability and growth, especially when it reappears after some setback for the client and integrates what occurred into the plan for continued movement.

Establishing goals and supporting their implementation may produce heightened self-doubt in those clients with little experience in stable relationships, with feelings of self-contempt, or with little social and emotional support. Feelings of inadequacy or of threat to the client's previous way of coping are not uncommon when people have been placed in dependent positions, are extremely vulnerable, and are asked to act in their own behalf (see Estroff, 1981). Case managers must learn to confront these feelings when they appear not as indicators of their own or their clients' failure or inadequacy. Rather, the fears and doubts that clients experience must be incorporated into the direction plan as matters to be discussed and objectives for which implementation has to be created.

The direction plan can never be more important than the person whose life is reflected in it. The client, therefore, must always be the center of case managers' attention. When such patterns as breaking appointments or subverting goals are routine, they cannot be denied. Confronting the behavior, in terms of goals rather than diagnosis or the case manager's judgments, makes it possible to incorporate self-destructive behavior into the array of obstacles to be overcome as articulated in the direction plan. Where case managers, perhaps with input from team members or supervisors, find negative behavior patterns preeminent in their contact with individual clients, they may choose to elevate the relationship problems to top priority. This involves pointing out that present ways of living and behaving obstruct any movement toward positive goals. The challenge here requires defining the situation as a problem or contradiction for the client, with the case manager sustaining allegiance to the person through her or his commitment to the positive goals and strengths the client demonstrated in setting up stabilizing goals.

In the advocacy/empowerment case management approach, defining goals, identifying needs, and setting forth implementation plans is an interactive process. On the one hand, there are the array of resources or barriers to them in the environment. On the other hand, there is the client's self-concept or perception of his or her own identity. As these come together, the client's concept of himself or herself and the depth and degree of self-confidence—a reflection of the existing trusted social support available outside the formal provider system—will structure the options that the client perceives as applicable to his or her life. The advocacy/empowerment-oriented case manager must recognize that the client is the center of this interactive process, not the array of options that appear to be available or the activity of choosing.

Movement toward self-determined goals and needs proceeds as a reflection of the interaction between the client's self-concept or identity and the array of existing options to be confronted. Can the client genuinely see himself or herself taking advantage of option X, Y, or Z or acting on advocacy strategy A, B, or C? Or are these options external to the client's range of plausibility or what the client deeply feels are his or her own real options? *The advocacy/empowerment case manager must develop an understanding of what the client perceives and feels about himself or herself, of how the person understands his or her identity. This forms the basis for assessing the client's range of plausibility, of what really can occur in the present. How the client perceives himself or herself now shapes what perceptions he or she can have of options and of future development.*

The case manager's work on validation, discussed earlier, will become central to the ongoing process, along with the level of social support the client experiences from informal networks. Can the client imagine himself or herself doing only strategy A or using only option Z, and even then, only with the case manager's continuing support? This level of knowing the clients or of entering their reality (see Freire, 1968; Rose & Black, 1985) challenges the advocacy/empowerment case manager, particularly when the case manager has worked very hard to produce options or possibilities that the client has not yet been able to incorporate or even envision as applicable to his or her life. The test emerges at this point: Is the client really the driving point of the practice? Or will the differing case manager's and client's perspectives on choosing options need to become a further part of the direction plan? The questions posed here are among the many that demonstrate the importance of supervision for advocacy/empowerment case management practice (see later). There are no answers that transcend the specific individuals involved, thus requiring consistent reflection and evaluation of the implementation of advocacy/empowerment practice principles.

Direction Plan Specifics

The direction plan can comprise any number of specific pages since each page is designed to elicit response for a specific direction or goal. Table 20–1 contains finances, housing, and social supports and friends, similar to the personal plan discussed in the Kisthardt and Rapp article (Chapter 5). But others might include informal systems or social networks, family, mental health, vocational training, and drug or alcohol rehabilitation. Certainly, the direction plan can also be used to identify areas related to relationships with others, including the case manager, or behavioral problems that interfere with goal attainment.

Because the direction plan is intended as a guide rather than a blueprint and because its use depends on the case manager–client relationship, the components or order of the problem or goal areas can be rearranged to suit specific needs. It seems reasonable, for example, to have home health care be a separate planning page for long term care case management while hospital-based case management might need more space for detailing the specifics of coordinated, high tech inpatient care and its litany of tests, results, machines, physicians, and decisions that must be made. The direction plan pages presented come from the intensive case management program in Suffolk County, New York. This program is targeted at high risk populations with psychiatric hospital experience, usually people with multiple hospitalizations.

The first section of the direction plan for every area contains straightforward questions about the client's present situation. Part of the present situation should include the client's strengths, or what the client brings to the situation. It is projected that considerable time and focus will be required of the case manager in determining how this factor is expressed, obscured, or doubted by clients, but it is an important aspect of the direction plan. If little else is forthcoming from the client, when she or he sets forth goals that are desired, as requested by the second column of the plan, the desire to attain a different situation—where positive—can be listed as a strength that is expressed as motivation.

The remaining sections of the direction plan are self-evident. The third section attempts to identify resource acquisition problems and target them for elaboration and advocacy interventions, where appropriate. It also serves as a basis for exploring with clients how they perceive themselves in relation to social and economic factors that influence the quality of their lives. The fourth section generates movement, communicates possibility, yet also creates a basis for reality testing and time-frame perception. For example, the need for safe, affordable housing in a community where none exists cannot be translated into immediate results. Creative short-term solutions will have to be pursued along with housing advocacy. The impact of unavailable resources as an externally imposed problem must be clear to the client.

The remaining sections prioritize and specify needs and the division of labor between the client and case manager in relation to implementation of the plan's goals. Monitoring and review are vehicles for assuring continuity and delineating benchmarks of movement for acknowledgment. Every entry, whether an initial statement or a small refinement or a major change, is recorded as it is decided, with a copy of all transactions for the client.

APPROPRIATENESS, ADEQUACY, AND ACCESS

In constructing a client's direction plan, advocacy/empowerment case managers always look first to informal networks in the community for appropriate resources and supports. The community must not be seen as a barrier, but as a potential resource (see Kisthardt and Rapp, Chapter 5). Use of formal service providers as a first resort can impede, if not contradict, the desired outcome of supporting clients to live as autonomously or interdependently in informal networks as possible (for each individual).

Where formal provider systems are required or desired, for example, in income maintenance or in home health care, the principle of conscious, knowledgeable participation remains. The same principle applies to all service provider interactions: The dignity, validity, and self-determination of clients precede professional convenience at all times. Pragmatically, this requires that informed consent be genuine rather than a facile, bureaucratic process; that every interagency meeting about a client take place with the client and his or her designated representative present or with the client's authorization.

The commitment to a client-driven practice requires an examination of three characteristics of services: appropriateness, adequacy, and access. These three factors must be kept separate in the mind of the advocacy/empowerment case manager. Considerations concerning service providers' domain or turf might cause them to prefer that the three areas be blended into each other. If a service provider can reduce evaluation of its services from questions of appropriateness to clients' goals and needs to issues of access or quantity, the qualitative question implied in the appropriateness issue is coopted into more simple, quantitative measures.

For our purposes, appropriate and inappropriate are designations that derive from the clients' goals and needs as they are developed in the case management direction plan. When we recall that needs and goals are not defined in accord with either service providers' practice models or service delivery patterns and that the people who use advocacy/empowerment case management services are seen as participating subjects rather than diagnostic categories, objects to be managed, or consumers, the issue of appropriateness becomes more apparent.

CASE STUDIES

A home health care agency does not want to take the time to explain to an elderly client exactly what services are being delivered, how those services relate to his hospital discharge plan, or how those services are being billed. Mr. Peters, the 73-year-old client, is told that all services are covered by insurance and not to worry. The treatment plan was drawn up by the discharging team at a local hospital who also arranged for the agency to deliver home health care as specified in the plan. With a premium on efficiency in delivery, taking time to talk to the recipient and involve him as an active participant, or to engage caregivers as vital participants can be seen as too costly by the provider.

A continuing treatment program tries to prevent a case management client from reducing her attendance at its program and replacing it by seeking support at a self-help group.

A person being discharged to a transitional community residence from a psychiatric hospital is told that he must attend a day treatment program five days per week and sit in on group therapy in the home as conditions for acceptance into the supervised residence.

These types of requirements are generally necessary to produce optimal reimbursements for providers and often are appropriate to that end—only. They do not come from drawing out clients' concepts of their own goals and what is necessary to achieve them.

Appropriateness deals with the level of problem definition or clients' goals and the "fit" between client's goals/needs and providers' services. Adequacy simply measures quantity. Adequacy can be applied either to appropriate or inappropriate resources, benefits, or services. For example, if a person becomes eligible for supplemental security income (SSI), how adequate is the amount of money provided each month in relation to paying for the monthly cost of living safely and decently? How adequate is the SSI entitlement when measured against the Bureau of Labor Statistics standards? In New York, the rate of SSI for a single person living alone can be less than 50 percent of what is needed to live in safe housing, eat minimally nutritious meals, use transportation to get to see family or find employment, and so on. Conversely, in some areas there are more than adequate amounts of certain treatment services, some of which can be inappropriate to clients whose goals call for learning to live more independently. In these same areas, there may be completely inadequate supplies of supported housing or independent housing appropriate to clients' goals to live stable, positive lives in communities.

The issue of access to services further complicates the situation. Most simply, access relates to whether services or resources are made available in ways that clients can use them. For people whose disability restricts them to wheelchairs, for example, are there ramps available at outpatient medical clinics? Can a client who wants to work on increasing his or her independence reduce the amount of time spent each week at a partial hospitalization program or a vocational skills training center? Are language specialists available to assist those whose primary language is different from a provider? Access, like adequacy, interacts with appropriateness. Easily accessible, but inappropriate services, even when in adequate supply, do not reduce the burden to case managers who want to operate from an advocacy/empowerment perspective. In fact, such a situation may make the case managers' lives more complicated and tensions with providers more pronounced.

The advocacy/empowerment client-driven focus mandates that appropriateness of resources, benefit or entitlement programs, or services becomes the pivotal factor in determining use. Case managers must be sure not to shape their evaluation of the appropriateness of providers' services because of sufficient adequacy or easy accessibility. Confusion of these factors can subtlely rearrange case managers' priorities because of ease of access or comparative availability of inappropriate services. When that occurs, the value of the advocacy/empowerment design gets coopted into provider-driven practice.

In relation to clients, this same issue arises in another form. Clients who are unsure of themselves can extend validity or appropriateness to providers because they have not yet developed sufficient trust in their own assessment of what they need or how a resource may or may not support their goals. Case managers have to confront this possibility, including making referrals where the case manager has some skepticism about a provider's appropriateness to a particular client. Where the client determines that the service is appropriate, case managers make the referral and link the client with the resource. The client's experience is reviewed and jointly evaluated as part of case management direction planning and ongoing evaluation. It becomes part of the direction plan monitoring process.

ADVOCACY/EMPOWERMENT CASE MANAGEMENT PROCESS

A number of the articles in this volume have presented case management as a job that usually comprises five functions: needs assessment, care planning, linkage or referral, monitoring, and advocacy. An implied linear progression seems to organize the tasks discretely and sequentially: One identifies clients, does a needs assessment, makes a plan, refers the client, monitors progress, and, on occasion and where necessary, does limited advocacy. Behind this notion is a basic broker model of case management or a provider-driven model.

Things do not go quite so smoothly for most case management clients. Appropriate resources, in adequate supply and easily accessible to people, do not routinely exist. Many case managers would assert that they never exist for most case management clients. Furthermore, the advocacy/empowerment commitment, to full self-determination in the context of being a valid, whole human being—despite the severity of handicapping conditions, creates the basis for extending the advocacy/empowerment case management practice from a simple sequence of tasks, or a linear model, to a more dialogical process (Freire, 1968; Rose & Black, 1985).

Phase I: Introduction and Engagement

People referred for case management services frequently have no knowledge of the services, why they were referred, who referred them, or what to expect. Empowerment cannot even be used as a guide without all of this information being communicated directly to the client at first contact. Uncertainty about the case management referral suggests that the following aspects be included in the earliest phase of client contact:

1. Introduction of the case manager together with presentation of a business card and any written brochures or materials describing the case management program and its sponsor. Where the case manager is part of a team, all staff members' names should be given out if they might have direct contact with the client.
2. Case managers inform the person about all aspects of the referral. If the client was involved, and a signed consent form was used, that should be given directly to the person to see. If a written referral exists, that can be shown directly to the person. We introduce client-driven practice by sharing providers' information about the person and putting him or her in control of information. The person's response to the referral is elicited and elaborated along with the person's agreement or disagreement with the referral or its reasoning.
3. The purposes of the case management program and its practice principles are discussed. Emphasize the client-centered commitments of the practice, confidentiality, and direction- or goal-focused work.
4. Case managers should be certain that accurate information remains with the client and review the person's thoughts about becoming involved. Where clients choose, family members or other significant people can become part of the process and gain access to both the case manager and the materials he or she has given out.
5. With the person's informed agreement to become a client, preliminary discussion occurs about the direction plan, and appointments are prepared for beginning its use. Any forms the client has to sign, such as eligibility forms or informed consent forms are explained with copies given to the person. If the client is not clear or unable to focus, regardless of the reason, the responsibility for repeatedly coming back to achieve clarity and an informed decision rests with the case manager.

It is expected that these tasks can be accomplished in a two-week time frame, with a range of 1 to 4 face-to-face meetings. But, as with the direction plan, no concrete, undifferentiated and predetermined time frame exists. The circumstances of a client's referral to case management may influence the process in the initial phase; e.g., a client in a crisis or in an acute care setting may respond differently from someone living at home with no crisis at hand. The key factors in the initial phase include the client's understanding of the case management function, the auspices of the case management program, how the case manager can be reached, and the commitment to confidentiality.

Phase II: Direction Plan Building

Rather than face people with the potentially overwhelming task of planning for their entire life, the direction plan breaks down the universe of interacting factors in people's lives into viable segments (see Freire, 1968, on "limit-situations"; and Rose & Black, 1985). Each direction area can be assessed with the client, goals can be established, and implementation steps can be set forth. The process requires constructing a dialogue with the client centered around the client's life; to move from the often seemingly impermeable status as object that is known and acted on toward becoming a subject with the supports necessary to acquire or produce positive outcomes. The direction plan intends to communicate to clients the belief that they can grow and act positively in their own established interests; that they can act to transform their situations and self-concepts when provided with the assistance and supports they need. The key variables in the direction plan building process are guided, supported, and purposive movement and continuity between goals, purpose, implementation, and evaluation.

Phase III: Direction Plan Implementation and Monitoring

Obviously, a direction plan cannot be a treatment plan or a service plan. Both of those instruments, in whatever form they take, are provider-driven tools that chart the itinerary of a client by providers' offerings and domain interests. The direction plan, like the personal plan in the Kisthardt and Rapp model, starts with the person. Where services are needed to accomplish clients' stated goals or implement steps toward goal attainment, appropriate referrals and linkages are made. In each referral situation, the client acts as informed authorizing agent by knowing the reason for each referral, what she or he can expect from the service, and the purpose of the referral in relation to specific goals in the direction plan. In other words, the client transforms the adaptive, incorporative consumer role into an active participation. The client becomes a self-conscious coproducer of his or her own resource utilization. Clients not only become active producers of their direction plans, or architects of their own development, but they become engineers as well. The direction plan specifies what steps have to be taken, by whom, and when. It also calls for regular monitoring and critical reflection by the client and case manager. With some success in this experience, case managers will assess the level and extent of their involvement—or the intensity and duration of contact. Key variables continue to be guided, supported movement, with purpose and direction deriving from clients' goals. This phase also includes accomplishment and movement toward increased autonomy.

Phase IV: Phasing Out

Case management clients often need to know that they can move away from case management services, but be able to reconnect quickly and for short-term contact as needed. Building on the replacement of formal system relationships by informal social supports, case managers use the goal-framing process from the direction plan to disengage the relationship through a process mutually determined with the client. Inactive status, with decreased face-to-face contact, can be planned without a set time period that applies to every client. Active involvement of members of the client's support system may participate in the termination process as part of an evaluative process.

SUPERVISION

Advocacy/empowerment case management practice requires extensive supervision. Two primary reasons for this include the necessity for developing case management practice from the client-driven, advocacy/empowerment paradigm and the need to construct a process for supporting the case managers and for eliciting their active participation in organizational decision making. Creating genuine organizational supports for case managers' input into program policy and strategy formulation prevents burn out and cynicism. Parallel to the principle of involving clients in their own direction plans, case managers have to become involved participants in the supervisory and administrative process that guides their work.

In the advocacy/empowerment design presented here, supervision can be looked at from two dimensions: quality assurance and accountability or utilization review. The quality assurance dimension assures the application and implementation of the advocacy/empowerment paradigm, or the dimension of responsibility for directing and evaluating the substance of case management practice. The utilization review dimension, or the accountability dimension, reflects the activities of maintaining client contacts, certifying the use of supervision, maintaining rational caseloads, keeping appropriate records, participating in appropriate meetings, and scheduling training.

Within these two task areas, supervision becomes an essential ingredient in staff development. For this reason, supervisors as well as any administrative staff with program responsibility must be actively familiar with the advocacy/empowerment paradigm and with the field of practice (e.g., aging, mental health, or health) in which the case management program exists. Supervision and staff development are interactive dimensions to the concept of staff growth and productivity. More formal supervision, face to face between supervisors and case managers, occurs weekly. The agenda for this supervision comes primarily from the practice of the case managers. They present problems or difficulties they experience in their work, either directly with clients or with people from the client's network, or from their interactions with providers. Supervision in the advocacy/empowerment design occurs in teams or groups, even for models where the case managers maintain their own caseloads. Preferably, case management practice will be implemented through a team approach where two or more staff share a common caseload and produce their own daily process of sustaining client contact or develop that process with their supervisors.

Material for supervision is elaborated through supervisory leadership, with discussion focused on applying the principles of advocacy/empowerment practice to the case specific situations introduced by the case managers. Staff receive support for discussing their feelings about their work; for identifying their frustrations; for talking about their own self-confidence; and for bringing into the dialogue material about the working relationships among team members. The purpose for these realms of concern is recognition of the subject dimension of the staff; of the broader concern with staff than their functioning.

Supervision at the direct practice level includes involving case managers as active contributors to their own development, eliciting suggestions to broaden practice options, validating case managers' efforts and initiatives, and constructively criticizing case managers' work and exploring alternative approaches in the light of the theoretical framework. Supervisory tasks at the indirect practice level include elaborating on the questions case managers have in relation to working with providers, formulating appropriate strategies for optimizing working relationships or reducing unnecessary friction with agencies, or developing a possible advocacy position for the case management program to adopt as policy or action. In all cases, supervisory and administrative staff must "take the heat" in supporting line workers attacked by service providers, family members, or others. Advocacy requires line support, as noted by Intagliata (1982; see Chapter 3).

At the conclusion to supervisory meetings, a focus summary (see Table 20–2) completed by supervisors and team members links descriptive material covered by team members to the themes or basic assumptions found in the advocacy/empowerment conceptual framework. Staff use the focus summary to identify the case managers' and the supervisors' practice concerns in terms of the advocacy/powerment paradigm. The program director reviews the focus summaries regularly to develop an appraisal of staff strengths and areas for continued growth. He or she uses the focus summaries to guide his or her own supervision of the supervisors. Together, this administrative group uses the organized material from the aggregate of focus summaries to suggest

TABLE 20-2. FOCUS SUMMARY-SUPERVISION

Case Managers Participate in:

1. First case synopsis–problem presented:

   Practice suggestions made and follow-up plan:

   Value-based issues identified:

   Themes requiring attention:

2. Second case synopsis—problem presented:

   Practice suggestions made and follow-up plan:

   Value-based issues identified:

   Themes requiring attention:

3. Third case synopsis—problem presented:

   Practice suggestions made:

   Value-based issues identified:

   Themes requiring attention:

4. Identified problems requiring follow-up

ongoing weekly staff development sessions. These sessions come from the work of the case managers, but filtered through the themes contained in the advocacy/empowerment paradigm. The concrete questions that arise in the course of practice are elicited from case managers in a descriptive form and returned to the staff in another form, the conceptual material that guides practice development. As with supervision, staff development issues exist at both the direct practice and interorganizational levels. The program director and the supervisors take leadership initiative in staff development with active input from line staff in planning for and chairing specific sessions.

A WORD ABOUT ADMINISTRATION

People with administrative responsibility in advocacy/empowerment case management programs must have thorough knowledge of the paradigm and contribute to its implementation.

Administrative staff have a qualitative, substantive leadership role to play in addition to their accountability for organizational operations. The absence of this role will cause the programs to drift into provider-driven models of case management. This will occur because client-driven bases for articulating resource deficits, providers' obstacles to appropriate service design, or issues related to either adequacy or accessibility will be misunderstood in favor of interorganizational domain agreement. The capacity for articulating advocacy issues and creating advocacy strategies rests entirely on the degree of substantive involvement of program administrators.

Creating a base for developing and implementing advocacy strategies produces a supportive working environment for the case managers. The line staff must know that they will be supported and that the issues they raise in their direct work with clients can be advanced through organizational support. Intagliata developed this point clearly in Part I.

The capacity to engage in advocacy strategies depends on the location of the case management program in the interorganizational field. Without a thorough knowledge of any particular interorganizational environment, making recommendations about locating an advocacy/empowerment case management program can be hazardous. However, we believe that these programs must be directly associated to public agencies and have direct line accountability to administrative officials who are not service providers, but funding-stream directors, regulators, or overseers. For example, the intensive case management program in Suffolk County, New York, directly reports to the regional director of the State Office of Mental Health (which pays for the program). It might also have been located in the office of the county director of community mental health. When case management programs become immersed in interprovider domain agreements, their capacity to function as client-driven services suffers.

EVALUATION

The Wilson article (in the program evaluation section earlier) emphasizes several critical points for advocacy/empowerment case management evaluation. The central conceptual issue for case management and for evaluation design involves the degree to which practice models capture and assess system functioning as directly related to client outcomes. Does the design assign responsibility for resource deficits? Can it incorporate the meaning of a grossly inadequate supply of safe affordable housing to stabilizing vulnerable people? Does it understand the differences between appropriateness, adequacy, and access to services? Can the design meet the test of evaluating system "impact," as Bachrach (1982) demands?

Wilson makes several contributions, especially reminding us that individual client outcomes cannot be equated with outputs of providers. Differentiating between outputs and outcomes allows the advocacy/empowerment case management program to design its evaluation to account for its dual responsibilities. Client outcomes can then be seen in terms of both client and system functioning as well as from their interaction. Efficiency in delivery of inappropriate services cannot be equated with effectiveness. The advocacy/empowerment approach to evaluation must capture the appropriateness, adequacy, and access dimensions to practice and to clients' lives.

TRAINING AND QUALIFICATIONS

Lengthy discussion about educational prerequisites for case management exist, particularly in relation to case managers in the mental health field. The basis for the discussion centers on the degree to which different case management models assume that clinical practice belongs in case management. As can be seen from the various models of case management, there are different perspectives on this point. For the advocacy/empowerment model, staff trained in generalist practice or with field work experiences in such places as shelters for battered women and children, psychosocial rehabilitation or supported housing programs are preferable to staff trained with psychodynamic theoretical foundations and office-bound psychotherapy practice models.

Advocacy/empowerment case management practice takes place where clients live, work, or attend programs, not in offices, behind desks or professional masks. It also empowers clients and engages advocacy issues at the client, organizational, or systems levels, thus prior education or experience in these areas would be advantageous. Educational requirements relate more to legitimation and eligibility for different grade or pay levels than they apply to predictors of future performance.

The discussion earlier should indicate that the crucial educative functions for advocacy/empowerment case management occur in supervision and staff development. Preservice training, which should be done in groups wherever possible, has one task—to begin the process of building an occupational identity as an advocacy/empowerment case manager within an organizational identity of an advocacy/empowerment program. The remainder of preservice training or other informational training, even including such essential information as legal rights, entitlements, and benefits, has to become part of the case managers professional identity building process. In this regard, time must be set aside by administrators and supervisors to discuss all specific training content in the context of the advocacy/empowerment paradigm of case management practice.

Advocacy/empowerment case managers learn through integration of ideas and resource materials with their role and its guiding principles: Integrative learning cannot be equated with aggregative or accumulative learning, where students ingest information in isolated packages, as receptive objects. Advocacy/empowerment training requires involvement, engagement, and creative input from the learners as a way of modeling the practice expected of the case managers.

In contrast to typical thinking about training, the qualified and developing advocacy/empowerment case manager will not be created by the perfect curriculum or training regimen—or from the accumulation of isolated bits of information, even where the input segments are relevant and useful. In parallel fashion, the perfect client outcome will not be attained by the well-constructed service plan. The training responsibility for the advocacy/empowerment program involves processing information, transforming it into personal and team use and applicability within the advocacy/empowerment concept, replacing information provision with dialogue, and developing active knowledge and growing self-confidence.

Advocacy/empowerment staff development intersperses outside information with the practice-based process described earlier, one that parallels the case manager–client relationship. The case managers, rather than imported experts, are the center of the educational/staff development process. Dialogue, focused on advocacy/empowerment concepts, principles, and application is the desired process outcome. Strengthening staff involvement, supporting staff self-confidence, and acknowledging staff achievement are the desired effects.

Social work can assume leadership in numerous fields of practice by expanding its psychosocial philosophies to elaborate the dual practice commitments embodied in advocacy/empowerment case management. The profession can just as easily continue on a path in the opposite direction, toward increasingly private practice, office-bound modalities. Each of the practitioners in the field will be faced with the dilemmas posed by the working conditions in the public sector, the risks in advocacy work, and the potential threats to job security that can come from "shaking the boat." But social work cannot simply watch or rationalize oppression; benign or avid neglect for our roots are too closely tied to the client constituencies that have historically justified our existence. We need to generate new practice models, based on emerging practice paradigms to guide our way back to our roots. Hopefully, the issues raised in this book will support that movement.

REFERENCES

Bachrach, L. 1982. Assessment of outcomes in community support systems: Results, problems and limitations. *Schizophrenia Bulletin*. 8:39–60.

Cnaan, R. A., et al. 1988. Psychosocial rehabilitation: Toward a definition. *Psychosocial Rehabilitation Journal*. 11(4):61–77.

Collopy, B. J. 1988. Autonomy in long term care: Some crucial distinctions. *The Gerontologist.* 28(Suppl.):10–17.

Freire, P. 1968. *Pedagogy of the Oppressed.* New York: The Seabury Press.

Intagliata, J. 1982. Improving the quality of community care for the chronically mentally disabled: The role of case manager. *Schizophrenia Bulletin.* 8:655–674.

Rose, S. M., & Black, B. L. 1985. *Advocacy and Empowerment: Mental Health Care in the Community.* London/Boston: Routledge & Kegan Paul.

Bibliography

American Hospital Association, Council on Patient Services. 1987. *Case Management: An Aid to Quality and Continuity of Care* (Mimeographed). pp. 1–11.

Anthony, W. A., & Blanch, A. 1989. Research on community support services: What have we learned? *Psychosocial Rehabilitation Journal.* 12(3):55–81.

Anthony, W. A., & Liberman, R. P. 1986. The practice of psychiatric rehabilitation: Historical, conceptual and research base. *Schizophrenia Bulletin.* 12(4):542–559.

Austin, C. B. 1983. Case management in long-term care: Options and opportunities. *Heath and Social Work.* 8:16–30.

Azzarto, J. 1986. Medicalization of the problems of the elderly. *Health and Social Work.* 11:189–195.

Bachrach, L. 1982. Assessment of outcomes in community support systems: Results, problems and limitations. *Schizophrenia Bulletin.* 8:39–60.

Capitman, J. A. 1986. Community-based long-term care models, target groups and impacts on service use. *The Gerontologist.* 26:389–397.

Capitman, J. A., Haskins, B., & Bernstein, J. 1986. Case management approaches in coordinated community oriented long-term care demonstrations. *The Gerontologist.* 26:398–404.

Cnaan, R. A., et al., 1988. Psychosocial rehabilitation: Toward a definition. *Psychosocial Rehabilitation Journal.* 11(4):61–77.

Collopy, B. J. 1988. Autonomy in long term care: Some crucial distinctions. *The Gerontologist.* 28(Suppl.):10–17.

Ehrenreich, J. H. 1985. *The Altruistic Imagination: A History of Social Work and Social Policy in the United States.* Ithaca, NY: Cornell University Press.

Estroff, S. 1981. *Making It Crazy.* Berkeley: University of California Press.

Franklin, J. I., et al., 1987. An evaluation of case management. *American Journal of Public Health.* 7:674–678.

Freire, P. 1968. *Pedagogy of the Oppressed.* New York: The Seabury Press.

Gough, I. 1979. *The Political Economy of the Welfare State.* London: Macmillan Press, Ltd.

Harris, M., & Bergman, H. C. 1987. Case management with the chronically mentally ill: A clinical perspective. *American Journal of Orthopsychiatry.* 57(2):296–302.

Harris, M., & Bergman, H. C. 1988. Capitation financing for the chronically mentally ill. *Hospital and Community Psychiatry.* 39:68–72.

Henderson, M., & Collard, A. 1988. Measuring quality in medical case management programs. *Quality Review Bulletin.* February:33–39.

Intagliata, J. 1982. Improving the quality of community care for the chronically mentally disabled: The role of case management. *Schizophrenia Bulletin.* 8:655–674.

Johnson, P. J., & Rubin, A. 1983. Case management in mental health: A social work domain? *Social Work.* 28:49–54.

Kane, R. A. 1988. Case management: Ethical pitfalls on the road to high-quality managed care. *Quality Review Bulletin.* 14(5):161–165.

Kanter, J. S. 1987. Mental health case management: A professional domain? *Social Work.* 32:461–462.

Lamb, R. H. 1980. Therapist–case managers: More than brokers of services. *Hospital and Community Psychiatry.* 31:762–764.

Libassi, M. F. 1988. The chronically mentally ill: A practice approach. *Social Casework.* 88–96.

Loomis, J. F. 1988. Case management in health care. *Health and Social Work.* 13(3):219–225.

Lourie, N. V. 1978. Case management. In APA (Ed.), *The Chronic Mental Patient: Problems, Solutions, and Recommendations for Public Policy.* Washington, DC: American Psychiatric Association, pp. 159–164.

Mathmatica Policy Research, Inc. 1986. *The Evaluation of the National Long-Term Care Demonstration: The Final Report.* Princeton: Mathmatica Policy Research, Inc.

National Association of Social Workers, 1987. *Policy Statement on Case Management.* Silver Spring, MD: NASW.

Ozarin, L. D. 1978. The pros and cons of case management. In APA (Ed.), *The Chronic Mental Patient: Problems, Solutions, and Recommendations for Public Policy.* Washington, DC: American Psychiatric Association, pp. 165–170.

Parrish, J. 1989. The long journey home: Accomplishing the mission of the community support movement. *Psychosocial Rehabilitation Journal.* 12(3):107–124.

Reamer, F. G. 1985. Facing up to the challenge of DRGs. *Health and Social Work.* 10:85–94.

Rose, S. M. 1972. *Betrayal of the Poor: The Transformation of Community Action.* Cambridge, MA: Schenkman.

Rose, S. M. 1979. Deciphering deinstitutionalization: Complexities in policy and program analysis. *The Milbank Quarterly.* 57:429–460.

Rose, S. M., & Black, B. L. 1985. *Advocacy and Empowerment: Mental Health Care in the Community.* London/Boston: Routledge & Kegan Paul.

Rose, S. M., & Steffens, N. D. 1986. *Reorganizaing Mental Health Care in The Netherlands: An Interorganizational Analysis* (Mimeographed). Rotterdam: Erasmus University, Institute of Social and Preventive Psychiatry.

Rubin, A. 1987. Case management. *Encyclopedia of Social Work.* Silver Spring, MD: National Association of Social Workers.

Seltzer, M. M., Ivry, J. & Litchfield, L. C. 1987. Family members as case managers: Partnership between the formal and informal Support Networks. *The Gerontologist.* 27:722–728.

Stroul, B. A. 1989. Community support systems for persons with long-term mental illness: A conceptual framework. *Psychosocial Rehabilitation Journal.* 12(3):9–26.

Turner, J. C., & TenHoor, W. J. 1978. The NIMH community support program: Pilot approach to a needed social reform." *Schizophrenia Bulletin.* 4:319–349.

Warren, R. L., Rose, S. M., & Burgunder, A. F. 1974. *The Structure of Urban Reform.* Lexington, MA: D. C. Heath.

Weick, A., et al. 1989. A strengths perspective for social work practice. *Social Work.* 34:350–354.

Wilson, S. F. 1989. Implementation of the community support system concept statewide: The Vermont experience. *Psychosocial Rehabilitation Journal.* 12(5):27–40.

Wood, J. B., & Estes, C. L. 1988. "Medicalization" of community services for the elderly. *Health and Social Work.* 13:35–42.

Credits

Index